HEALTH 95/96

Sixteenth Edition

Editor

Richard Yarian

Richard Yarian is a health educator with extensive training in the area of biomedical health. He received his B.A. in biology from Ball State University. Before leaving Ball State University he also received both an M.A. and an Ed.S. in the area of health education. He continued his academic training at the University of Maryland where he received his Ph.D. in biomedical health. Following completion of his doctoral program, he became an assistant professor at the University of Maryland and taught courses in the areas of personal health, stress management, drug abuse, medical physiology, and cardiovascular disease.

Cover illustration by Mike Eagle

Annual Editions

A Library of Information from the Public Press

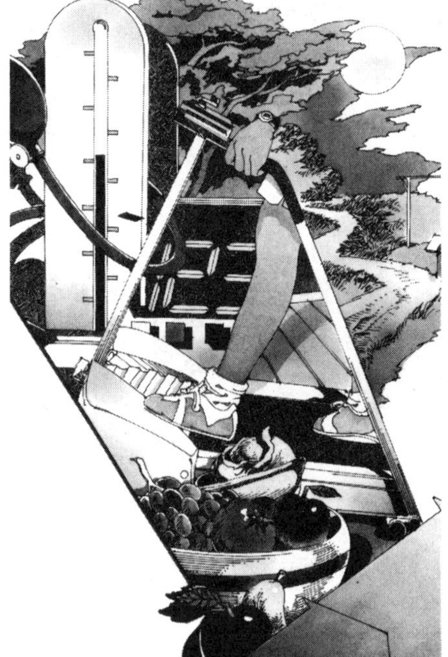

Dushkin Publishing Group/
Brown & Benchmark Publishers
Sluice Dock, Guilford, Connecticut 06437

The Annual Editions Series

Annual Editions is a series of over 65 volumes designed to provide the reader with convenient, low-cost access to a wide range of current, carefully selected articles from some of the most important magazines, newspapers, and journals published today. Annual Editions are updated on an annual basis through a continuous monitoring of over 300 periodical sources. All Annual Editions have a number of features designed to make them particularly useful, including topic guides, annotated tables of contents, unit overviews, and indexes. For the teacher using Annual Editions in the classroom, an Instructor's Resource Guide with test questions is available for each volume.

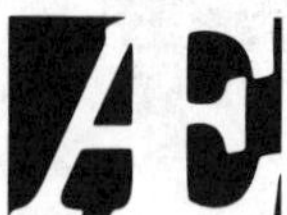

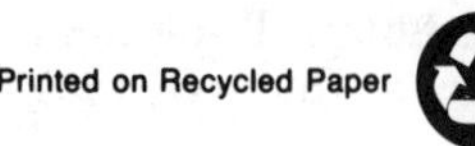

VOLUMES AVAILABLE

Africa
Aging
American Foreign Policy
American Government
American History, Pre-Civil War
American History, Post-Civil War
Anthropology
Archaeology
Biology
Biopsychology
Business Ethics
Canadian Politics
Child Growth and Development
China
Comparative Politics
Computers in Education
Computers in Business
Computers in Society
Criminal Justice
Developing World
Drugs, Society, and Behavior
Dying, Death, and Bereavement
Early Childhood Education
Economics
Educating Exceptional Children
Education
Educational Psychology
Environment
Geography
Global Issues
Health
Human Development
Human Resources
Human Sexuality
India and South Asia
International Business
Japan and the Pacific Rim
Latin America
Life Management
Macroeconomics
Management
Marketing
Marriage and Family
Mass Media
Microeconomics
Middle East and the Islamic World
Money and Banking
Multicultural Education
Nutrition
Personal Growth and Behavior
Physical Anthropology
Psychology
Public Administration
Race and Ethnic Relations
Russia, the Eurasian Republics, and Central/Eastern Europe
Social Problems
Sociology
State and Local Government
Urban Society
Violence and Terrorism
Western Civilization, Pre-Reformation
Western Civilization, Post-Reformation
Western Europe
World History, Pre-Modern
World History, Modern
World Politics

Cataloging in Publication Data
Main entry under title: Annual editions: Health. 1995/96.
1. Hygiene—Periodicals. I. Yarian, Richard, *comp.* II. Title: Health.
613'.05 81–643582 ISBN: 1–56134–358–7

Sixteenth Edition

Printed in the United States of America

Editors/ Advisory Board

Members of the Advisory Board are instrumental in the final selection of articles for each edition of Annual Editions. Their review of articles for content, level, currentness, and appropriateness provides critical direction to the editor and staff. We think you'll find their careful consideration well reflected in this volume.

To the Reader

In publishing ANNUAL EDITIONS we recognize the enormous role played by the magazines, newspapers, and journals of the *public press* in providing current, first-rate educational information in a broad spectrum of interest areas. Within the articles, the best scientists, practitioners, researchers, and commentators draw issues into new perspective as accepted theories and viewpoints are called into account by new events, recent discoveries change old facts, and fresh debate breaks out over important controversies.

Many of the articles resulting from this enormous editorial effort are appropriate for students, researchers, and professionals seeking accurate, current material to help bridge the gap between principles and theories and the real world. These articles, however, become more useful for study when those of lasting value are carefully *collected, organized, indexed,* and *reproduced* in a *low-cost format*, which provides easy and permanent access when the material is needed. That is the role played by *Annual Editions*. Under the direction of each volume's *Editor*, who is an expert in the subject area, and with the guidance of an *Advisory Board*, we seek each year to provide in each *ANNUAL EDITION* a current, well-balanced, carefully selected collection of the best of the public press for your study and enjoyment. We think you'll find this volume useful, and we hope you'll take a moment to let us know what you think.

America is in the midst of a health revolution that is changing the way millions of Americans view their health. Traditionally, most people delegated responsibility for their health to their physicians and hoped that medical science would be able to cure whatever ailed them. This approach to health care emphasized the role of medical technology and funneled billions of dollars into medical research. The net result of all this spending is the most technically advanced and expensive health care system in the world. Unfortunately, health care costs have risen so high that millions of Americans can no longer afford health care, and even among those who can there is limited accessibility to many of the new technologies because the cost is prohibitive. Despite all the technological advances, the medical community has been unable to reverse the damage associated with society's unhealthy lifestyle. This fact, coupled with rapidly rising health care costs, has prompted millions of individuals to assume a more active role in safeguarding their own health. Evidence of this change in attitude can be seen in the growing interest in nutrition, physical fitness, and stress management. If we as a nation are to capitalize on this new health consciousness, then we must devote more time and energy into educating Americans in the health sciences so they will be better able to make informed choices about their health.

Health is such a complex and dynamic subject that it is practically impossible for anyone to stay abreast of all the current research findings. For this reason Americans have generally come to rely on the public press for information on major health issues. Unfortunately, the information presented in some health articles is questionable at best and, in many cases, it is totally inaccurate. If consumers are to make wise decisions about their health based on information such as this, then they must possess the skills necessary to sort out fact from conjecture. *Annual Editions: Health 95/96* was designed to aid in this task. It presents a sampling of quality articles that represent current thinking on a variety of health issues and serves as a tool for developing critical thinking skills.

The articles selected for this volume were carefully chosen on the basis of their quality and timeliness. Because this book is revised and updated annually, it contains information that is not currently available in any standard textbook. As such, it serves as a valuable resource for both teachers and students. The book itself is divided into topical areas that are commonly covered in introductory health courses. The nine topical areas are: *America's Health and the Health Care System*, *Contemporary Health Hazards*, *Stress and Mental Health*, *Drugs and Health*, *Nutritional Health*, *Exercise and Weight Control*, *Current Killers*, *Human Sexuality*, and *Consumer Health*. Because of the interdependence of the various elements that constitute health, the articles selected were written by naturalists, environmentalists, psychologists, economists, sociologists, nutritionists, consumer advocates, and traditional health practitioners. The diversity of these selections provides the reader with a variety of points of view regarding health and the complexity of the issues involved.

Annual Editions: Health 95/96 is one of the most useful and up-to-date publications currently available in the area of health. Please let us know what you think of it by filling out and returning the postpaid article rating form on the last page of this book. Any anthology can be improved. This one will be—annually.

Richard Yarian

Richard Yarian
Editor

Contents

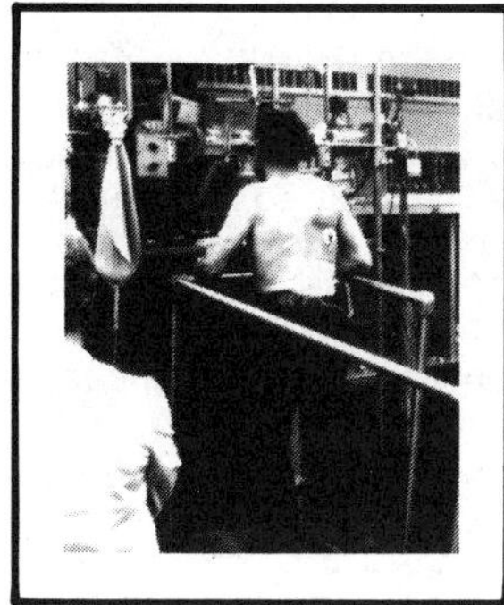

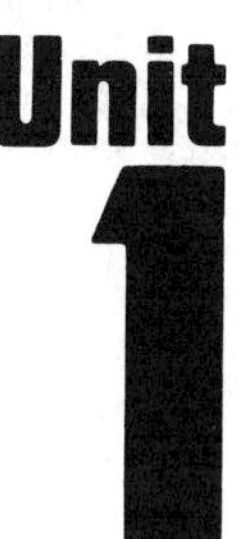

America's Health and the Health Care System

Six selections discuss the current state of health care in today's society by focusing on self-care, health care costs, and the health care industry.

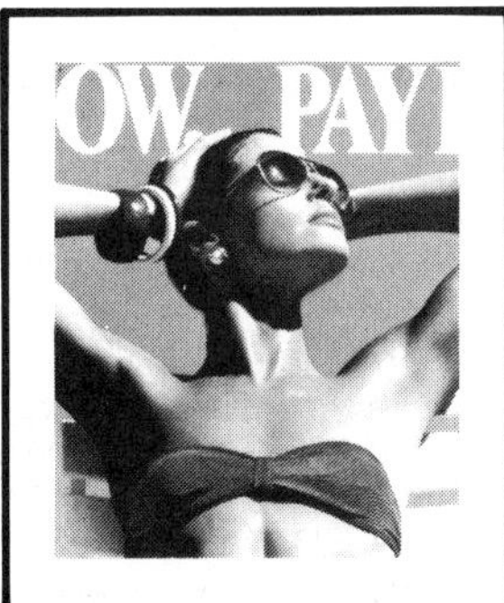

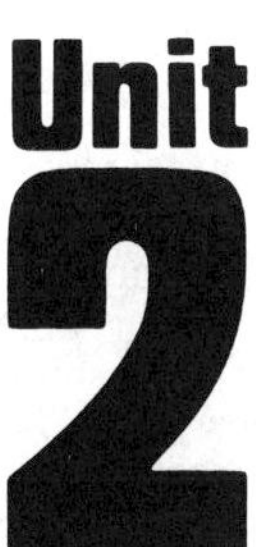

Contemporary Health Hazards

Six articles examine hazards that affect our health and are encountered in today's world.

The concepts in bold italics are developed in the article. For further expansion please refer to the Topic Guide and the Index.

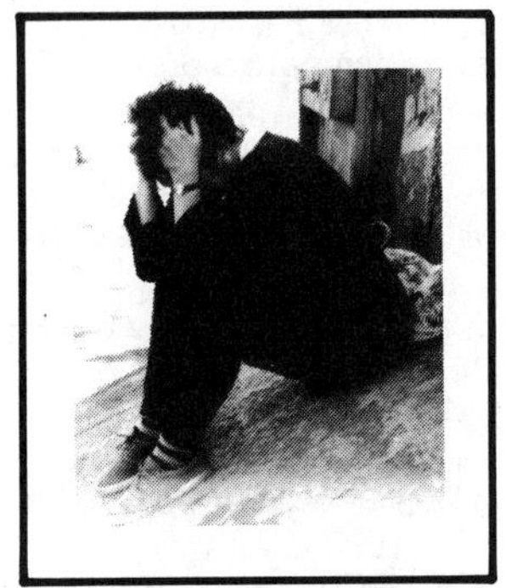
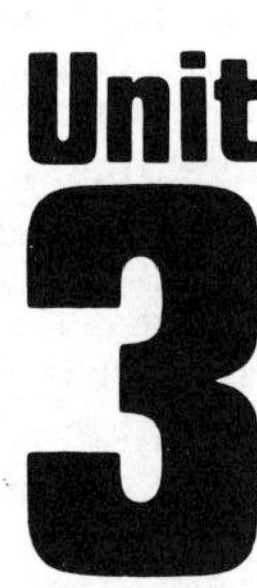

Unit 3

Stress and Mental Health

Five selections consider the impact of stress and emotions on mental health.

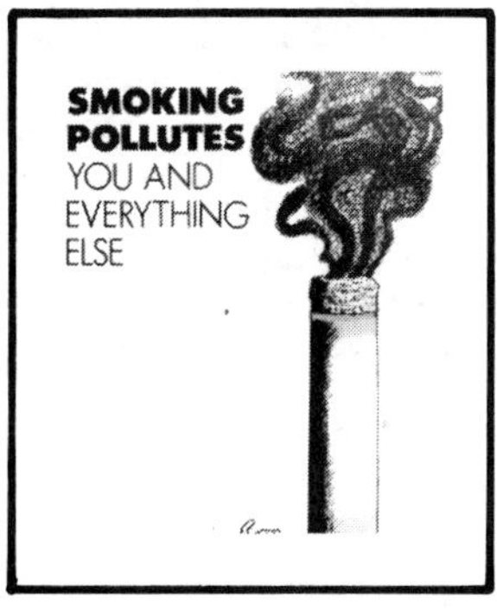

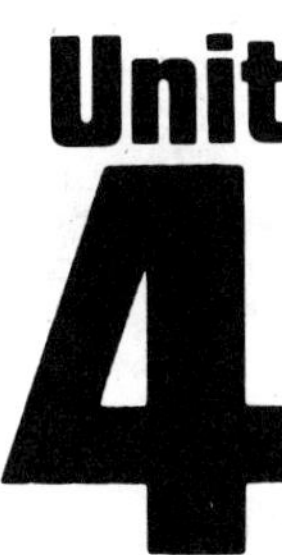

Unit 4

Drugs and Health

Seven articles examine how drugs affect our lives. Subjects discussed include the dangers of tobacco, alcohol, and the potential hazards of over-the-counter medications.

The concepts in bold italics are developed in the article. For further expansion please refer to the Topic Guide and the Index.

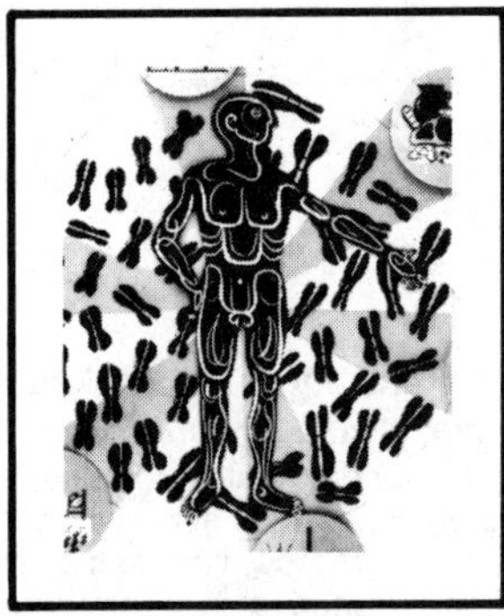
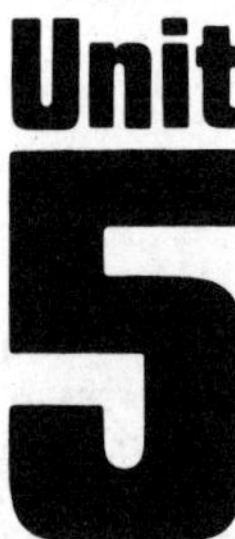

Unit 5

Nutritional Health

Six articles discuss the effects of diet and nutrition on a person's well-being. The topics include the link between diet and disease, fat in the diet, and the latest on vitamins.

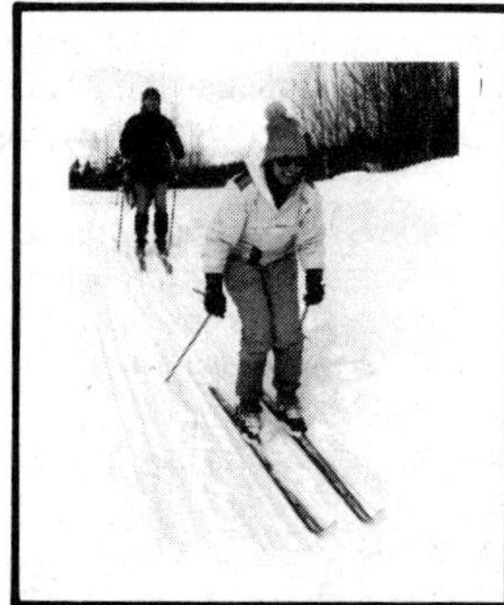
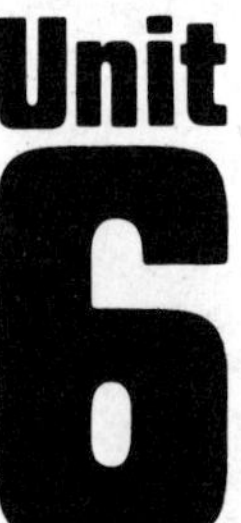

Unit 6

Exercise and Weight Control

Six articles examine the influences of exercise and diet on health. Topics discussed include walking as an effective exercise, how to prevent the most common sports injuries, and dieting myths.

The concepts in bold italics are developed in the article. For further expansion please refer to the Topic Guide and the Index.

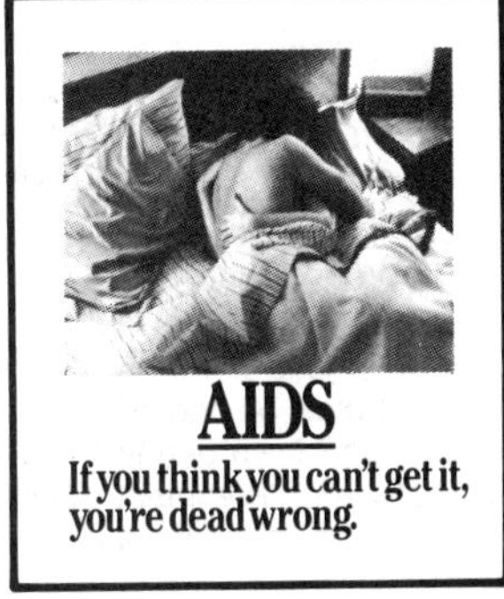

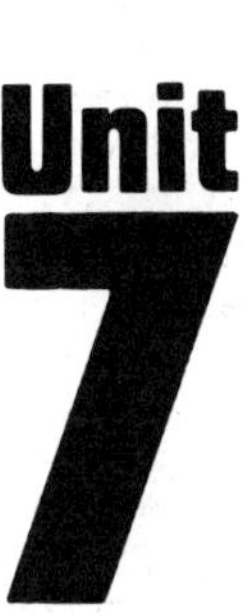

Current Killers

Five selections examine the major causes of death in the Western world. Heart attack, stroke, cancer, and AIDS are discussed.

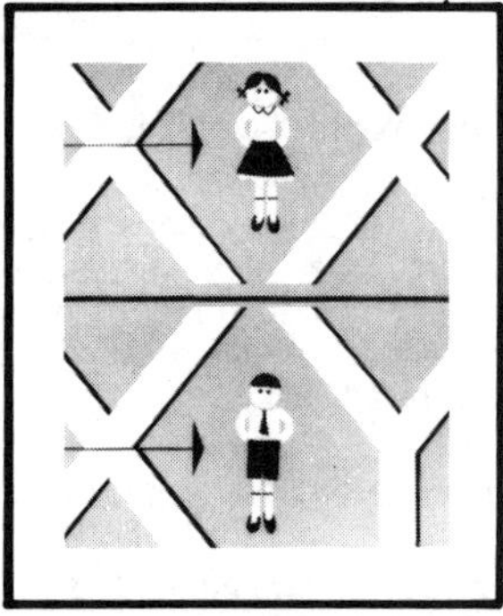

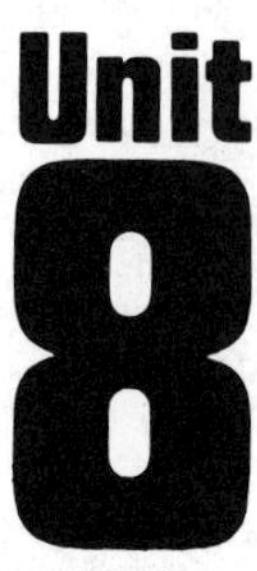

Human Sexuality

Five articles discuss the most recent research on human reproduction and sexuality. The selections consider sex differences, birth control, and sexual myths.

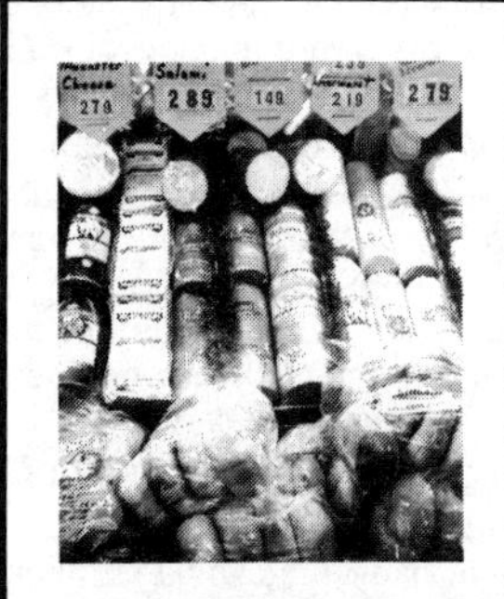

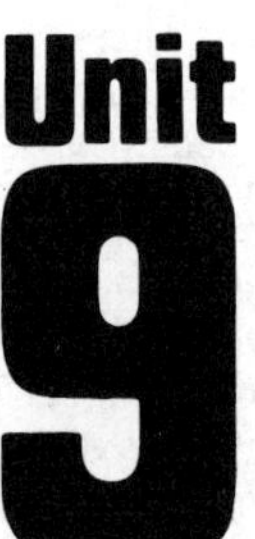

Consumer Health

Six selections examine how food labeling, cholesterol testing, and food and drug interactions relate to consumer health.

The concepts in bold italics are developed in the article. For further expansion please refer to the Topic Guide and the Index.

Topic Guide

This topic guide suggests how the selections in this book relate to topics of traditional concern to health students and professionals. It is very useful for locating articles that relate to each other for reading and research. The guide is arranged alphabetically according to topic. Articles may, of course, treat topics that do not appear in the topic guide. In turn, entries in the topic guide do not necessarily constitute a comprehensive listing of all the contents of each selection.

TOPIC AREA	TREATED IN:
Abortion	45. New, Improved and Ready for Battle
Addiction	21. Kicking Butts 22. Alcohol and Tobacco 23. Alcohol in Perspective
AIDS (Acquired Immune Deficiency Syndrome)	11. Sleeping with the Enemy 41. Confronting the AIDS Pandemic 46. It's Not Just AIDS
Alcohol	22. Alcohol and Tobacco 23. Alcohol in Perspective 24. Does Moderate Alcohol Consumption Prolong Life? 26. Mediterranean Diet 39. Rating Your Risks for Heart Disease
Birth Control/ Contraception	44. Choosing a Contraceptive 46. It's Not Just AIDS 51. Preventing STDs
Blood Fats/Serum Cholesterol	26. Mediterranean Diet 27. New Thinking about Fats 38. Cholesterol 39. Rating Your Risks for Heart Disease
Cancer	2. Future of Medicine 3. Heal Thyself 5. Timing Is Everything 7. Beach Bummer 10. Return of the Germ 11. Sleeping with the Enemy 22. Alcohol and Tobacco 23. Alcohol in Perspective 24. Does Moderate Alcohol Consumption Prolong Life? 26. Mediterranean Diet 27. New Thinking about Fats 28. Taking Vitamins 29. Salt Shake Out 37. Trace Your Family Tree 40. Stopping Cancer in Its Tracks 45. New, Improved and Ready for Battle 49. Sunscreens 50. Something Fishy
Cardiovascular Disease	3. Heal Thyself 5. Timing Is Everything 13. Stress 23. Alcohol in Perspective 24. Does Moderate Alcohol Consumption Prolong Life? 26. Mediterranean Diet 28. Taking Vitamins 34. Losing Weight 35. Best Shape of Your Life 38. Cholesterol 39. Rating Your Risks for Heart Disease
Cholesterol	*See* Blood Fats
Consumer Health	7. Beach Bummer 10. Return of the Germ 18. One Pill Makes You Larger 19. OTC Drugs 47. 'Nutrition Facts' 48. Taking Control of Your Disease 49. Sunscreens 50. Something Fishy 51. Preventing STDs 52. Food News Blues
Depression	16. Out of the Blues 17. Depression 21. Kicking Butts
Dietary Fat	25. How's Your Diet? 26. Mediterranean Diet 27. New Thinking about Fats 30. Snack Attack 35. Best Shape of Your Life
Dietary Fiber	25. How's Your Diet? 26. Mediterranean Diet
Dietary Minerals	29. Salt Shake Out 47. 'Nutrition Facts'
Dietary Salt	25. How's Your Diet? 29. Salt Shake Out
Drugs	5. Timing Is Everything 9. Allergies 17. Depression 18. One Pill Makes You Larger 19. OTC Drugs 20. Placebo Effect 21. Kicking Butts 22. Alcohol and Tobacco
Environmental Health Hazards	7. Beach Bummer 8. Uninvited Guests 9. Allergies 49. Sunscreens 50. Something Fishy
Exercise	14. Does Tension Cause Hypertension? 15. Energy! 26. Mediterranean Diet 31. Revive Sore Muscles 32. 10 Most Common Sports Injuries 33. Which Exercise Is Best for You? 34. Losing Weight 35. Best Shape of Your Life 38. Cholesterol 39. Rating Your Risks for Heart Disease
Food Labeling	47. Nutrition Facts
Food Poisoning	8. Uninvited Guests 10. Return of the Germ 50. Something Fishy

TOPIC AREA	TREATED IN:
Genetics	2. Future of Medicine 15. Energy! 17. Depression 21. Kicking Butts 34. Losing Weight 35. Best Shape of Your Life 37. Trace Your Family Tree 39. Rating Your Risks for Heart Disease
Health Care Costs	1. Wasted Health Care Dollars 2. Future of Medicine 3. Heal Thyself 4. When Doctors Jump the Gun 5. Timing Is Everything 6. Do Health Care Costs Matter? 41. Confronting the AIDS Pandemic
Hypertension	14. Does Tension Cause Hypertension? 23. Alcohol 29. Salt Shake Out 33. Which Exercise Is Best for You?
Immunity	5. Timing Is Everything 9. Allergies
Infectious Illness	8. Uninvited Guests 10. Return of the Germ 11. Sleeping with the Enemy 41. Confronting the AIDS Pandemic 46. It's Not Just AIDS
Longevity	24. Does Moderate Alcohol Consumption Prolong Life? 34. Losing Weight 37. Trace Your Family Tree 40. Stopping Cancer in Its Tracks
Lyme Disease	10. Return of the Germ
Medical Concerns and Ethics	1. Wasted Health Care Dollars 2. Future of Medicine 3. Heal Thyself 4. When Doctors Jump the Gun 5. Timing Is Everything 18. One Pill Makes You Larger 19. OTC Drugs 20. Placebo Effect 28. Taking Vitamins 48. Taking Control of Your Disease
Medical Technology	2. Future of Medicine 4. When Doctors Jump the Gun
Mediterranean Diet	26. Mediterranean Diet 27. New Thinking about Fats
Mental Health and Stress	13. Stress 14. Does Tension Cause Hypertension? 15. Energy! 16. Out of the Blues 17. Depression 18. One Pill Makes You Larger 36. Body Mania 38. Cholesterol 39. Rating Your Risks for Heart Disease
Nutrition	15. Energy! 26. Mediterranean Diet 27. New Thinking about Fats 28. Taking Vitamins 30. Snack Attack 34. Losing Weight 38. Cholesterol 47. 'Nutrition Facts'
Omega-3 Fatty Acids	26. Mediterranean Diet 27. New Thinking about Fats
Osteoporosis	26. Mediterranean Diet 29. Salt Shake Out 33. Which Exercise Is Best for You?
Personality and Disease/Type A Personality	13. Stress
Radiation	7. Beach Bummer 49. Sunscreens
Rape	12. What Every Woman Needs to Know
Sexual Behavior	11. Sleeping with the Enemy 42. Mating Game 43. Indispensables 46. It's Not Just AIDS 51. Preventing STDs
Sexually Transmitted Diseases (STDs)	11. Sleeping with the Enemy 41. Confronting the AIDS Pandemic 44. Choosing a Contraceptive 46. It's Not Just AIDS 51. Preventing STDs
Sports Medicine	31. Revive Sore Muscles 32. 10 Most Common Sports Injuries
Stress	13. Stress 14. Does Tension Cause Hypertension? 15. Energy! 18. One Pill Makes You Larger 33. Which Exercise Is Best for You? 36. Body Mania 38. Cholesterol
Tobacco and Health	21. Kicking Butts 22. Alcohol and Tobacco 38. Cholesterol 39. Rating Your Risks for Heart Disease
Vitamins	25. How's Your Diet? 28. Taking Vitamins 38. Cholesterol 47. 'Nutrition Facts'
Weight Control	26. Mediterranean Diet 30. Snack Attack 33. Which Exercise Is Best for You? 34. Losing Weight 35. Best Shape of Your Life 36. Body Mania 39. Rating Your Risks for Heart Disease

America's Health and the Health Care System

Americans are healthier today than at any time in this nation's history. Americans suffer more illness today than at any time in this nation's history. Which statement is true? They both are depending on the statistics you quote. According to longevity statistics, Americans are living longer today and, therefore, must be healthier. Still other statistics indicate that Americans today report twice as many acute illnesses as did our ancestors 60 years ago. They also report that their pains last longer. Unfortunately, this combination of living longer and feeling sicker places additional demands on a health care system that, according to experts, is already in a state of crisis. How severe is the health care crisis? What has caused it? Who is responsible? What can and should be done to solve it? This unit will attempt to explore these questions and present some possible solutions along the way.

From the discovery of the smallpox vaccine and penicillin to the first heart transplant, the marriage of modern medicine and science has seemed a perfect match. Over the last 30 years, Americans have witnessed some remarkable scientific breakthroughs that have revolutionized the diagnosis and treatment of a variety of illnesses. While these medical advances have served to establish America as the leader in medical technology, waste, inefficiency, and greed have so corrupted the system that despite the advances, millions of Americans can no longer afford basic health care.

Why have health care costs risen so high? The answer to this question is multifaceted and includes such factors as hospital costs, physician's fees, insurance costs, pharmaceutical costs, and health fraud. It could be argued that while these factors operate within any health care system, the lack of a meaningful form of assessment has permitted and encouraged waste and inefficiency within our system. Clearly, ours is not the only health care system plagued by waste and inefficiency, but values as high as 20 percent are outrageous and earn the United States the dubious distinction as the most wasteful and inefficient health care system among industrialized nations. The buzzword within the health care industry lately has been cost containment.

Is cost containment a viable solution to our escalating health care costs? William Baumol's article "Do Health Care Costs Matter?" presents an interesting point of view regarding escalating health care costs. Baumol argues that rising health care costs are an inevitable and ineradicable aspect of a developed economy, and efforts to control costs are as foolhardy as they are impossible. He argues that because the nature of health care is labor intensive relative to other products and services, the cost per unit of service is bound to rise in a growing economy.

Physician's fees account for approximately 19 percent of the total amount spent on health care. While this figure may not appear excessive, it also is a multidimensional factor that involves much more than simply the cost of the service rendered by a doctor. The fee-for-service that doctor's charge has risen in response to reimbursement through third-party payment plans such as Medicare and private health insurance.

The third-party payment plan has not only reduced incentives to keep prices affordable, but it has changed the very nature of medicine itself. Today private physicians must spend increasing amounts of time and money on the business aspect of their medical practice just to keep up with the increasing demands of third-party reviews, regulations, and paperwork. Many private physician's clerical staff members outnumber their clinical staff. This cost is passed on as fee-for-service, but contributes nothing to the quality of health care. Another expense incurred by the private physician that is passed along in the fee-for-service is the cost of malpractice insurance. The threat of malpractice has also led to wasted health care dollars through the practice of defensive medicine, in which physicians order unnecessary medical tests for their patients as a hedge against litigation.

Frequently, physicians choose to employ "cutting edge technologies" in both diagnosis and treatment as a means to demonstrate that they are attuned to the latest advances in medicine. Unfortunately, this rush to employ the latest technology can drive up the cost of health care, with no appreciable benefit to the patient. This issue of "jumping the gun" on new technologies is dealt with in the article "When Doctors Jump the Gun."

Evidence is mounting that certain medical conditions, including localized prostate cancer, cataracts, gallstones, cardiomyopathy, and uterine fibroids, which are usually treated through surgical interventions, may improve on their own when doctors simply monitor these conditions. This approach, discussed in the article "Heal Thyself," not only saves money but appears to enhance the quality of life and may extend the longevity of the patient.

Another new approach to the practice of medicine that may reduce costs by increasing the effectiveness of some medical interventions is "chronotherapy." Chronotherapy is the treatment of illness according to circadian rhythms. Evidence is mounting that circadian variations in symptoms and in the ability of tissues to absorb certain drugs can dictate how effective a particular drug is in treating a specific disorder. Obviously the more effective the treatment is, the fewer medical resources the patient will use, and the more money that can be saved or spent on other items or services. "Timing Is Everything" by William Hrushesky discusses why chronotherapy should become a more utilized form of therapy for patients suffering from allergies, arthritis, asthma, and cancer.

Hospitals have also contributed to the high cost of health care in the United States. Statistics indicate that they account for approximately 38 percent of all health care expenditures. Because hospitals account for such a high percentage of health care dollars, reducing hospital costs could significantly reduce the cost of health care.

The one area of health care costs that is often considered immutable is the cost of medical technology and pharmaceuticals. Americans pay substantially higher prices for pharmaceuticals and diagnostic tests than in any other industrialized country. The manufacturers argue that this practice is necessary if they are to continue to pour large sums of money into research and development in order to satisfy the stringent guidelines established by the Food and Drug Administration (FDA). Perhaps it is time to let the rest of the world contribute their fair share to these costs.

For years researchers and health care officials believed that high-tech medicine would reduce medical care costs by providing safer, less expensive procedures. Unfortunately, in many cases just the opposite has been true. It could be argued that the reason that technological advances have not resulted in lower health care costs is because our health care system does not include a means for evaluating outcomes and determining which medical procedures are most effective. "The Future of Medicine: New Anatomy Lesson, Please" discusses how computers, telecommunications, and robotics could be utilized to transform our bloated, costly, health care system into a much more efficient and effective system.

Over the last few years, complaints regarding not only the inequities, but the economic costs of the American health care system have risen dramatically. Many experts argue that the American health care system is in such a financial mess that the only viable solution is a complete restructuring of the system. Others, however, contend that the current system can be preserved by instituting reform legislation. While nothing is certain regarding health care reform, the political climate is ripe for such reform.

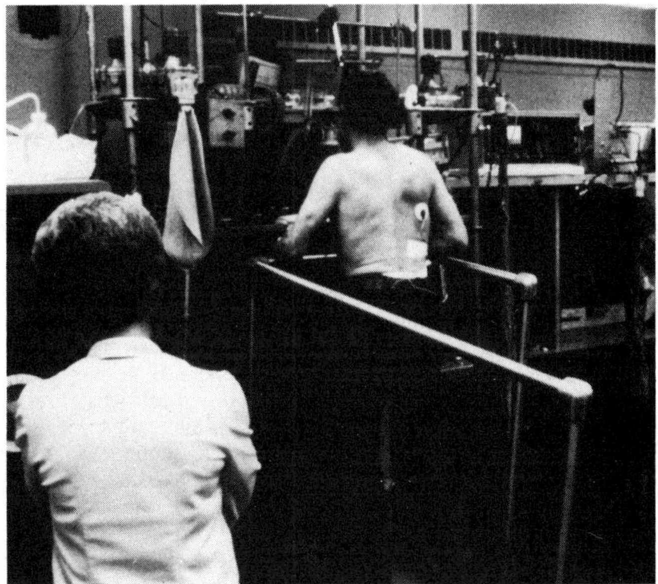

While it is easy to find fault with our health care system, the real challenge is to find solutions that can control the costs and yet provide high quality health care for all. Critics of nationalized health care argue that this form of health care limits patients' choices and results in a rationing of services. "Wasted Health Care Dollars" discusses why our health care is so expensive and suggests that perhaps the best solution is to scrap our current system and start anew.

America is about to undergo a revolution in the health care system, ushered in by excessive health care costs. At this time the future of the American health care system is uncertain, but one thing is clear—change is coming.

Looking Ahead: Challenge Questions

Is health care just another commodity? Should it be treated differently from other consumer services?

Is quality health care a right or a privilege?

How have third-party payments contributed to the rising cost of health care in America?

What can you as an individual do to help reduce health care costs? Give specific actions that can be taken.

How have hospitals contributed to the rising cost of health care?

If medical interventions must be limited for economic reasons, who should have the authority to decide "how much" and "for whom"?

WASTED HEALTH CARE DOLLARS

The U.S. is spending enough to bring every citizen high-quality, high-tech medical care—if we stop squandering our resources.

Less waste, longer lives
"Look at the rest of the industrial world. On average, they spend half as much as we do on health care. They cover everyone and live longer. It's waste. There's no other explanation." —Alan Sager, health economist, Boston University School of Public Health

Of the $817-billion that we will spend this year on health care, we will throw away at least $200-billion on overpriced, useless, even harmful treatments, and on a bloated bureaucracy. We are no healthier than the citizens of comparable developed countries that spend half what we do and provide health care for everybody. In fact, by important measures such as life expectancy and infant mortality, we are far down the list.

If the wasted money could be redirected, the U.S. could include those now shut out of the system—without increasing the total outlay for health care and without restricting the availability of $100,000 bone-marrow transplants or $40,000 heart operations to those relatively few who need them.

"I can't imagine a system that's more dysfunctional than the one we have now—more expensive, not doing the job, with more waste," says Dr. Philip Caper, an internist and medical policy analyst at Dartmouth Medical School. Although the total amount of waste in our health-care system is difficult to estimate, researchers have now examined many of the system's components, with consistent results. For a wide range of clinical procedures, on average, roughly 20 percent of the money we now spend could be saved with no loss in the quality of care. By restructuring the system, we could also save almost half of the huge amount we now spend on administrative costs (see "The $200-Billion Bottom Line"). A more efficient system would also make it much easier to detect health-care fraud—a problem that the U.S. General Accounting Office has estimated to cost tens of billions of dollars a year.

While these facts are well known to students of the health-care system, they've been remarkably absent from the debate that's developing over health care in this election year. Politicians and lobbyists for health-care providers have presented the public with a daunting choice: If we want to provide every American with access to health care, they say, we'll either have to pay much more into the system or accept lower-quality medical services.

However, such scenarios assume that the current price structure for medical care, and the current patterns of treatment and hospitalization, will remain fixed. They needn't, and they shouldn't. Our health-care system is so inherently wasteful and inefficient that a complete overhaul is an option worth contemplating. It may, in fact, be the only option that makes sense.

The waste in the system comes from many sources. We receive a great deal of care that we don't need at all. The care we do need is delivered inefficiently. And the futile effort to control a runaway system has created a huge bureaucracy that by itself sucks up more than a hundred billion dollars a year.

30 years of increases

By now, it's hardly news that health costs have spiraled out of control. Health care now consumes about 16 percent of state and local tax revenues. In the years since 1986, private businesses have spent about as much on health care as they earned in after-tax profits. For small businesses, insurance has become unaffordable; three of four concerns employing 10 or fewer people simply don't provide health bene-

This report [Part 1 of a 3-part series] examines the forces behind the current crisis in health-care costs. The next two reports in this special series will look at the possible solutions [see *Consumer Reports,* August and September, 1992].

One approach to cost control, pioneered by health maintenance organizations, is to "manage" medical care in detail. The management can include such practices as restricting patients to a single primary-care doctor who must approve all specialist referrals; penalizing doctors who order too many tests or procedures; and preapproving elective hospitalizations. In our next report, we'll rate HMOs and examine how well managed care actually contains costs.

Another approach is to set overall spending limits and stick to them, while otherwise leaving doctors and hospitals to practice as they see fit. That's what other industrialized countries, including Canada, do in various ways. Part three of our health-care series, [in] the September issue, will take a close look at the Canadian system, among others, and will analyze the criticisms that have been leveled against it by U.S. health-care providers and insurers.

Finally, we'll outline the health-care reform proposal that Consumers Union favors as providing the best combination of universal access, quality care, and cost containment.

fits. At any given time, roughly 35 million Americans—most of them employees of small businesses or their dependents—have no health coverage at all.

Over the last 10 years, Government and private business, appalled to see health care absorbing an ever-growing portion of their revenues, have tried to get a grip on its costs in various ways. But costs have risen as fast as ever. "As quickly as payers patch the system up, the providers find the spaces between the patches," says Maryann O'Sullivan, director of Health Access, a California consumer coalition.

Our health-care system doesn't just allow prices to rise—it practically demands that they do. Although some recent reforms have had a modest effect, the system has traditionally allowed doctors to order whatever procedures they want, and has paid both doctors and hospitals whatever they think they should get.

In both respects, the American system stands alone in the developed world. Though the particulars of their systems differ, Canada, Japan, and the Western European countries all have adopted universal, standard payment schedules set by direct negotiation with doctors and hospitals. In addition, most have set an overall ceiling on national medical expenditures. As a result, not a single developed country other than the U.S. devotes more than 10 percent of its gross national product to health care. The U.S. broke that barrier in 1985; this year, the nation will spend 14 percent of the GNP on health.

It wasn't always so. Back in 1960, the U.S. spent a modest 5.3 percent of its GNP on health care, about the same as other industrialized nations like Canada or Germany did at the time. What changed everything was the advent in 1965 of Medicare, which ultimately had implications far beyond the over-65 population it served.

Before Medicare, private insurance companies covered the population less extensively than they do today. All the insurers left treatment completely to the doctor's discretion and provided reimbursement for any test or treatment a physician ordered. But because a large percentage of people had only hospital coverage, and no insurance to cover doctors' bills, physicians tended to keep fees at affordable levels.

In 1965, Congress enacted Medicare, the vast, Government-financed

High-tech without high costs

Although they control health-care costs much more effectively than the U.S., other developed countries still provide high-tech care to those who need it. Between 1988 and 1990, Canada, France, Australia, and Israel all did more bone-marrow transplants per capita than the U.S.

THE $200-BILLION BOTTOM LINE

To date, no one has come up with a comprehensive price tag for the cost of unnecessary medical care, overpriced procedures, and inefficient administration in the U.S. health-care system. After extensive review of the literature, however, we believe that $200-billion is a conservative estimate of the amount the health-care system will waste this year. Here's why.

Of the $817-billion projected to be spent on health care this year, about one fifth—$163-billion—will go for administrative costs. Except for a fraction of a percent spent on research, the rest—roughly $650-billion—will go to actual patient care. Physician and hospital services together make up most of that total, with the rest going to dentists, nursing homes, drugs, and various other expenses.

By our estimates, at least 20 percent of that $650-billion, or $130-billion, will be spent on procedures and services that are clearly unnecessary.

Many researchers have now attempted to quantify the rate at which specific procedures are used unnecessarily. Twenty percent represents a rough average of the rates found in major studies, and is a figure that several leading researchers in this field told us was a good approximation for the rate of unnecessary care.

Twenty percent also seems to be a conservative estimate of the rate of unnecessary hospital days, even though changes in Medicare and private-insurance policies make it difficult to estimate that number precisely.

Finally, as Dr. John Wennberg of Dartmouth and his colleagues have demonstrated repeatedly, the rate at which physicians use a given procedure can vary four- or five-fold between one location and another. The supply of hospitals and physicians also varies greatly. Except in extreme cases where people lack access to basic medical care, people living in low-use or low-supply areas seem to be just as healthy as those in high-use or high-supply areas.

Dr. Wennberg and his colleagues argue that areas with abundant doctors and hospitals could provide significantly fewer health-care services without harmful consequences. Similarly, the high rates of procedures done in many areas could be cut back without overall harm. This sort of adjustment happens automatically, they note, in industrialized countries that control costs by capping the amount of money available for health care.

If overuse of medical services wastes $130-billion a year, administrative inefficiency adds about $70-billion. Projecting from 1991 estimates by the General Accounting Office, the U.S. could save roughly $70-billion this year by switching from our fragmented and inefficient insurance system to a single-payer system—one in which all citizens receive health care from private doctors and hospitals that are paid by a single insurance entity. The savings would come roughly equally from insurance-company overhead and hospital and administrative costs.

Adding those two figures together—$130-billion plus $70-billion—gives an estimate of $200-billion for the annual waste in the U.S. health-care system. This estimate, however, leaves out several important elements: Physicians' fees and the cost of technology, drugs, and procedures. If those costs were brought into line with reimbursement standards in other countries, the savings would be greater.

Moreover, we have not added in the cost of outright fraud—a factor that the General Accounting Office estimates could eat up a full 10 percent of the total health-care budget.

Some physicians cheat the system by ordering unnecessary tests and procedures—a type of fraud that is included in our estimates of unnecessary care. Other types of fraud, however, would not have been caught in the studies of unnecessary care that have been done. These include billing for services never rendered, falsifying reimbursement codes to collect more than the usual payment for a service, and submitting inflated bills for supplies and medical devices.

Since we have not counted the cost of these fraudulent practices—or of the high price scale for health-care providers in the U.S.—our $200-billion figure is truly a minimum estimate.

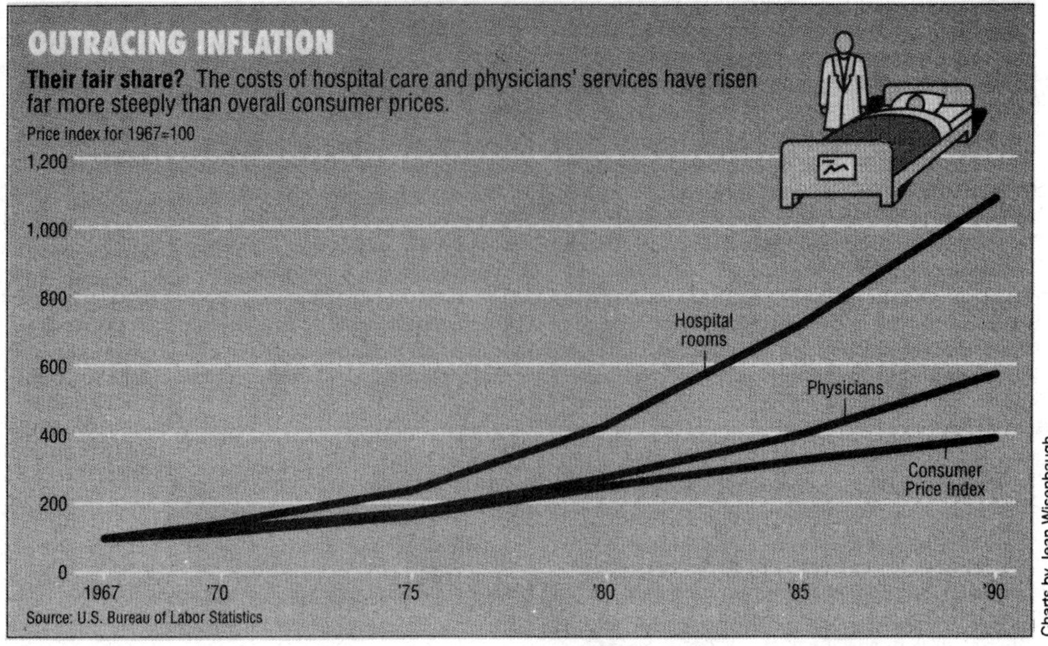

program of social health insurance for the elderly, along with the less extensive Medicaid program, in which the Federal Government shares costs with the states. In order to overcome the powerful, sustained opposition of doctors and hospitals to what they called "socialized medicine," Congress made a fateful—and, in retrospect, very expensive—decision. Under Medicare, all doctors were paid on the basis of their "usual and customary" fees for a given service (the system that Blue Shield was already using).

This approach, which allowed each individual physician to name his or her own price, soon became universal throughout the insurance industry. So as more and more employers began offering major-medical plans that covered doctors' bills, they bought into a system with no effective constraints on costs. Predictably, doctors' fees began a rapid upward climb.

***A freeze or a meltdown?* In 1986, in the midst of a Medicare freeze on physicians' fees, doctors increased their services enough to collect 15 percent more from Medicare than they had the year before.**

Hospitals profited as well. Under Blue Cross, which had dominated hospital insurance, hospitals were paid only a daily room charge, plus additional fees for various services, tests, and supplies. Under Medicare, however, the hospitals were not only able to collect their actual charges; for the first time, they were allowed to build the cost of capital improvements into their rates. Hospitals, which had been receiving Federal subsidies for growth since the late 1940s, now got another incentive to expand.

After Medicare, U.S. health-care expenditures turned more sharply upward. For a time—perhaps a decade or more—no one seemed to notice or care. But over the past 10 years or so, as costs have become truly staggering, the system has begun to change. Medicare has set limits on physicians' fees for several years, and private insurance companies have begun reviewing many procedures doctors perform before they will pay for them. Medicaid budgets have been steadily cut back, to the point where many states now pay doctors and hospitals less than the cost of delivering care.

Experience has shown, however, that attempts to manage the health-care system a piece at a time are likely to fail. Physicians and hospitals can charge their privately insured patients more to make up for Medicare's fee restrictions. And doctors and patients alike have resisted efforts by insurance companies to determine what is appropriate and necessary treatment, having grown used to a system that has provided as much medical care—to the insured population, that is—as anybody wants.

No sense of limits

Having operated for years under a system that sets virtually no limit on what can be done or what can be charged, both doctors and patients have been seduced by the idea that, when it comes to treating sickness, it's necessary to do "everything."

"We want more. We want more time with the doctor. We want more procedures. We want more pills," says Randall Bovbjerg, a health-policy analyst at the Urban Institute in Washington, D.C. "We can't sit and watch the course of a cold; we go and buy tons of things we aren't even certain will make it better."

"Imagine if we sold auto-purchase insurance and said, go and buy whatever car you want and we'll pay 80 percent of it," says James C. Robinson, a health-care economist at the University of California, Berkeley. Under those conditions, a lot of people would go buy a Mercedes.

Much of the time, physicians will order more tests and procedures out of a genuine desire to do whatever they can for their patients. "Doctors look at one patient at a time and think, 'If I've done one thing, what else can I try?' " says Ann Lennarson Greer, a medical sociologist at the University of Wisconsin. "They're not inclined to think about overall costs." Several studies, in fact, have asked doctors if they knew the costs of hospital tests and services they routinely ordered—and found many had only a vague idea at best.

But while extra tests and treatments drive up the cost of medical care, they may do so with no real benefit to the patient. New diagnostic technologies, in particular, are especially likely to be overused; unlike surgery or invasive procedures, they "don't require the clinician to take any real risk," Greer says. Thus, the use of computerized tomography (CT) and magnetic resonance imaging (MRI) scans, two expensive, relatively new imaging technologies, has grown explosively in recent years. Yet no one has clearly defined when they are useful and when they are a waste of time and money.

"The original CT scanner proved to be an absolute revolution in the treatment of patients with head injury," says Dr. Mark Chassin, a physician who is senior vice president of Value Health Sciences, a private firm that analyzes the use of health-care services. "We produced hundreds of these things and they got out in the community. They were used for people with head trauma—terrific—but they also were used for people with headaches, dizziness, and all sorts of other vague symptoms." Diagnostic imaging, says Dr. Chassin, is a prime example of how "we continue to invest in technology in an absolutely irrational way."

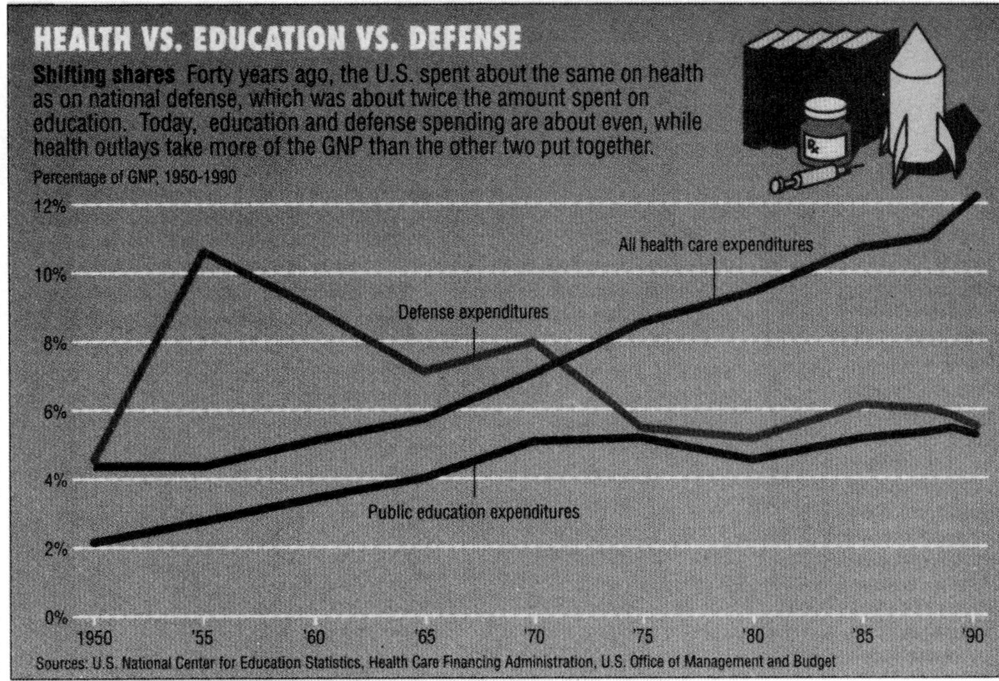

The law of induced demand

Medical care is totally unlike services delivered by other professionals. When clients hire an architect or a lawyer, they generally know what they need and roughly how much it's going to cost. But in medicine, physicians make virtually all the decisions that determine the cost of care. The patient, ill and uninformed, is in no position to do comparison shopping—nor motivated to, if insurance is paying the bill.

And the more doctors do, the more they get paid—a situation that's tailor-made for cost escalation. "It's the easiest thing in the world to increase the volume [of things a doctor does]," says Dr. Philip Caper, the Dartmouth internist. "Just do a few more tests. There's always a rationale. Schedule three doctor visits instead of two, and reduce the time you spend on each visit."

The creation of medical "need" by those who then profit from it is called induced demand, and it's rampant. Most obvious is the problem of "self-referral," in which physicians will refer patients for treatment at facilities in which they have a financial interest. In Florida, where at least 40 percent of physicians have such investments, a study by professors at Florida State University found that physician-owned laboratories performed twice as many tests per patient as independent labs. Similarly, in a study of private health insurance claims records for more than 65,000 patients, University of Arizona researchers found that doctors who had diagnostic imaging equipment in their offices ordered four times more imaging exams than doctors who referred patients elsewhere for the tests.

Occasionally, self-referral can turn into actual fraud. A recent report by the General Accounting Office—which estimated that fraud may account for as much as 10 percent of all health-care costs—cited several examples in which self-referral had been abused. In one California case, the owners of mobile medical laboratories allegedly gave kickbacks for referrals to physicians who sometimes used phony diagnoses. The case, which is still being investigated, involves an estimated \$1-billion in fraudulent billings.

In other cases, however, physicians may increase the demand for their services without even being aware of it. When it comes to American medical care, supply seems to create demand almost automatically. Actuarial studies have shown that in areas with the greatest supply of physicians, people simply go to the doctor more often.

If more physicians create more demand for medical care, we can look forward to a flood of it in the near future. The per capita supply of practicing physicians is expected to increase 22 percent between now and the year 2000.

The phenomenon of induced demand applies to hospitals, too. Dr. John Wennberg, a physician who is professor of family and community medicine at Dartmouth Medical School, was curious as to why people in Boston went to the hospital more frequently than people in New Haven. When he studied the problem, he found a simple answer: Boston has more hospital beds to be filled—one-third more than New Haven on a per capita basis.

Surprisingly, Dr. Wennberg found that physicians in Boston and New Haven were completely unaware of the discrepancy. When he asked doctors in New Haven whether they felt their area was short of hospital beds, they said they didn't. In fact, at any given time, about 85 percent of hospital beds in New Haven were filled—precisely the same percentage as in Boston.

The likely explanation, according to Dr. Wennberg, is that physicians almost unconsciously will refer their patients to the hospital if space is available, stopping only when the local hospitals' capacity is nearly used up. If many beds are empty, doctors will be more likely to refer patients with borderline conditions, such as gastroenteritis or acute low back pain, for which hospitalization is optional but not imperative. By doing so, of course, they drive up the cost of care.

An unnecessary burden

With so many incentives to overtreat patients, it seems inevitable that a sizable fraction of American medical care must be simply unnecessary, if not downright harmful. But how large a fraction? In the late 1970s and early 1980s, researchers at the Rand

Growth without limits

The Health Industry Manufacturers Association, a medical-equipment trade group, predicts a 7.4 percent annual growth rate for health technology throughout this decade—unless "negative scenarios," such as more safety regulation and cost containment, take effect.

Medical Red Flags

IS THIS TREATMENT NECESSARY?

Over the past decade or so, an entire industry has sprung up to identify overused and unnecessary medical treatments. The players range from academic researchers to policy analysts to private entrepreneurs that have insurance companies as their clients.

Some treatments, by virtue of their cost or their ubiquity, have attracted particular attention from the watchdogs. These treatments, listed below, are hardly the only sources of unnecessary care in the system. Nor, of course, does a procedure's presence on the list mean that it is always used unnecessarily—or even that that is usually the case.

Nevertheless, if your physician does suggest that you have one of these procedures, you'd be well advised to think twice. You might want to seek a second opinion, if possible, or question your doctor closely on the possible alternatives to the suggested treatment.

Cesarean section. About one in four U.S. births is completed surgically, a rate that may be twice the ideal. In this country, obstetricians routinely perform cesareans when the baby is breech, or for the vaguely defined diagnoses of "prolonged labor" or "fetal distress." Hospitals that have systematically set out to eliminate unnecessary cesareans have cut their rate at least in half without any apparent risk to mothers or babies. (See CONSUMER REPORTS, February 1991.)

In recent years, the electronic fetal monitor, a device for tracking the fetal heart rate during labor, has come to be used routinely in American hospitals—and has contributed to the high cesarean-section rate. Since abnormal fetal heart rates are associated with oxygen deprivation, it was assumed that prompt, automatic detection would enable doctors to intervene early enough to prevent fetal brain damage—for example, by performing a cesarean section on the mother.

But since the fetal monitor's introduction, no fewer than nine comparative studies, involving tens of thousands of women, have failed to demonstrate the hoped-for benefit. Monitored women do have a higher rate of cesarean sections and other costly interventions. But their babies fare no better than those of women monitored by the traditional means, in which a nurse simply checks the fetal heartbeat periodically with a stethoscope.

Hysterectomy. After cesarean section, this is the second most common major surgery in the U.S. Value Health Sciences, a firm that applies the Rand Corp.'s methodology for insurance-industry clients, calls 27 percent of hysterectomies unnecessary, the highest percentage of all procedures it evaluates. Rates of hysterectomy also vary greatly throughout the country, an indication that physician practice and preference play as much of a role as objective need in the decision to perform the operation. Many gynecologists still routinely recommend hysterectomy for fibroids, uterine prolapse, and **heavy bleeding; alternative treatments are available for all three conditions. (See CONSUMER REPORTS, September 1990).**

Back surgery. Value Health Sciences has reported that 14 percent of proposed laminectomies, the most common type of back surgery, are unnecessary. Occasionally, some material from a ruptured disc will press on spinal nerves and cause disabling or painful symptoms that require surgical correction, says Dr. Charles Fager, a neurosurgeon at the Lahey Clinic in Burlington, Mass. But usually, back pain yields to bed rest, the passage of time, physical therapy, or a combination thereof. "I only operate on one out of every 25 or 30 people I see," says Dr. Fager. Some surgeons aren't so finicky. Dr. John Wennberg of Dartmouth Medical School has traced sudden "epidemics" of back surgery to the arrival of a new neurosurgeon in a locality.

Magnetic resonance imaging. This powerful new imaging technique, which produces detailed pictures of internal organs without exposing the patient to radiation, is still so new that doctors are working out its best uses. In the process, they'll inevitably use it when they don't need to. Some groups of physicians have invested in MRI machines, creating the added temptation to profit by referring their patients for the test. Also, because MRI is virtually risk-free, it's especially likely to be overused as a defensive measure.

Experts stress that MRI procedures, which cost about $1000 apiece, should be ordered only when a patient's symptoms suggest he or she may have a condition that cannot be diagnosed definitively in any other way.

Prostate surgery. Dr. Wennberg and his colleagues at Dartmouth have shown that surgery for noncancerous enlargement of the prostate is among the most variable of procedures. They have also looked closely at what happens to men who get the surgery and those who don't. For many men, medical therapy can relieve symptoms. For

Redlined jobs
Many health-insurance companies won't sell policies to people working in barbershops, car washes, convenience stores, grocery stores, hospitals, nursing homes, doctors' offices, law offices, parking lots, or restaurants.

Corp., a think tank in Santa Monica, Calif., began to find out.

Using an elaborate process for developing a consensus among nationally recognized medical experts, the Rand team came up with an agreed-upon list of "indications" for various procedures. They then checked the actual medical records of thousands of patients who had received the procedures, to see whether they had been treated appropriately. The definition of "appropriate" care was starkly simple: Based on the patient's condition and expert opinion, the likely benefit of the procedure must have been greater than the risk involved in doing it.

Even with their elaborate analysis, the Rand researchers were not able to tell in every case whether a given procedure had been appropriate or not. They divided their cases into three groups: Those where the procedure had been "appropriate," those where it was "inappropriate," and those where its use was "equivocal," the largest group. Despite this degree of uncertainty, however, others, putting off surgery isn't particularly dangerous, though the urinary obstruction caused by the condition can be uncomfortable.

When patients in a health maintenance organization were fully informed in advance of the risks and benefits of surgery, in a study that Dr. Wennberg designed, 80 percent of men with severe urinary symptoms chose to postpone the operation.

Clot-busting drugs. These drugs, when administered within four to six hours of the onset of a heart attack, can break up the blood clot blocking the coronary artery and thus greatly reduce the damage to the heart muscle. The largest comparative study done to date, of 41,000 patients worldwide, has found that all currently available clot-busting drugs are about equally effective in preventing fatal heart attacks—but one, streptokinase, has the lowest incidence of the most dangerous side effect, cerebral hemorrhage.

Of the two drugs used in the U.S., streptokinase also happens to be by far the cheaper—about $200 per dose compared to $2000 per dose for its genetically engineered competitor, tissue plasminogen activator (TPA). Nevertheless, TPA commands a majority of the U.S. market, apparently thanks to aggressive marketing by its manufacturer, Genentech.

For a person having a first heart attack, there's no reason to be treated with the more costly drug. Second treatments with streptokinase, however, are unsafe, since the first treatment can set up the mechanism for an allergic response to any future injection.

Rand found clear evidence of inappropriate overtreatment. Among the results:

- Of 1300 elderly patients who had an operation to remove atherosclerotic plaque from the carotid artery, nearly one-third—32 percent—didn't need it.
- Of 386 heart bypass operations, 14 percent were done unnecessarily.
- Of 1677 patients who had coronary angiography—an X-ray examination of blood flow in the arteries nourishing the heart—17 percent didn't need it.

So striking were the results that Rand's methods for determining appropriateness have since been put to commercial use. Value Health Sciences, which now employs some of the original Rand researchers, has extended the methodology to several dozen high-volume medical procedures. A number of major insurance companies and health maintenance organizations now use this program to flag unnecessary procedures.

Value Health's results confirm the original Rand findings. Its review system has found very high rates of unnecessary usage for certain procedures: hysterectomy, 27 percent unnecessary; surgery for an uncomfortable wrist ailment called carpal tunnel syndrome, 17 percent; tonsillectomy, 16 percent; laminectomy, a type of back surgery, 14 percent. Similar results have come out of studies done by other investigators, who have examined procedures from preoperative laboratory screening (60 percent unnecessary) to cesarean section (50 percent unnecessary) to upper gastrointestinal X-ray studies (30 percent unnecessary).

The uncertainty principle

Physicians can inadvertently contribute to the cost of unnecessary medicine even when they have only their patients' best interest in mind. Lay people tend to think of medical care as a straightforward proposition: For Disease A, prescribe Treatment B. That's not the way it is in real life. To practice medicine is to be afloat in a "sea of uncertainty," says Dartmouth's John Wennberg.

Every symptom can be investigated by a huge array of tests; for many diseases, physicians have a wide range of treatment choices. And doctors often base their choices as much on folklore and intuition as on science.

"Doctors really hate risks," says Ann Lennarson Greer, the Wisconsin sociologist. "They have certain procedures that seem to work for them, and they'd prefer to keep doing them, especially in areas where there's a lot of uncertainty."

This innate conservatism is reinforced by the isolation in which most doctors practice, says Greer, who has spent more than a decade studying why doctors and hospitals behave as they do. A physician can spend his or her entire career within a single referral network, based at a single hospital. These local colleagues, Greer has found, are the principal influence on a physician's decisions about how to diagnose and treat diseases or whether or not to adopt new technology. But they may not be the most reliable source.

A phenomenon called "small area variations," which was discovered by Dr. Wennberg early in his career, is a striking demonstration of just how unscientific medical practice really is. In the late 1960s, he had moved to Vermont to work as a health administrator and educator. Once there, he soon stumbled across a curious geographic pattern to a common operation, tonsillectomy.

"In Stowe, the probability of having a tonsillectomy by age 15 was about 70 percent," Dr. Wennberg recalls. "If you lived in Waterbury, over the hill from Stowe, it was about 10 percent." Indeed, there turned out to be a 13-fold difference in the local rates of tonsillectomy between the most and least surgery-happy Vermont communities he studied.

Medical uncertainty and the isolation of doctors largely explain those bizarre disparities. Dr. Wennberg discovered that doctors in Stowe, who talked mostly to each other, believed that if you didn't take tonsils out early, they'd become chronically infected and cause no end of trouble. Doctors in Waterbury, who didn't talk to the doctors in Stowe, held the opposite (and, as it turned out, correct) viewpoint: If left alone, most kids with frequent sore throats would eventually outgrow them.

This phenomenon turned out to be true of a lot more things than tonsillectomies. In Portland, Me., Dr. Wennberg found, 50 percent of men had prostate surgery by the age of 85; in Bangor, just 10 percent did. The rate of heart surgery was twice as high in Des Moines as it was in nearby Iowa City.

Subsequent studies by a number of researchers, working throughout the country, have shown that the use of all kinds of medical procedures varies dramatically from region to region. In fact, Dr. Wennberg has found the only procedures that *don't* show such variations are those few for which there is basically only one accepted treatment, such as hospitalization for heart attack or stroke.

Serving the rich
In 1988, Beverly Hills had one internist for every 566 people. Compton, a poor Los Angeles community, had one internist per 19,422 people.

Inefficiency experts

The waste in the system goes far beyond the provision of unnecessary care. Even when medical treatments are necessary, they're frequently done with no regard for efficiency.

Milliman and Robertson, a Seattle-based consulting firm, advises hospitals and other health-care organizations on ways to cut costs without compromising the quality of care. The firm's actuaries and physicians have examined thousands of individual medical records to develop guidelines on how long patients should stay in the hospital for such common conditions as childbirth or appendectomy—provided they're in generally good health and have no complications. Applying those guidelines to actual current records from a dozen urban areas across the country, the firm's actuaries concluded that 53 percent of all hospital days weren't necessary, including all the days spent in the hospital by the 24 percent of patients who didn't need to be there in the first place.

Where readers placed the blame

Asked to name the biggest contributor to the cost of health care, 23 percent of our readers incorrectly picked malpractice suits (see the box at right). An equal number named hospital costs, which *are* the biggest factor. Doctors' fees and health-insurance companies came in third and fourth in the survey.

As a private, commercial firm, Milliman and Robertson is in business to identify overuse for its clients, and might have a bias in favor of finding what it's paid to find. However, other studies by academic researchers have also found high rates of inappropriate hospitalization. A recent Rand Corp. review of published studies, most of which used data from the early and mid-1980s, estimated that 15 to 30 percent of hospital use was unnecessary.

The current rates of unnecessary hospitalization are difficult to estimate, since the system is in flux. The overall number of hospital days per thousand Americans—a standard measure of hospital utilization—has dropped over the last decade, in response to efforts by Medicare, health maintenance organizations, and private insurers to contain costs. But there are still large regional variations in hospital use, suggesting that waste still exists in the system.

Past experience shows it's possible to lower the number of days people spend in the hospital with no ill effects. In 1984, Medicare created financial incentives for hospitals to discharge patients as soon as possible, and not to admit them at all unless strictly necessary. The incentives worked; in two years, the average number of in-patient days per Medicare recipient fell 22 percent.

That sharp decline apparently had no real impact on the health of the patients involved, according to several statistics. The rate at which discharged patients need to be readmitted to the hospital shortly after leaving—an important index of low-quality care—has actually gone down for Medicare patients since 1984. Some care that used to be provided in the hospital can now be done at home, at much lower cost.

A medical arms race

Despite the efforts over the past decade to keep the costs of hospitalization down—by limiting hospital admissions, length of stay, and in-patient costs—our national hospital bill continues to rise. In 1990, hospitals soaked up 38 percent of national health expenditures (twice as much as doctors) and collectively earned a profit of $7-billion. Hospital administrators have proven how nimble health-care providers can be in getting around virtually any effort to rein them in.

For many years, hospitals expanded at a rate well beyond the national need, with the Government's help. During the 1950s and into the 1960s, the Federal Government provided subsidies to build new hospitals, and a decade later, Medicare allowed hospitals to pay for their capital improvements by charging higher fees. The result was a spate of hospital-building that had little relationship to clear community needs. New facilities and new wings were built, beds needed to be filled, and the law of induced demand kept them occupied—imposing a high cost on the health-care system and providing a high profit for the hospitals themselves.

When Medicare started to crack down on costs in 1984—paying hospitals a fixed fee to take care of each patient, based on his or her diagnosis—the hospitals reacted swiftly. Fewer Medicare patients were admitted, and those that were admitted stayed in the hospital for a shorter time. But the hospitals compensated by boosting their outpatient, psychiatric, and rehabilitation services, for which Medicare had set no cost limits. Although charges for hospitalization dropped, the costs for those other services ate up those savings, and more.

Hospitals also stepped up their efforts to attract privately insured patients to make up for the money they were losing on Medicare and Medicaid. Having built the capacity for many more beds than the nation needs, hospitals now tried to fill them—and to fill them with patients who had generous insurance policies and needed lots of medical services. "Hospitals make money by delivering services," explains William Erwin, who is a spokesman for the American Hospital Association. "If you don't need much done to you, the hospital isn't going to make money on you."

Attracting patients to a hospital isn't the same as attracting customers to a new restaurant or hardware store. Consumers decide on their own when and where they want to eat out or buy some drill bits. When they're sick, their doctors decide when and where to hospitalize them. So hospitals must market on two fronts: They must appeal directly to privately insured patients, and they must keep their admitting doctors happy.

To induce physicians to admit patients, hospitals resort to everything from first-year guaranteed incomes to subsidies for initial practice expenses. The effort pays off. In 1990, according to an annual survey by Jackson and Coker, an Atlanta physician-recruiting firm, the average doctor generated $513,000 in in-patient hospital revenue.

Another way to keep doctors happy is to provide them with state-of-the-art medical equipment. As a bonus, hospitals can then tout their up-to-date technology directly to consumers. Uwe Reinhardt, a Princeton University health economist, likes to paint the following scenario in his lectures:

"Imagine that you're a young couple in Chicago, stuck in a traffic jam in the Loop, and you see a billboard that says: 'Mount Sinai: The Cheapest Place in Chicago, Have Your Baby Here.' Then you go on and you see another billboard that says, 'Holy Mercy: The Only Place with a Glandular Schlumpulator, Have Your Baby Here.' Where are you going to go?"

Some regulatory efforts were made in the 1960s and 1970s to restrain hospitals from acquiring excessive amounts of expensive technology, with mixed success. In any case, Federal support for that effort was discontinued during the Reagan years. The rationale was that "unleashing competition" among hospitals would allow the free market to operate and help keep the cost of medicine down.

The irony, though, is that competition actually drives costs *up* where hospitals are concerned. The hospitals gain no competitive advantage by controlling costs, since their customers—doctors and patients—don't pay for their services anyway. In-

THE 'CRISIS' THAT ISN'T

MALPRACTICE: A STRAW MAN

Ask physicians to explain why the cost of health care goes up continually, and you're likely to hear complaints that the U.S. malpractice system encourages unnecessary "defensive" medical care. The public seems to have bought this argument. In a recent survey, CONSUMER REPORTS subscribers guessed that malpractice tied with hospital costs as the biggest factor driving the cost of health care.

Is malpractice such a villain?

It's true that malpractice costs are higher in the U.S. than in other countries. And in the mid-1980s, malpractice claims—and, accordingly, insurance premiums—did take a sharp upward swing. There was much talk then of a malpractice "crisis." But that crisis now seems to have abated, as have previous ones. Malpractice is a cyclical phenomenon: Periodically, the incidence of claims rises, then falls back.

At the moment, malpractice claims have been in one such downswing. The rate of claims has declined steadily since the peak of the last "crisis" in 1985. So have malpractice insurance premiums. In 1990, according to Medical Economics magazine's annual survey of physicians, doctors' malpractice premiums on average consumed only 3.7 percent of their practice receipts—although the percentage may be double that for high-risk (and high-paid) specialties, such as obstetrics, surgery, and anesthesiology. The U.S. Department of Health and Human Services puts the total cost of malpractice at less than 1 percent of total health outlays.

But then, no one argues that the direct cost of malpractice insurance is the main factor driving up the cost of care. Instead, it's assumed that physicians, fearing malpractice suits, are forced to practice "defensive medicine" just to protect themselves in the event of a lawsuit.

Defensive medicine undoubtedly exists, and doctors themselves feel that the threat of malpractice forces them to do more tests than are truly necessary. But quantifying the cost of defensive medicine is a slippery matter. The American Medical Association made a stab at it in the 1980s, and decided that the total cost of medical malpractice, including premiums and defensive medicine, was about 17 percent of physicians' earnings.

However, the AMA estimate was based on physicians' own reports of what they considered defensive practices, such as doing more diagnostic tests, sticking with the safest possible treatments, telling patients more about treatment risks, and keeping more complete records.

As that list suggests, one problem with defining defensive medicine—let alone measuring it—is that it's difficult to distinguish from care delivered for other reasons. Is a doctor doing an unnecessary test out of fear of a lawsuit, or because the medical culture values doing "everything," or simply to reassure an anxious patient? Did an obstetrician perform an unnecessary cesarean for legal protection, for scheduling convenience, or to earn a higher fee?

"You mostly get anecdotes when you're talking about defensive medicine," says Randall Bovbjerg, an analyst at the Urban Institute in Washington, D.C., who has worked on several malpractice studies.

That's not to say there isn't a malpractice crisis, however. "The greatest single problem about malpractice is that there's a lot more of it out there than anyone is dealing with," says Bovbjerg. "Patients are getting avoidable injuries and no one is stopping it."

Documentation for Bovbjerg's claim comes from a study conducted by Harvard University researchers for the state of New York. The researchers reviewed a random sample of New York hospital records in 1984 and found that 3.7 percent of patients suffered "adverse events," slightly more than one-quarter of which could be attributed to actual negligence.

Of those who suffered negligent injuries, only about one-eighth ever filed malpractice claims, and only about one-sixteenth ever recovered any damages. Conversely, the study found many cases in which patients filed malpractice suits with no clear evidence of negligence.

Costs aside, the current malpractice system is at best only an imprecise means of controlling the quality of medical care.

stead, hospitals compete only on the basis of perceived quality, and end up vying to see which one can secure and promote the newest well reimbursed technology, whether the technology is needed or not. Several hospitals in an area may have their own neonatal intensive care units, MRI machines, or cardiac care centers, when only one would serve the population equally well (see "The Cardiac Money Machine"). This year, despite the recession, hospitals plan to increase spending on new equipment by 15 percent, according to a survey by Shearson Lehman Brothers.

To attract the well-insured population, hospitals also provide amenities that have nothing to do with actual health care but add to the bill, including cable TV, private rooms and baths, gourmet menus, and the like. Baylor University Medical Center in Houston spent $18-million on the Tom Landry Sports Medicine and Research Center, complete with 7000-square-foot dressing rooms lined with oak lockers, and a 10-lane pool with underwater computerized video cameras used to analyze its patrons' swimming strokes.

Hospitals have also become more and more consciously concerned with projecting an upscale image that they hope will bring in an affluent clientele. Entries in a recent contest held by the Academy of Health Services Marketing, an organization of hospital marketing executives, reveal the new focus. For instance, the Southern Regional Medical Center in suburban Atlanta got Rosalynn Carter to endorse its maternity service after her grandchild was born there—as part of a successful campaign "to increase gross revenue . . . by marketing to a target market of insured, higher-income women, ages 25-49," according to the contest submission.

The trend is troubling, because there's clear evidence that the total cost of health care rises in areas where many hospitals begin to compete for the same pool of well-insured patients. Health economists James C. Robinson and Harold S. Luft of the University of California, Berkeley, examined data from 5732 hospitals nationwide, and found that costs per admission were 26 percent higher in hospitals that had more

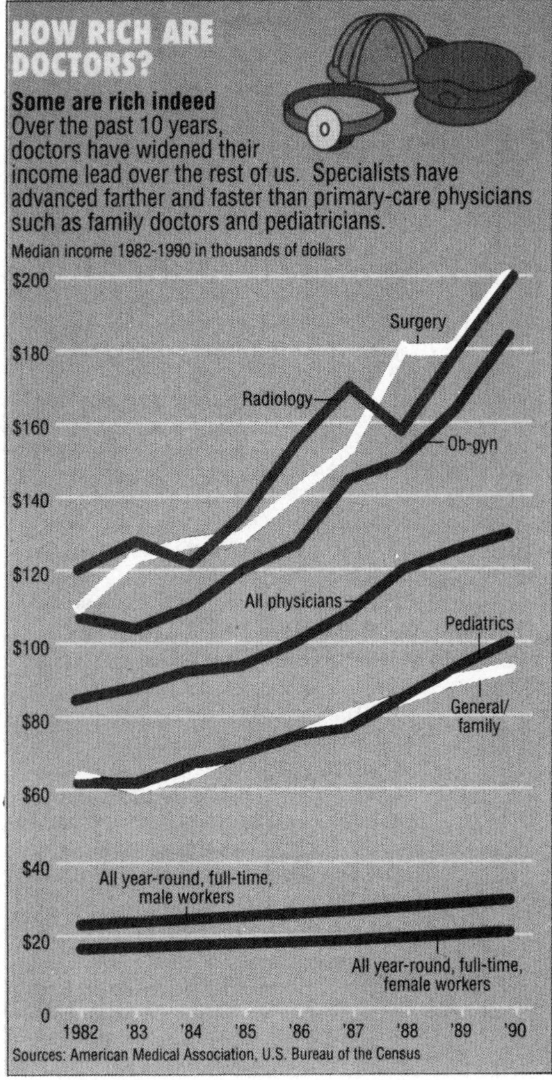

than nine competitors within a 15-mile radius. In a smaller-scale study of 747 hospitals, they found that those in competitive areas allowed patients to stay in the hospital longer after surgery—something that tends to please both patients and doctors, but with a high cost and no clear medical benefit.

More specialists, high costs

Just as American hospitals lead the world in high-priced technology, American physicians are heavy purveyors of expensive treatments and diagnostic tests—and reap great personal rewards for using them. Doctors in the U.S. earn much higher incomes relative to their fellow citizens than do doctors in other countries. According to figures from the Organization for Economic Cooperation and Development, in 1987 U.S. doctors earned 5.4 times more than the average worker. In Germany, the multiple was 4.2; in Canada, 3.7; and in France, Japan, and the United Kingdom, 2.4.

Historically, the highest fees have gone to doctors who perform concrete procedures, such as surgery, endoscopy, or diagnostic imaging. So-called evaluation and management services—in which doctors may examine and question the patient and prescribe a treatment, but don't actually do a specific procedure—haven't paid nearly as well.

In 1990, for instance, internists charged a median of $110 for a comprehensive office visit for a patient they hadn't seen before, according to a survey by Medical Economics magazine. Such a visit involves taking a medical history, doing a physical examination, and talking with the patient about his or her current condition. It can take up 45 minutes of the doctor's time. By contrast, the same survey found internists charged a median fee of $126 for spending 10 minutes to examine the bowel with a flexible fiberoptic device called a sigmoidoscope.

While individual physicians have great leeway in deciding what they will charge for a given procedure, insurance companies have established computerized databanks that help them determine whether or not the fee is "usual and customary" for that procedure. By this standard, a doctor whose fees are at the very top of the local scale may not receive full reimbursement. But there's no track record of cost for new procedures. With the help of medical specialty societies and the AMA, physicians have secured very high rates of reimbursement for new treatments.

"When something is in development, it's new, it's experimental, only a few physicians use it, there's some risk involved, and the price gets set accordingly," explains Joel Cantor, a program officer at the Robert Wood Johnson Foundation. "Then the technology diffuses and gets easier to use. More physicians get good at it. But the price never goes down."

The classic example is the extraction of cataracts and implantation of artificial lenses in the eye. This undeniably useful technology was introduced in the early 1980s and became a standard procedure by the end of the decade. During that time, however, many ophthalmologists became wealthy by charging $2000 or more for a cataract extraction that could be done in about an hour.

Primary-care physicians, such as general internists, family practitioners, and pediatricians, don't do procedures like that. Instead, they spend their days in office visits, which have long-established, and thus lower, "usual and customary" fee profiles.

As a result, their incomes are much lower than those of specialists. In 1990, the median income for general family practitioners was $93,000, and for pediatricians, $100,000, according to the American Medical Association's annual survey. Median income for surgeons and radiologists, on the other hand, was $200,000. Senior specialists can earn much, much more. Cardiovascular surgeons in group practice averaged about $500,000 in 1990, according to a study by the Medical Group Management Association.

Medical-school students, who must pick a residency program in their senior year, are painfully aware of these economic distinctions. In addition, they're trained in an academic environment that has long rewarded specialists with prestige and research grants. Young physicians, who leave medical school with a huge debt load, are increasingly turning to specialization. Overall, about one-third of U.S. physicians are in primary care. But among 1987 medical school graduates who have now completed their internships and residencies, only one-fourth have gone into primary care, according to data from the Association of American Medical Colleges.

A fed-up Ohio family doctor, responding to a survey by his professional society, the American Academy of Family Physicians, summarized his feelings this way: "Why bother with 60- to 70-hour work weeks, constant phone calls, all night emergency room visits, poor reimbursements, demanding patients, the need for instant exact decisions . . . concerning a million possible diseases, when you can 'specialize' in one organ, get paid $500 for a 15-minute procedure, only need to know a dozen drugs and side effects, and work part time?"

Do we really need our luxurious quantities of cardiologists, dermatologists, neurosurgeons, and urologists? Other countries get along fine with about a 50-50 ratio between primary-care doctors and specialists. The evidence is that we could, too.

A team from the New England Medical Center recently looked at patients who got their usual care from primary-care physicians (internists or family doctors) or from specialists (cardiologists and endocrinologists). The groups were not identical; the specialists tended to have older patients with more medical problems. But even after that difference was factored in, the specialists ran up higher bills, on average, than the primary-care doctors. They put more patients in the hospital, prescribed more drugs, and performed more tests. Yet an analysis still in progress appears to show that the two groups of patients had similar health outcomes.

The medical profession itself acknowledges the imbalance. The principal professional journal for internists, the Annals of Internal Medicine, said in a 1991 editorial: "Given the number of subspecialists already in practice, there are not enough highly specialized cases to go around. . . . We cannot continue to practice this way when cost containment is the dominant health policy issue of our times."

This year, Medicare began an effort to even out the economic imbalance between primary care and specialty physicians. The new program, known as the Resource-Based Relative Value Scale (RBRVS), is essentially a standard, national fee schedule, adjusted for geographic variations in the cost of practice. It increases the reimbursement for evaluation and management services, and greatly reduces the reimbursement for procedures. Physicians, however, may find a way around this constraint, as they have around others. For one thing, doctors can always simply raise their fees for privately insured, non-Medicare patients—although some private insurance companies may eventually adopt a version of the RBRVS fee schedule.

Since the mid-1980s, doctors have also manipulated the reimbursement system by "unbundling" services—that is, charging for two or more separate procedures instead of one. For instance, instead of billing $1200 for a hysterectomy, a doctor can collect $7000 by billing separately for various components of the operation. Commercial services conduct seminars to teach doctors how to maximize reimbursement in this way. But unbundling can cross the line into outright, prosecutable fraud, according to the General Accounting Office's health-care fraud report.

Supplier-side economics

Just as the providers of care have profited hugely over the years, so have those who supply the providers—the pharmaceutical companies and the makers of medical equipment and devices. They can charge top prices for their products, secure in the knowledge that the system will reimburse them. The pharmaceutical industry has been one of the nation's most profitable industrial sectors; it operates with an average profit margin of 15 percent and has given an average annual return to investors of 25 percent over the last decade.

Companies that latch on to new medical technologies can also earn huge profits. In spite of the current hand-wringing over health-care reform, health-care stocks as a group increased in value by fully 50 percent in 1991.

"A lot of people in health care are making a lot of money," says Stephen Zuckerman, a senior research associate at the Urban Institute in Washington, D.C. "They're not unhappy with the current system."

Curiously, the debate over health-care costs in the U.S. tends to assume that the cost of drugs and medical technology is immutably fixed. But international comparisons demonstrate that this needn't be so. In Japan, for example, the national fee schedule pays $177 for a magnetic resonance imaging (MRI) exam, compared with an average charge of about $1000 in the U.S. Pharmaceutical prices, which vary widely from country to country, are also significantly higher in the U.S. than anywhere else.

Nothing for something

As costly as it is, our health-care system might be worth its price if it somehow ended up making us healthier than people in other countries. But it doesn't.

Of the 24 industrialized nations making up the Organization for Economic Cooperation and Development (OECD), the U.S. spends more than twice as much on health per capita as the average. And it devotes a far greater percentage of its gross national product to health care than any other country. Yet the other OECD countries—with the exception of Turkey and Greece, by far the poorest of the group—all have roughly as many doctors and hospitals per capita as we do.

As for health status, of the 24 OECD countries, the U.S. ranks:

- 21st in infant mortality.
- 17th in male life expectancy.
- 16th in female life expectancy.

Dr. Barbara Starfield of the Johns Hopkins School of Public Health compared the U.S. with nine industrialized European nations in three areas: the availability of high-quality primary care, public-health indicators such as infant mortality and life expectancy, and overall public satisfaction with the value of health care. In all three areas, the U.S. ranked at or near the bottom.

The problem, simply put, is that the system is geared to providing the services that can earn physicians and hospitals the most money—not the ones that will do the public the most good. The U.S. has four times as many $1.5-million magnetic resonance imaging devices per capita as Germany does. But at the same

The uninsured aren't welcome
From a hospital marketing consultant's brochure: "To promote cardiology services, savvy marketers select all those at higher risk for heart disease, who are between the ages of 35 and 65, privately insured . . . it's target marketing at its best."

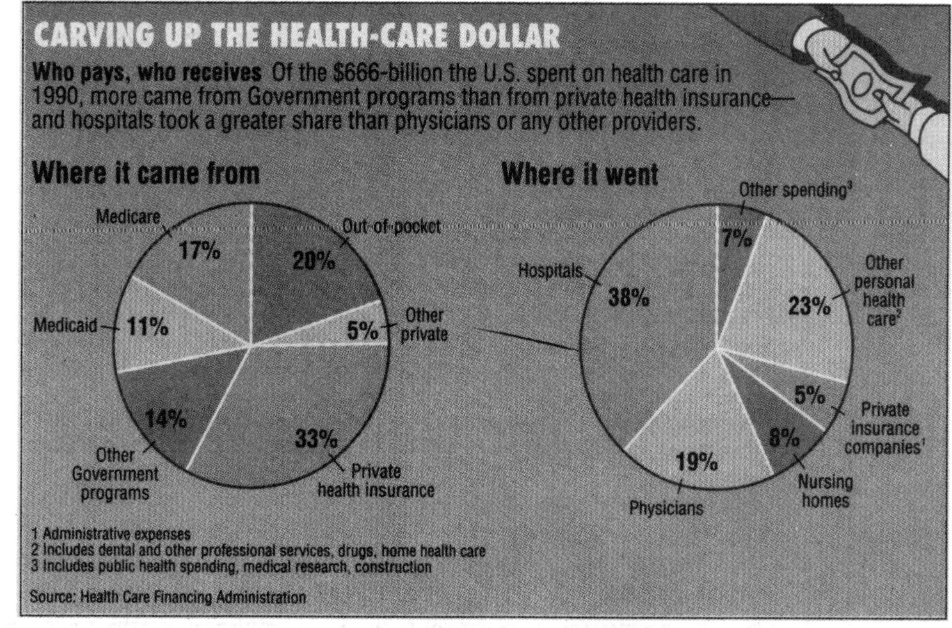

HIGH-TECH COMPETITION

THE CARDIAC MONEY MACHINE

People with heart and circulatory diseases, the leading causes of death in the U.S., have benefited enormously from medical and surgical advances over the past two decades. Until the late 1960s, doctors couldn't do much more than give them a little nitroglycerin or digitalis in the hope of extending their lives moderately. Then came **coronary bypass surgery, the first great treatment advance, in which blood vessels from elsewhere in the body are used to bypass diseased coronary vessels and restore more blood to the heart muscle. Next, in the 1980s, came balloon angioplasty, in which a balloon attached to a catheter is passed into the narrowed coronary vessel and inflated to crush the blockage against the wall of the coronary artery.**

The last decade has also brought new drugs to dissolve blood clots, to right irregular heartbeats, and to treat heart failure and high blood pressure; new imaging techniques; implantable electronic devices; and, as a last resort, new methods of heart transplantation.

All this, together with changes in diet and exercise habits, has had a dramatic effect. The death rate from heart disease in the U.S. has dropped roughly by half since 1950.

But the improvement has come at a very high cost. New technologies are expensive technologies, and the cardiac field is no exception. Coronary bypass surgery, for example, can easily run $30,000 or more for a single operation.

"It is just well-paid by everybody; even Medicare pays handsomely for it," says Ann Lennarson Greer, a medical sociologist at the University of Wisconsin. "The hospitals are crazy about bypass. Even if they're six blocks from a major heart center, they think they can't afford not to be in on it. People who get coronary problems, namely middle-aged men, tend to be among the best-insured people in our society."

(Uninsured patients may simply not get these costly procedures. One national survey found they were 39 percent less likely than the insured to get coronary angiograms—X-rays to evaluate the heart's blood supply—and 29 percent less likely to have bypass surgery.)

A growing profit center

Just how lucrative the cardiovascular field is was revealed in a 1990 report prepared by the Advisory Board Company, a Washington-based consulting firm, for its hospital clients. The report concludes that nearly one-quarter of all hospital revenues come from cardiology-related business, and of that, more than 80 percent comes from just four procedures—cardiac catheterization, angioplasty, bypass surgery, and heart-valve surgery. Not surprisingly, cardiovascular surgeons bring in the most revenue per in-patient hospital admission of any specialty—$10,942 in 1989, more than twice the average doctor's rate—according to an annual survey by Jackson and Coker, an Atlanta-based physician-recruiting firm.

The profit margins are as impressive as the revenues, according to the Advisory Board report: 70 percent for catheterization, 37 percent for angioplasty, and 40 percent for bypass, compared with overall profit margins for hospitals of less than 4 percent. And, to top it all off, the number of cardiac diagnostic and treatment procedures performed in the U.S. has been growing at an average annual rate of 12.7 percent.

The Advisory Board report uses a real, though unidentified, hospital to illustrate the profit potential. Wanting to increase its cardiology market share, the hospital invested $3-million in state-of-the-art equipment for catheterization and open-heart surgery. **The improved equipment (and additional support staff) attracted 25 new cardiologists to the hospital, who brought in hundreds of new patients for catheterization, angioplasty, and bypass. Within two years, the extra business had repaid the entire upfront investment and was adding $1.8-million a year in profits to the hospital's bottom line.**

This sort of return on investment has caused hospitals to look increasingly to cardiovascular care to fill their empty beds. In 1980, according to the Advisory Board report, there were 382,000 cardiac catheterizations performed in the U.S. and 340,000 treatment procedures, including bypass, angioplasty, valve surgery, and pacemaker implantations. By 1988, the volume of catheterizations had grown to 965,000 and the volume of procedures to 930,000.

Were all those procedures really necessary?

Doctors' dilemmas

The treatment of heart disease is a classic example of the way in which medical uncertainty produces variable, unnecessary care. Treatments for heart disease are advancing so rapidly that there's often little consensus on what to do or when to do it. What symptoms require a coronary angiography exam? Should a person with mildly uncomfortable angina and blockages in one or two vessels stick with drug treatment, or undergo angioplasty? If angioplasty has failed once, should it be repeated or should the patient get a bypass operation?

Medical journals are filled with debates on those questions. In the meantime, physicians must make daily treatment decisions with little guidance on which course is preferable—but knowing that they will be financially rewarded for ordering the maximum intervention.

Writing in the Journal of the American Medical Association, Dr. Thomas N. James of the University of Texas, Galveston, put it this way: "The same physician who decides whether a diagnostic or therapeutic procedure is to be done is too often also the one who does the procedure, interprets the findings (and decides whether additional procedures are indicated), and is paid for each step of the way.

This is not to say that such physicians are unskillful or that their decisions are necessarily made on the basis of personal gain, but the temptation is inescapably there."

Under those circumstances, it would be surprising if unnecessary procedures were not being done. The evidence is that they are:

- A study of pacemaker implantations in Philadelphia hospitals found that 20 percent were unnecessary and another 36 percent were problematic.
- A San Diego team found that, among patients who'd been hospitalized with mild heart attacks, 40 percent of those who got angiograms didn't need them. In addition to running up a bill ranging from $2000 to $3500, these patients were put at a slight risk of complications from the procedure itself.
- A team from Brigham and Women's Hospital in Boston examined the need for bypass surgery among 88 patients for whom it had been recommended. They advised against surgery for 74 of the 88. Among those 74, 60 accepted the second opinion and didn't have the operation. Over a follow-up period of more than two years, there were only two subsequent heart attacks, neither of them fatal, among this group—an outcome comparable to that of people who receive angioplasty or coronary bypass surgery.

Risky medicine

Despite findings like these, competitive and financial pressures conspire to encourage hospitals to build even more cardiac-care units. Consider the case of Manchester, N.H. Until 1985, Manchester residents who needed open-heart surgery had to travel to Boston or to Hanover, N.H., to get it. That year, a Manchester hospital, Catholic Hospital Medical Center, opened the first local open-heart surgery service. Within one year, the rate of heart surgery among residents of Manchester more than doubled.

What could explain the immediate jump in volume? An analysis by the Codman Research Group, a private health-care consulting firm, found that before the local program started, 90 percent of bypasses done on Manchester residents involved the transplantation of three or more arteries—a sign of serious and extensive disease. By 1988, however, over half the operations were single or double bypasses.

"They were clearly operating on less severely ill patients," says Dr. Philip Caper, Codman's chairman and a professor at Dartmouth Medical School. "The hooker is, nobody really knows whether they were better off. Some doctors think most single bypasses should almost never be done, because the risk is more than the benefit."

While coronary bypass can be lifesaving, it is an extremely traumatic procedure involving stopping and cooling the heart, hooking the patient up to a heart-lung machine, then restarting the heart. Handling an operation of this complexity requires a skilled and coordinated surgical team. That's why studies have repeatedly demonstrated that hospitals performing fewer than 150 open-heart procedures a year have higher death rates than those that perform more. In addition to driving up health-care costs, hospitals joining the cardiac gold rush may actually be putting their patients at serious risk.

That was the case in Phoenix in 1985, when the state of Arizona, in the spirit of deregulation, decided to abdicate its authority to control the introduction of new open-heart surgery programs. At that time, four Phoenix hospitals provided open-heart surgery. Almost immediately, seven more began programs. A computer-aided study of Medicare records performed by the Phoenix Gazette and the University of Arizona found that in the first year of deregulation, the local death rate from heart surgery increased by 35 percent. The average cost of the procedure, meanwhile, rose 50 percent.

time, the U.S. system short-changes the basic, low-tech care that has, over the years, proven effective at preventing disease.

The poor and uninsured are most likely to suffer from the imbalance. During the 1980s, while American hospitals were falling all over themselves to add costly, high-tech neonatal intensive-care units, the number of mothers unable to get basic prenatal care climbed, as did the incidence of premature births.

In most states, Medicaid now pays nowhere near the actual cost of delivering care; hospitals lose money on their Medicaid admissions. As a result, many doctors and some for-profit hospitals refuse even to accept Medicaid patients.

People with no insurance at all fare even worse. A group from the University of California, San Francisco, for example, looked at the hospital care given to sick newborn babies in the state's hospitals in 1987. Even though the uninsured babies were, on the average, the sickest group, they left the hospital sooner than insured babies and received fewer services while they were there. The Rand group has also shown that when California cut back on Medicaid coverage a decade ago, the health of people who lost their coverage declined dramatically.

"We've been sucked into believing that if we have a national health program, we're going to have rationing," says Dr. Philip Caper of Dartmouth. "The answer is, we have rationing already. Ask somebody who lost their health insurance, or can't get a bone-marrow transplant because they're on Medicaid. If that isn't rationing, what is?"

Hospitals that serve the poor and uninsured are suffering as well. The success of private hospitals in attracting well-insured patients has put an increasing burden on the public and not-for-profit hospitals still willing (or required) to accept all comers. A 1990 survey of 277 public and teaching hospitals found that 38 percent sometimes held patients overnight in the emergency room because no regular beds were available; 40 percent had turned away ambulances because of overcrowding.

Hospitals in California have even shut down their trauma centers as a way of barring the door against uninsured patients. "Hospitals find themselves jockeying for geography," says Bettina Kurowski, a vice president of St. Joseph Medical Center in Burbank, which closed its

Costs exposed, prices cut
After a state government survey revealed it was charging $14,000 more for heart bypass than a local competitor, St. Vincent Health Center in Erie, Pa., dropped its bypass price by $10,000—the first rate reduction in its 116-year history. Estimated annual savings: $5-million.

trauma center when its annual losses hit $1.5-million and threatened the financial survival of the hospital as a whole. "If you can be promised service areas that include freeways, and therefore get trauma cases covered by auto insurance, you can break even. If you don't include freeways, mostly you get penetrating [gunshot and stab wound] trauma, and those patients by and large don't have insurance."

Dissatisfied Americans **Pollsters asked citizens of 10 developed nations to rate their health-care systems. U.S. respondents were the unhappiest of the lot. Fully 60 percent said our system is in need of "fundamental changes."**

Red tape and red ink

Ultimately, our cumbersome, inequitable system of reimbursement raises the costs for all of us—insured and uninsured alike—and causes problems for physicians as well. "In order to preserve the mirage of a private system, we've created the most bureaucratic, regulated system of any in the world," says David Mechanic, director of the Institute on Health Care Policy at Rutgers University.

A key characteristic of the U.S. system is its obsession with making sure that patients get only what their insurance entitles them to, and nothing more. That means, for instance, that hospitals must keep meticulous track of everything used by a particular patient, down to individual gauze sponges or aspirin tablets—all adding to administrative costs. More important, the burden of dealing with multiple forms from a huge number of insurance companies requires a lot of clerical manpower.

Increasingly, too, doctors and hospitals have to answer to Government and private review panels that evaluate many aspects of the care they offer. Government reviewers work to ensure that Medicare and Medicaid patients are not being undertreated, while private insurers want to make sure that their patients are not being overtreated.

Hospitals in the U.S. spend fully 20 percent of their budgets, on average, on billing administration—compared to only 9 percent for Canadian hospitals. To run a health plan covering 25 million people, Canada employs fewer administrators than Massachusetts Blue Cross, which covers 2.7 million.

Our nation's more than 1200 private health-insurance companies add to the red tape by the necessary maintenance of their underwriting, marketing, and administrative staffs. This overhead consumed an average 14 cents out of every premium dollar in 1990, according to the Health Care Financing Administration.

Private physicians, too, have been forced to hire extra office help to cope with the ever-enlarging demands of third-party review, regulations, and paperwork. Drs. David Himmelstein and Steffie Woolhandler, internists at Harvard Medical School who are prominent critics of the U.S. health-care system, have calculated that the average office-based U.S. physician employs twice as many clerical and managerial workers as the average Canadian doctor. Dealing with the bureaucracy has become so intrusive that doctors have developed a name for it: the "hassle factor."

Dishonest physicians have also taken advantage of the system to bilk insurance companies. According to the General Accounting Office report: "This complex system itself becomes an impediment to detecting fraud and abuse. . . . a physician who bills for more office visits than can reasonably be performed in a day, for example, may not be detected if the billing is split among several payers."

Drs. Woolhandler and Himmelstein, who favor a Canadian-style system, have calculated that about 20 percent of U.S. health-care spending goes for administrative costs: insurance overhead, hospital and nursing administration, and physicians' overhead and billing expenses. Not surprisingly, the private health-insurance industry says this estimate is too high. However, industry representatives decline to offer their own figure.

Universal coverage and uniform fee schedules enable other countries to avoid most of the administrative expense of the U.S. system. The single-payer Canadian system, where all health-care costs are ultimately paid by the Government, devotes about 10 percent of expenditures to administration. The General Accounting Office calculates that if the U.S. were to adopt a single-payer Canadian-style system, we would save about $70-billion a year in insurance overhead and the administrative costs to doctors and hospitals.

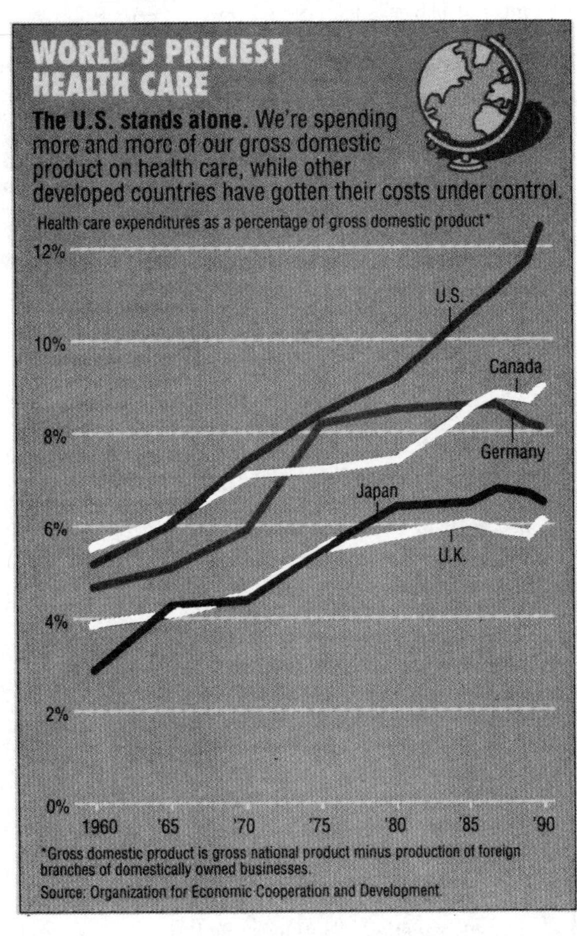

Enough for all

No matter what corner of the health-care system is examined—hospital costs, clinical procedures, administrative expenses—at least 20 percent seems to represent waste or inefficiency. If the system could be redesigned to get rid of this excess, it could, in effect, provide 20 percent more necessary service without costing any more than it does now.

Granted, devising a totally efficient system would be difficult, if not impossible, to accomplish. However, there is easily more than enough excess spending in our current system to take care of the roughly 14 percent of the population who are not currently under any public or private insurance plan.

THE FUTURE OF MEDICINE

New anatomy lesson, please

The business of medical care is under attack from all sides. Luckily, writes Alexandra Wyke, new technologies are set to transform medicine, eradicate most disease and hugely improve people's health

THE medical world is in a sorry state. Doctors and hospitals complain that they cannot satisfy what has become an unlimited demand for medical care. Medical breakthroughs are quickly taken for granted; eager patients soon want more. Even with the best available therapy, many sufferers are provided with only partial solutions. Some are left permanently disabled, unable to cope with everyday life. Meanwhile, such ordinary illnesses as the common cold remain virtually untreatable. And everywhere cash shortages are biting; patients grumble because they have to wait for treatment or because they get no treatment at all. The world is crying out for more, and better, medicine.

Since the discovery in the late 1930s of drugs that could kill bacteria, modern medicine has burgeoned into a multi-trillion-dollar business. With a few exceptions, doctors had been mostly powerless before antibiotics. They may have been adept at diagnosis, spotting a disease among a hotch-potch of complaints; or at prognosis, guessing what might happen to patients as a result of illness; but they could offer little in the way of treatment. Antibiotics changed all that. And explosive technological development after 1940 gave the medical profession enormous new powers to fight disease and sickness. Patients duly put their health care into the hands of these omnipotent doctors who, encouraged by medical manufacturers, prescribed liberally.

Yet there is, surprisingly, little or no evidence that modern doctors, pills or surgery have improved people's overall state of health. The increase in Americans' average life expectancy from 63 years in 1940 to 76 today (see chart 1) has been ascribed more to increased wealth, better sanitation, nutrition and housing, and the widespread introduction of the refrigerator than to modern medicine.

In 1992 the World Health Organisation (WHO) concluded that the world's population is not getting any healthier. The WHO study showed that people are reporting more frequent and longer-lasting episodes of serious and acute illness than they did 60 years ago. The world is still plagued by a string of nasty diseases, many of which afflict the growing elderly populations of richer countries. As for antibiotics, even they have become an overworked remedy. They may have saved millions of lives since they first appeared 50 years ago; but today some infectious diseases that were once curable no longer respond to treatment. Tuberculosis is reappearing in America and Europe because doctors have dished out antibiotics too carelessly, giving bacteria an opportunity to evolve drug-resistant strains.

The problem is not confined to rich countries. The burden of sickness is growing in poor countries, too, as populations explode, new diseases like AIDS take their toll, and heart disease and cancers strike those who manage to survive beyond middle age. After childhood disease, heart disease and cancer are the biggest killers in poor countries. Not surprisingly, the WHO thinks there is still considerable scope for the discovery of new drugs and medical techniques.

Mindful of their previous shortcomings, scientists have taken up the challenge: to discover effective medical products. The financial rewards, they know, could be huge; health care is one of the world's biggest industries. Luckily, too, they have new technological tools at their disposal. Biotech-

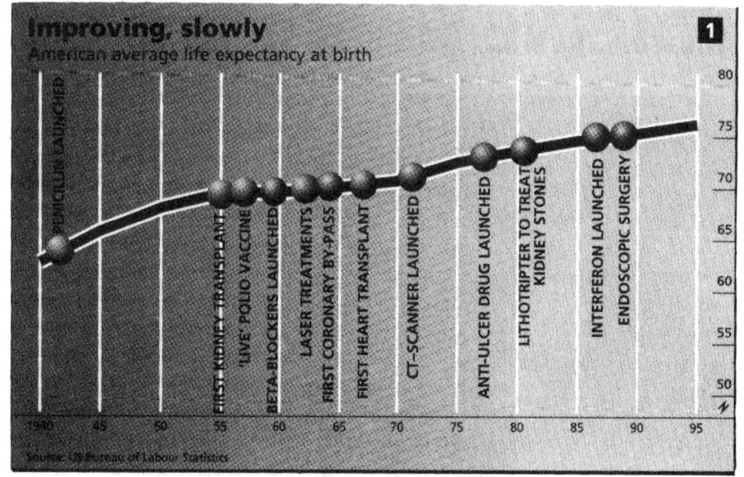

nology, faster and smarter computers, telecommunications and robotics are coming together to transform health care. New products are rolling out of laboratories at breathtaking speed. Here is some idea of what may be to come.

There will be drugs for hitherto untreatable diseases. There will be easy-to-use medical tests that predict a person's prospective state of health throughout his lifetime so steps can be taken to prevent diseases. There will be surgical robots operating with a precision that puts their human counterparts to shame. Doctors, nurses, hospitals and manufacturers will all be linked through a network of computers, telephones, optical fibres and satellite link-ups that a patient can plug into. The entire health-care business will be automated and closely monitored for cost and efficiency.

There will be more careful assessment of the benefits of medical treatment. Such benefits are obvious for procedures like mending broken bones, removing eye cataracts, or treating ulcers or bacterial infections. But the value of many other present-day treatments remains obscure; indeed, in many cases, no proper study of their effects on health has ever been done. And even when treatments can offer temporary help—such as removing a blood clot from a heart-attack victim—there is little change in a patient's underlying complaint, so that he stands a good chance of falling sick from the same disease again. In the meantime the surgery or pills that he has been given may have had harmful and not always well-monitored side-effects.

The new generation of medical products will change this by making it easier to measure health outcomes. Surgery will be less intrusive, less painful and safer. In some cases it will be performed without the knife. Patients will recover more quickly and need less hospital care. As for drugs, biotechnology will re-engineer them from mere palliatives into full-scale cures that tackle not just the ills of rich countries but those of poorer countries too.

These innovations have come at a good time for health-care businesses. In the past decade governments, insurers and employers in all rich countries have realised that they can no longer pay health-care bills that were growing enormously as populations became older and more demanding (see chart 2). In 20 years' time the proportion of most rich countries' populations aged 65 and over will have doubled to around 20-25%. Old people today consume a third of total health spending; the way things are going, by 2000 they will be consuming half.

Those who finance health care—ie, governments and insurance companies—are responding by demanding more information about the cost, effectiveness and quality of the services they are buying. They increasingly want health care to be "managed"—that is, delivered for a prepaid fee. They hope that this will get rid of medical tests and operations that are unnecessary; and persuade doctors to prescribe only the most cost-effective drugs or surgical procedures. New technologies may help. Computerisation will provide more information with which to manage costs. Even on the medical level, though many new technologies will be expensive, they will yield off-setting savings by reducing the need for hospitals, doctors and nurses.

The movement of most health-care systems towards managed care is clear, especially in America, where well over half the privately insured are now enrolled in managed-care plans. The Clinton administration's plan to reform America's health-care system through the creation of large health alliances that choose mainly among competing managed-care plans will be a further boost—if Congress adopts it, or something like it. Those who have made a fat living from America's bloated health-care system are certainly resigned to change.

The "Hillary factor", as some American circles have dubbed the change of mood in the health-care market, has already prompted insurers, hospitals, doctors and medical suppliers to regroup into health-care networks offering one-stop shopping for patients. According to David Vandewater, chief operating officer of Columbia Healthcare, a hospital chain based in Louisville, Kentucky: "The strat-

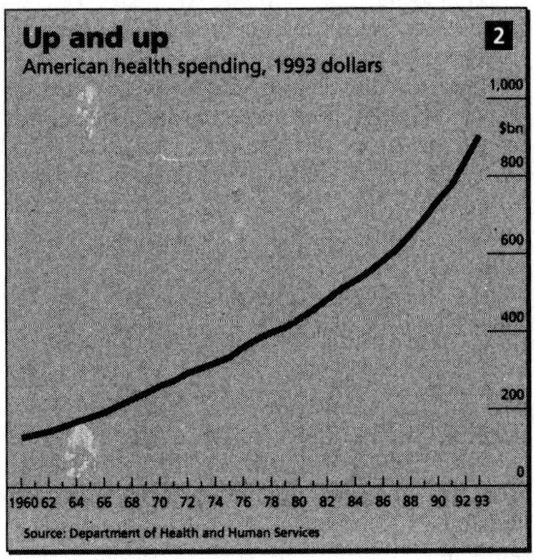

egy at Columbia is to establish a provider network, where we can offer anything the patient needs, be it diagnoses or skilled nursing facilities, not just hospitals." Sir Richard Sykes, chief executive of Glaxo, a British drug firm, agrees: "Ultimately Glaxo will have to manoeuvre itself from drug firm to health-care concern, from Glaxo to Glaxocare."

Throughout America competitive medical networks, whose success will be determined by their performance, efficiency and cost, are springing up. Every business in the health-care market is entering partnerships by acquisition or through alliances to deliver a comprehensive health service. In the past year Columbia Healthcare has merged with Galen Health Care and HCA, increasing the number of hospitals under its umbrella from 21 to 192. Columbia is also forging new associations with nursing homes and health maintenance organisations (HMOs), the flagships of managed care, which offer health services in return for a flat fee. Merck, the world's biggest drug company, recently paid $6 billion for Medco, a drug distributor. Merck made the acquisition after it concluded that the days of traditional pill manufacturers flogging their wares to gullible doctors were numbered.

In Europe too, managed care is arriving. Holland is shaking up its social-insurance system to introduce it. Germany is trying to inject more competition into the 1,000-plus sickness funds that insure most of its population. In Britain the government has created an "internal market" under which providers compete for business from purchasers. It is now pushing most general practitioners towards "fund-holding", which would give them set budgets out of which to pay for most hospital services and drugs for patients on their lists. Fund-holders are already proving effective at shopping around for the best and cheapest care. That is forcing hospitals to vie for doctors' business; many have appointed special sales representatives to plead their case on the basis of high-quality service or bargain deals.

Thanks to these changes, drug firms and other health-care suppliers, all of them under fire for making excessive profits on useless products, will become more dependent on R&D to produce new products. Doctors will have to demonstrate, with the help of computers, that their work is cost-efficient. Hospitals will be encouraged to treat more people as out-patients or even at home to curb health-care costs. Already in 1993 one in three hospital beds in America were empty each day.

Robotics and other new technologies are now poised to accelerate change—rapidly enough to come as a shock to many patients, let alone to the producers who will have to alter their ways. This survey offers a tour through some of the world's industrial and academic laboratories in order to spotlight the huge changes that technology is about to impose on health care—and their consequences.

Automating health care

Information technology takes medicine into the 20th century

SHINY machines may clutter doctors' surgeries and hospital wards, but when it comes to exploiting the information revolution health care is still in the Dark Ages. In the medical world communication means doctors writing (often illegibly) on scraps of paper that are stored in filing cabinets to be forgotten or lost. Consultants, junior doctors, nurses, pharmacists and even managers crowd around hospital beds, but their association with each other stops outside the ward. Family doctors practising outside hospitals rarely meet their peers inside. One result is unnecessary duplication. Today's health budgets are too tight to support such haphazard and wasteful practice.

Health-care systems are creaking under the growing mounds of documents, facts and figures they need to store and process. The mounds are becoming mountains as insurers and governments clamour for evidence that doctors do any good. Meanwhile doctors are finding it hard to absorb ever more information. An average American doctor spends nine hours a week educating himself. And for most doctors, integrating data generated in each hospital on each patient and applying the knowledge gained from reading journals has become an art as much as a science. The information can often be conflicting and few doctors have any idea how to resolve such conflicts.

Enter, belatedly, the computer. By becoming doctors' helpmates they can manage medical data, combine information sources and advise on trade-offs using something more than enlightened guesswork. Plummeting computer prices combined with rapid increases in computer power are allowing the development of information systems that can satisfy most doctors' needs at affordable prices. Paul Clayton, who is introducing an information system at Columbia Presbyterian Medical Centre, in New York city, reckons that within a decade all the data generated about the 50,000 in-patients admitted each year to his hospital and its 800,000 out-patient visits will be storable on magnetic disks for $63,000—or on optical disks for as little as $4,500. Already it is cheaper to store information on optical disks than on paper.

As computers become more mobile and smaller—with desktop workstations miniaturised into mobile clip-boards or dictating-machines—the risk of their physically intruding on a doctor's dealings with patients will decrease. According to Ifay Chang at IBM's Thomas J. Watson Research Centre, in Yorktown Heights, New York city, computers already deliver information in the integrated form that doctors require. Systems allowing people at different sites to collaborate via computers have already been designed. Computers should soon allow a surgeon sitting in Minneapolis to operate by proxy on a patient thousands of miles away.

Modern methods of compressing huge amounts of data will permit complex pieces of information, such as x-rays or even moving pictures of a surgical operation, to be sent across long distances via satellites or fibre-optic cable. High-definition television can provide imagery good enough for diagnoses that require subtle differences of colour or tone. The multimedia revolution will let medics and patients write to, talk to and see each other simultaneously.

Hospitals have already largely automated the prescription of drugs. A start has been made on a global medical database. The electronic Internet has helped patients to make contact with, and perhaps learn from, fellow sufferers. Several small firms now sell do-it-yourself diagnosis software that can run on most consumers' personal computers. Bigger changes loom ahead: notably the electronic storage of all medical records with systems that facilitate access, retrieval and information-sharing. That should provide enough information for computerised clinical decision-making to become the norm. Managed-care information systems will generate (and update) the value-for-money appraisals that insurers and governments now demand. They will also help doctors to take the right decisions.

Some doctors may not like the notion of machines monitoring their performance. But patients and those paying health-care bills will benefit hugely. Information technology should speed up delivery so that surgical waiting lists or hanging about in out-patient departments become things of the past. On the clinical side, even if information technology does no more than identify useless and unnecessary treatment, it could save lots of money.

A poor medical record

The writing and collection of patient records has changed little in response to the computer age, as doctors have been reluctant to abandon paper for electronics. The first generation of electronic medical-record systems required some computer know-how. InterPractice Systems, a joint venture between EDS (a subsidiary of General Motors created by Ross Perot) and Harvard Community Health Plan, a health-maintenance organisation, installed a mini computer in 1988 at a health centre in Burlington, Massachusetts. The system stores all the information on the centre's 8,000 patients, from the minute they walk into reception. The centre's 15 doctors each need a powerful Apple computer, however; terminals have also been installed in the examination room.

Computerised record-keeping systems will become simpler. Stanford University's Medical Computer Science Laboratory, among others, has compressed data collection down to a portable pen-based computer for roaming doctors that can store a complete set of patient records. When the computer "reads" what seem to be illegible scribblings, it flashes up on the screen its guesses of what was written. The system has graphics and a palette of 256 different colours, so doctors can draw the anatomy of the abdomen, say, and show where a pain is being felt. Most important, the electronic pad can communicate with a central computer, which is continuously updated with information entered by doctors wherever they are. The system still has teething problems, but the Stanford group hopes to test the pads in hospitals soon.

As patient records become digitised they also become easier to process. Clinical information systems (the most elementary form of data-processing designed to give patient data to those who need it) are spreading fast through hospitals and doctors' surgeries. IBM and Kaiser Permanente, America's largest HMO, are testing one such system in Colorado. Digitised patient records are shared through an information network among all of Kaiser's 400 doctors, employed in 17 health clinics. Eventually the electronic network will be linked to local chemists' shops, to laboratories and to hospitals, all of which will feed data into the system. Hewlett-Packard, DEC and AT&T are among other companies working on similar networks.

Multimedia can do more than computerise records. Linda Tetzlaff of IBM's Thomas J. Watson Research Centre is developing a system for parents who look after young children with leukaemia. A computer set up at home answers such questions as how to give drugs; what to do if the child has a seizure; or simply what a seizure is. The answers are given in writing, orally or on screen. There is an interactive link with a doctor in the clinic, who is kept up to date whenever a parent logs on with trickier queries that the computer cannot answer.

This kind of computer doctor can be "intelligent". The Imperial Cancer Research Fund in London is developing a system that signals whenever patients are allergic to particular drugs; and another that keeps track of recent reports on medical practice or changes in clinical guidelines. Stephen Pauker of Tufts University in Massachusetts is working on a system that looks at awkward clinical choices, such as whether somebody who has just had a heart attack should be operated on, whether to carry out a coronary by-pass operation on a patient who has cancer or the risks to a fetus if a pregnant woman with cancer is given radiation therapy.

Lots of gadgets are being developed to improve the quality of patient records and the information that can be extracted from them. Some feed directly into the health-care electronic network. Biocircuits of Sunnyvale, California, is testing a desktop analyser that measures hormone concentration or the presence of viruses in a pinprick sample of blood. Usually such tests have to be done in pathology laboratories, which take days to deliver the results; the Biocircuits device can be used in a few minutes.

Patients too will soon have products they can use to examine themselves. They can then feed their own reports into a home computer health diary. Separately, BioControl, an American firm based in Pennsylvania, and Omron, a Japanese firm based in Kyoto, have developed gadgets that can read the broad chemical content of blood when it is placed on the skin—without so much as a drop of blood actually being shed. According to Koichi Takizawa, a research director at Omron, it should be possible to miniaturise any hospital medical equipment, even body scanners. The difficulty, he says, is to adapt the information generated by such machines so that it is intelligible to patients. Next on Omron's list for miniaturisation is electro-cardiography, which measures the electrical action of heart muscle and gives information on the pumping action of the heart.

Aprex, a firm based in Fremont, California, has SmartCaps, which incorporate the simple electronics of a digital watch into a pill bottle-cap to record the time and date when the bottle is opened. This helps doctors monitor whether their patients are taking prescribed medicines. Aprex hopes to adapt SmartCaps so they can "talk" to doctors' information systems. Such a discourse could ensure that action is taken immediately if medication is being skipped.

For the future, Ted Shortliffe of Stanford University suggests that computers will be used to disseminate medical literature; to offer access to individual patient records, which is useful for tracking people when they move; to handle billing and general accounts; to bring specialists via interactive TV to inner cities, rural areas or poor countries where they are scarce; to give individuals, sick or healthy,

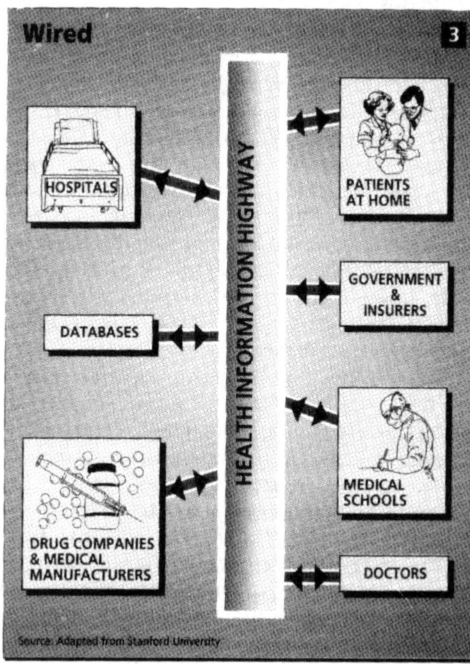

Source: Adapted from Stanford University

their medical bulletins plus a personal health database; to create databases on how well populations and patients do on particular medical regimes, which are also primed to give doctors advice; and to prepare clinical reports for drug regulators that have to approve the use of experimental medical products (see diagram 3). All this will have huge implications for patient privacy, a point to which this survey will return.

Saving money too

From Silicon Valley in California to NTT in Tokyo, computer and telecoms firms are piling into the health-care market because they see a chance to make big profits. Patients will usually welcome anything that improves their care; payers of health-care bills will also be keen if it helps to contain costs. And some recent studies have shown just how big the savings might be. In 1993 the Regenstrief Institute at the University of Indiana published the results of a trial that produced savings of over $800 per hospital in-patient when doctors used computers to order tests or to receive reminders. The figures suggested that the hospital concerned could save over $3m a year. The savings across the whole country could approach billions of dollars—for just one computerised procedure.

Until recently, little state- or federal-government support for such projects has been forthcoming. But President Clinton's plan for health-care reform refers explicitly to the cost savings that can be made by using information technology. The so-called "Gore-2" bill to promote an information superhighway (initiated by then-Senator Al Gore before he became vice-president) could speed up the wiring of America's health-care system. The government is encouraging the private sector to build the superhighway with promises of further deregulation. In return, however, the telecoms industry will be expected to provide free links from the highway to every American hospital and health clinic by the end of the decade.

The remaining obstacles to a super-efficient electronic-communication network for medicine are mostly practical. The cottage-industry approach of most doctors has been the cause of enormous inefficiencies in health care. It has also created an excess of medical languages. Consider the six teaching hospitals in Boston. Each has a different technique for creating medical records. Their doctors describe symptoms and remedies differently. In 1991 the Institute of Medicine, part of the National Academy of Sciences in Washington, DC, published a report on computer-based patient records that argued strongly for the creation of a single medical language. It triggered a huge global effort. Europe is perhaps more advanced than America, through the Advanced Informatics in Medicine (AIM) programme based in Ghent, Belgium.

Even the most conservative believe that by 2010 computers will enable health-care workers to work more efficiently. But the computers' contribution will not end there. Their enormous processing power and the new channels of communication they have created are about to trigger an even more profound revolution—in the hospital operating theatre.

(continued)

A trip to the theatre

Why there will be fewer doctors and hospitals

FROM their origins as barbers, surgeons have accepted illness or even death as an unfortunate side-effect of their craft. Surgeons have rarely been criticised even though much surgery seems primitive. Surgeons cut big holes in bodies in order to repair them. To do good, they plead, they have to do harm. Yet how much better it would be if surgery were less violent. Patients would suffer less and recover more quickly. And for those worried about costs, less violent surgical treatment ought also to be less expensive. As John Wickham of the department of minimally-invasive therapy at Guy's Hospital in London puts it: "Open surgery with its hands-in approach will appear quite gross when viewed by the standards that will be set in the next 20 years."

Two technological advances, image-guided therapy and robotics, are behind the forthcoming revamp of the operating theatre. By hooking up conventional medical tools to computers, image-guided therapy offers surgeons the ability to see into and through patients' bodies. Surgeons should then do less damage to their patients. Of the several research groups round the world working on these technologies, including the University of Grenoble and the National Cancer Centre Research Institute in Tokyo, the largest is led by Ferenc Jolesz of Brigham and Women's Hospital and Harvard Medical School in Boston, Massachusetts. Dr Jolesz's sponsors are General Electric, which is funding most of the project, IBM, Sun Microsystems, Kodak, Zeiss and Thinking Machines Corporation. Dr Jolesz says that image-guided therapy "enhances reality" by improving upon the naked eye; and unlike virtual reality, it depicts a real patient.

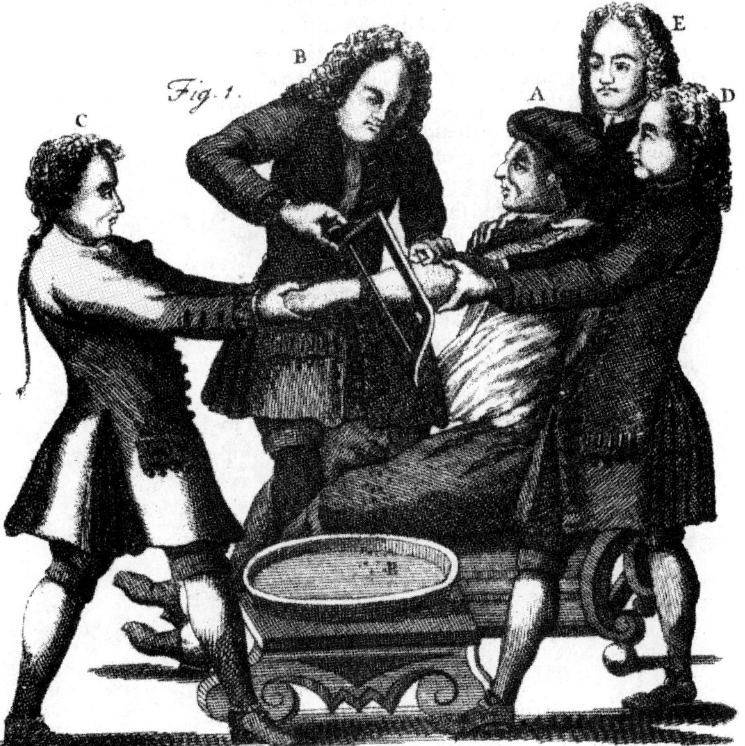

Shouldn't we try aromatherapy, first?

Since the discovery of X-rays at the end of the 19th century, doctors have used medical images to peer inside bodies. Pregnant women are delighted when ultrasound gives them a glimpse of their fetuses, even though the images are usually fuzzy. More distinct pictures come from X-ray computerised tomography (CT) and from magnetic resonance imaging (MRI), which provide two-dimensional slices of a patient's body. Although MRI cannot "see" bone in the way that CT can, it picks up everything else including skin, blood vessels and even cartilage with a resolution of 0.5-1mm, the dimensions in which surgeons usually work. MRI can also differentiate the heart from the kidney or cancers from healthy tissue.

Seeing like Superman

Medical imaging is typically used by doctors to make a diagnosis: the existence of a brain tumour, say, or a fractured bone. With powerful computers, according to Dr Jolesz, it can be put to even better use by giving the surgeon in the operating theatre supernatural sight. But several technological leaps have to be made to get this far. By putting sliced CT/MRI images of the body on top of one another, a computer can construct a see-through three-dimensional model of a patient, exposing his flesh and bones. Like Superman, the computer can choose just how far it wants its CT/MRI eyes to penetrate below the surface of the skin.

The next trick is to bring computerised images into the operating theatre. The problem here is "registering", matching life to image. A real patient will not stay in exactly the same position as when a CT/MRI scan was taken. Tiny errors in registering can have devastating results. A displacement of a millimetre can make the difference between hitting and missing a blood vessel. Using fancy computer footwork, several research groups have worked out ways of improving registration. One, developed by Ron Kikinis, of Brigham and Women's Hospital, is to relay a video of the patient to the computer, which then blends the CT/MRI image with a video image of the live patient. The video camera is fixed to certain visual features of the patient. If the patient moves, the CT/MRI image moves in concert with the video image as the camera repositions itself.

To many surgeons this sounds like gobbledygook. In practice, says Eric Grimson, of Massachusetts Institute of Technology, a surgeon will be able simultaneously to see a live patient and an overlaid detailed image of his internal anatomy. Mr Grimson is developing, with the help of a firm called TASC, a transparent panel rather like a teleprompter that will be placed above the patient during the operation. A three-dimensional image of the patient will be projected on to the panel. The surgeon can be wired into the system too. As he moves his head the image will reflect the new angle from which he is viewing the patient. If scalpels are loaded with light-emitting devices they can be registered too, so that the computer follows the surgeon's movements and projects them on to the panel. The surgeon can dig with greater precision and safety because he can follow where the scalpel is in parts of the body he could not normally see.

Even open-body surgery offers a limited view. A surgeon can see only the surfaces of the parts of the body that he has laid bare; he has little idea of what lies below. Dr Jolesz gives an example of a child with a brain tumour that was close to the part of the brain that controls movement. Normally the surgeon, after consulting a few MRI slices, would have cut the quickest route through to the tumour to remove it. But this time the surgeon asked for a computerised registration. Knowing the exact position of the tumour and the other parts of the brain's anatomy, the computer showed the safest way to the tumour. Without the computer, the surgeon would have had to open up a large part of the brain.

Image-guided therapy has also proved effective in surgical planning. Court Cutting, a plastic surgeon at New York University's Medical Centre, has, with Russell Taylor at IBM, used CT images of the deformed skull of a girl and, helped by a computer, determined the best breaks and alignments needed to match her skull to a computerised model of an average skull. Without a computer masterplan, surgeons have to cut and paste the skull together in the operating room. Because the face swells under surgery the outcome is not always clear. Not surprisingly, several operations are usually necessary before surgeon and patient are happy. In computer-assisted surgery fewer are needed.

Image-guided therapy promises more even than this. The recent introduction of keyhole surgery has made many operations less harrowing. Endoscopes (thin, flexible rods) are inserted through a small incision in the body to give an inside view—literally. Long, thin appliances carrying miniature surgical tools, working through other man-made portholes, then carry out the operation.

Endoscopy still involves some violation of the body. The ideal operation would be done with what is called "trackless" surgery, in which operations are conducted without touching the body at all. Ultrasound waves can be focused on diseased tissue, for example—leaving the rest of the body unscathed. But first surgeons would need to see inside people to know where to point their deadly beams. Working blind they could, as with present-day invasive surgery, end up damaging healthy parts of the body as well.

Dr Jolesz's group is now putting the final touches to a grand plan: to remove a breast tumour without making a single cut. Image-guided therapy marks out the breast tumour, which can then be destroyed by zapping it with ultrasound. However, says Dr Jolesz, trackless surgery should be immensely powerful in getting rid of brain and other cancers too. In fact image-guided trackless surgery should be so simple that it can be performed by a doctor thousands of miles away from the treated patient. Because everything is computerised, there is no need for direct patient contact and the operation can be executed through a network of satellites. (As such it has earned the soubriquet "Nintendo medicine.")

First, though, several important adaptations must be made. The MRI and CT images are, like photographs, just a historical record. During surgery much can change—there can be unexpected bleeding or organs can be accidentally knocked and moved into the knife's position. What is needed to cope with this is real-time imagery. General Electric has now built an MRI machine that scans a patient while an operation is going on. The first one has just been installed in the basement of Brigham and Women's Hospital. Dr Jolesz and his team are adapting the computer so it can generate real-time, three-dimensional, moving MRI images from the data produced by the new machine. The group hopes to be ready for its first trackless operation in the next few weeks.

The cost of all this technology is, of course, high. The GE machine plus all its extras comes to a cool $40m-50m. But, says Dr Jolesz, if it improves the chances of survival, decreases pain, or does away with the need for anaesthetics or hospitalisation, the investment should be worth making. Trackless surgery still has its limitations. It can be used only in "ablative" procedures, in which the surgeon's job is to destroy a body's rotten fabric. For stitching or mending, new trackless tools must be invented; they seem some way off. But another scientific field, robotics, is also producing new challenges to old surgical habits.

Robodoc takes charge

Seven years ago William Bargar, an orthopaedic surgeon, and Howard Paul, a veterinary surgeon, both from the University of California, Davis, approached IBM with a problem. To complete a hip-replacement surgeons must hollow out a specially shaped cavity in the thigh-bone designed to take the prosthesis. The tighter the fit, the better the chances of success. But the hammer and broach that surgeons now use to make the cavity are primitive—and operations can sometimes disappoint. Surely, they thought, IBM could design a robot to do a better job? IBM's answer was Robodoc, which is now being developed by Integrated Surgical Systems in Sacramento, California.

The skills demanded of a surgical robot are different to those needed on a factory floor. In the factory efficiency and speed are the priorities. In the operating theatre it is precision and safety. In the case of Robodoc, it must mill out a cavity matching the desired prosthetic shape to within a few thousandths of a centimetre and place the cavity within 0.05 centimetres of the desired position in the thigh-bone, which could otherwise fracture. This fine placement can be done using image-guided therapy: CT scans of the thigh-bone are registered to the live patient.

The robot, which is linked to the main computer, positions itself using information obtained from CT and then mills the cavity in the thigh-bone, which is held immobile in a clamp. A separate computer attached to the robot monitors its movements, checking with the CT model that the robotic drill is in the right place. This makes Robodoc 20 times more accurate than a human doctor. As a bonus the computer can, with the help of CT data, plan the ideal-shaped prosthesis to fit into the thigh-bone. Before, this was done mostly by pot luck.

Clinical trials of Robodoc should be concluded by 1995. Preliminary results show that patients treated by Robodoc recover faster than those oper-

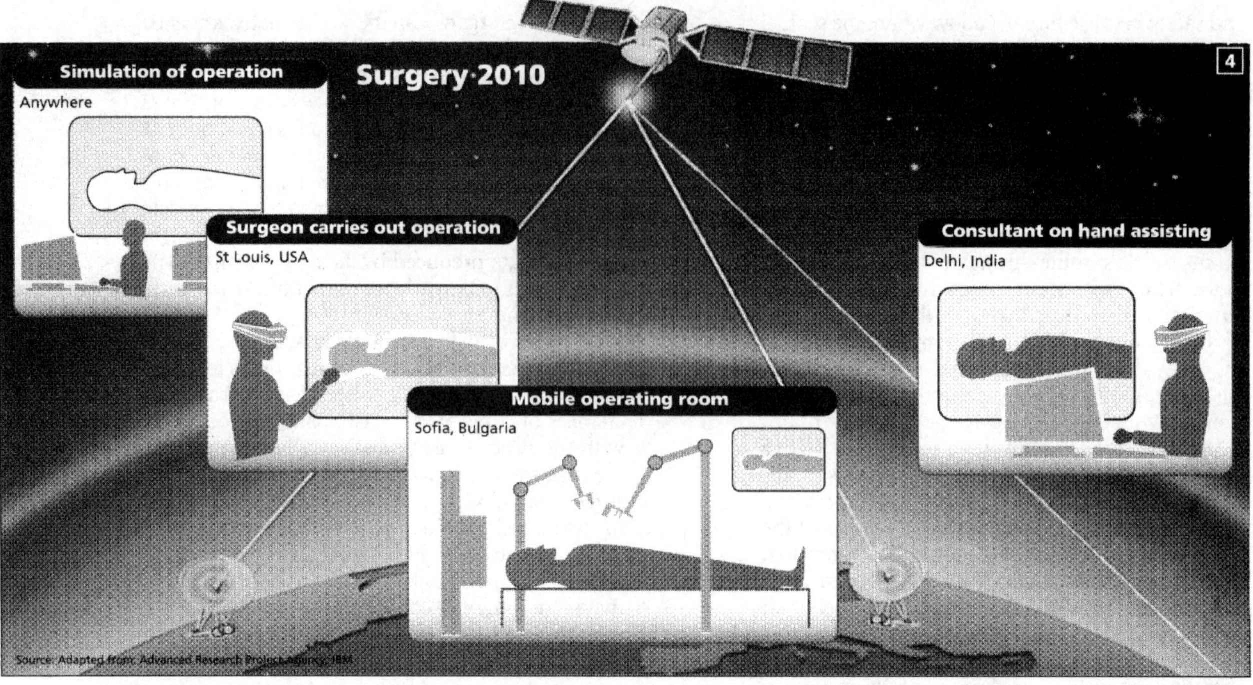

ated on by humans. Though designed for use by surgeons, Robodoc is so simple to use that eventually technicians might do most hip-replacements. According to Bela Musits, who left IBM to run Integrated Surgical Systems, the Robodoc will be priced to be equivalent to the cost of normal hip-replacements. But there should still be significant cost savings because patients should recover more quickly.

The three-dimensional accuracy and easy reproducibility of automated procedures, says Mr Wickham of Guy's, have still to be fully exploited. Mr Wickham was partly responsible for the development of the first surgical robot in 1989. It removes a diseased prostate (a male gland that helps make semen) via the urethra (the tube connecting the bladder to the exterior). The task is delicate because the gland has to be sliced off a little at a time. Thanks to its precision, the robot can perform the task in 20 minutes, a third of the time it takes a human. It too is being tested in clinical trials.

Mini-robots are another possibility. Electric motors less than a millimetre in size, made by etching tiny gears and mechanisms on a silicon crystal, power tiny surgical devices or tractors bearing cameras. Such a miniature battalion can be swallowed and, when instructed by remote control, perform delicate operations in the gut, eliminating the need for invasive surgery.

Perhaps most exciting of all is the prospect of "tele-presence surgery", where surgeons can operate at a distance from patients using robots guided by remote control. So far only a few researchers have got anywhere near setting up a remote surgical system. The Technical University of Karlsruhe, in Germany, is one; another is the American Defence Department. The Pentagon is taking a keen interest because of the chances of improving the treatment of wounded soldiers on the front line (in past wars, up to 90% of deaths of those injured at the front line happened because the wounded did not reach a hospital in time). Electronic advances in health care could bring a remote doctor to a casualty's side.

Sponsored by the Defence Department, Philip Green of Telesurgical in Redwood City, California, has developed robotic precision instruments that can give to remote controls the same feelings of contact and cutting as if a surgeon were using the scalpel himself. Colonel Richard Satava, of the Advanced Research Projects Agency, dreams that "with medical informatics and networking, and mechanically driven doctoring, the physician can see, feel and interact at a remote site from the patient. Surgeons will be able to operate in dangerous and inaccessible areas, from war zones to third-world countries, without the expense and time of travelling there."

So far remote surgical operations have been conducted only on animals. But last June, at Fort Gordon, Georgia, the United States Army Medical Department conducted a field training exercise of a medical battlefield that might exist at the end of the decade—including remote surgery (see diagram 4).

Once the paramedic has reached a wounded soldier at the front lines, he can have a tele-consultation with experts around the battlefield to agree on a decision to operate. To bring the expertise of the surgeon, who could be anywhere, to the wounded soldier, a tele-operation system, which is installed in an ambulance and acts as a mobile operating room, can go immediately to the soldier. The surgeon, watching on a three-dimensional monitor, performs the operation using a central master controller that manipulates remote robot forceps, scalpels and needles while tele-consulting with a paramedic in the ambulance who has prepared the patient for surgery. "There is very little difference", adds Colonel Satava, "between a wounded soldier and a patient, so all these technologies have a civilian use as well."

(continued)

Engineering health

COMPUTERS, telecommunications and robots may make doctors and hospitals more efficient and safer. Biology will take medicine to places that are not even dreamed of—yet. In the past two decades scientific discoveries have turned biology from being a discipline dedicated to the passive study of life into one that can alter it at will. Biologists today believe that by tinkering with people's genes, the units of heredity, they will eventually be able to eliminate most of the diseases that now plague the world. Tomorrow, such extraordinary ambitions may seem modest, as scientists start to work on improving a person's genetic lot in life.

It all started in the early 1970s, when scientists first learnt how to clone and engineer genes. In cloning, a single gene is isolated from millions of others. Before this, scientists were confronted with the genetic equivalent of noise. Now they were free to study the structure and function of gene entities in isolation. By the end of the decade, Genentech, in San Francisco, had launched the first-ever genetically-engineered drug, human insulin. What Genentech had done was to take the cloned gene coding for human insulin and transfer it to bacteria. Genentech had synthesised a new life-form, a bug capable of making a protein foreign to itself. For centuries selective breeding has produced novel crops or cattle, but always with unpredictable results. With genetic engineering, scientists can be surer of outcomes: that a particular bacterium will produce insulin, say.

Scientists now have a rag-bag of new tricks to help them probe nature. Mike McCune of SyStemix in Palo Alto, California, an experienced geneticist, points to four other bits of cleverness crucial to the progress of biotechnology, as the new field of biology became known. On the McCune list are the cloning of pure antibodies, polymerase chain reaction, differential hybridisation and multiparameter flow cytometry. Without going into the details of what this jargon means, all four aim broadly at the same goal: to provide a better understanding of what makes nature tick. This knowledge is now being put to good effect, with the discovery of powerful new medicines.

Biotechnology has made big promises before, without delivering on its early hype. But as Glaxo's Sir Richard Sykes points out:

> Just the past year has seen a paradigm shift in modern biology, because it is revealing so much information about the basic mechanisms of disease for which drugs can be developed. In the past, pharmaceutical firms relied on serendipity to find new drugs. In future that is not the way to go if the idea is to produce medicines of value.

The rest of the drug industry feels the same way. According to Steve Burrill, a biotechnology buff, in the year to June 1993 drug firms formed around 100 strategic alliances with small biotech firms to tap into their know-how—twice as many as in the previous year. Research successes have fuelled a huge expansion of the biotechnology industry. In 1993 Mr Burrill counted 1,300 biotech firms in America, 200 in Britain, and 400 elsewhere in Europe. Mr Burrill reckons that by 2010 biotechnology firms' sales will have grown ten-fold compared with 1993, to some $100 billion. Because of the long lead-times involved, products began to trickle out of biotech R&D laboratories only about five years ago. Two drugs already have sales in excess of $1 billion a year, because they are so good at what they do: Amgen's EPO, which prevents anaemia during kidney dialysis, and its Neupogen, which decreases the incidence of infection in cancer patients undergoing chemotherapy. But these two seem dull compared with what the next generation of biotech products will bring.

Views differ about where biotechnology's biggest contribution will be made. But for a 2010-plus outlook the overwhelming vote goes to human genetic engineering.

The gene genie

Genetic engineering could eradicate most disease

On September 14th 1990, after years of foot-dragging, America became the first country to allow new genes to be introduced into people. On that day French Anderson, Michael Blaese and Ken Culver, all at the National Institutes of Health (NIH), used a gene drug to treat a four-year-old girl with severe combined immunodeficiency (SCID), a rare and dreadful disease, whose sufferers once had to live inside a sanitised plastic bubble. Those with SCID lack a gene that controls the production of an enzyme known as adenosine deaminase (ADA), which plays an important role in the body's immune defences. Dr Anderson put copies of the ADA gene into the girl's white blood cells. In early 1991 a nine-year-old girl with ADA deficiency was also treated under the gene therapy programme. In May 1993 the two young girls appeared at a press conference looking happy and healthy. The striking results achieved in these two cases have spurred on the use of "gene drugs".

ADA deficiency is one of 4,000 known disorders that result from a single genetic flaw. Most are as rare as SCID; a few, such as cystic fibrosis, are quite common. "But the grand strategy of gene therapy", says an NIH booklet, "also envisages a much broader use of the new techniques to include assaults on heart disease, diabetes and other major health problems that are influenced by the functioning genes." The development of such diseases depends on how a person reacts to environmental factors, such as pollution or smoking. However, the body's susceptibility to them is imprinted in a mix of bad genes inherited from parents. Gene therapy tries to correct these genetic faults to abolish or at least reduce the spread of disease. Dr Anderson, now at the University of Southern California School of Medicine in Los Angeles, says that "it can be used to treat disease, but its primary value will be in prevention." Genetic screening at birth can tell what diseases a person is susceptible to—so genetic protection can be given to prevent the diseases appearing in later life.

In 1993 a lot of progress towards this goal was made. The Centre d'Etude du Polymorphisme Humain (CEPH), in Paris, published the first genetic map of a human genome, the totality of human DNA. Before then, only 2% of the genome had been mapped. What the French did was to establish landmarks (marker genes) among the 100,000 genes that stretch along the human genome. This helps to track down genes that cause most inheritable diseases; patients suffering from such diseases often also inherit distinctive marker genes that are absent in healthy people. With the new map researchers can quickly isolate genes closely associated with the markers to determine which ones cause a disease. The map will also help to obtain a more detailed account of the human genome itself. Thanks to the global efforts of the Human Genome Project, it is hoped that by 2010 the structure and function of almost all human genes will be understood.

Even without the map, in 1993 the genetic causes of several diseases were found. A gene that leads to Huntington's disease, a form of dementia, was found after years of searching. Scientists are close to tracking down genes that cause breast cancer. Tests to screen several diseases were also invented in 1993. Oncor, a tiny biotechnology outfit in Gaithersburg, Maryland, launched a genetic testing service for breast cancer that uses computers to interview patients about family cancer history. It also screens for gene markers associated with breast cancer. As soon as genes that cause breast cancer are found, these too will be screened for to predict a person's chances of contracting the disease. Those with bad test results could opt to take the radical step of having their breasts removed. In time, however, they may get gene drugs that prevent the disease from occurring altogether.

Some 250 patients are now being treated with 12 different gene drugs in 74 approved trials around the world: the majority are for cancer, the rest for single-fault genetic diseases, which include haemophilia. The results of several trials are trickling in. Patients with abnormally high levels of cholesterol have, after receiving gene drugs, seen their cholesterol levels fall. Three out of eight patients with terminal brain cancers have experienced a reduction in the size of their tumours. Nobody has reacted adversely to any of the drugs, except for one cystic-fibrosis patient who had breathing difficulties for a few hours. That may have been because the drug was administered through the trachea.

Such technical problems of delivery, which is currently laborious and painful, are slowly being sorted out. There is still some worry about the safety of the delivery system, because viruses, even though inactive, are involved. The virus is a vehicle that carries gene drugs to cells in patients' bodies. Apart from the treatment of cystic fibrosis, the therapy has been administered by extracting bone-marrow cells from the patient, treating them with a virally-packaged form of the gene drug in the laboratory, and then returning them to the body. In 1993 Vical, a biotechnology firm in San Diego, found that by combining fat with DNA, it could bypass this procedure and inject genes direct into the bloodstream, much like any conventional drug. Dr Anderson is also working on injectable gene drugs. Researchers are trying to refine delivery systems so that they are longer-lasting and require only a single shot in a lifetime. It is still early days to be sure of the results, but most of the signs emerging from the research are encouraging.

So encouraging, indeed, that Daniel Cohen of CEPH reckons that by 2010 gene doctors will have found a way of dealing with most diseases caused by single gene defects. Over the next 50 years most common serious diseases will also succumb to gene therapy. And 50 years, he adds, is almost no time at all in the history of medicine (penicillin is now 50 years old). These are inspiring goals.

More controversially, gene doctors also want to shape human destiny. So far they have confined themselves to delivering genes to the somatic cells that make up most of the body. Germ cells in the testes and ovaries are not affected; the new genes are not passed on to the next generation, which remains as vulnerable as its parents to disease. But germ-line gene therapy would correct a genetic defect in the reproductive cells of a patient; offspring would also be corrected and disease could be eradicated.

Human genetic engineering could also enhance or improve "good" traits—for instance an extra copy of the human-growth-hormone gene could be added to increase height. On December 31st 1993 a scientific journal, *Nature Genetics*, published an article by CEPH that examined two genes in a group of 338 French people over 100 years old. They found that the centenarians had different levels of genes compared with younger people. A person carrying the right gene variants had twice the chance of reaching old age. This was the first time that genes had been linked to longevity. It follows that gene therapy might extend life-expectancy. And though scientists still do not understand enough about the genetic processes that make humans intelligent or beautiful, it might eventually be possible to tailor people to taste.

Some scientists believe that nature will act as a brake on genetic tinkering, because the human genome might be able to accommodate only a limited number of extra genes. It would also be hard to deal wtih multi-gene traits. As with the genie in Aladdin's lamp, people may be offered a fixed number of wishes: a cure for cancer, a height-inducer or whatever. Once their wishes are used up their genetic make-up will be unalterable—at least by their own hand. Yet no matter how they are dressed up, such uses of gene therapy will have moved medicine from the business of curing or caring into the more ethically dubious areas of life-enhancement and eugenics: two issues to which this survey will return later.

(continued)

In 2010

THIS whirlwind tour of the progress being made in medical science in the laboratory scarcely does justice to the scale of today's changes. It has not touched upon the headway made in transplanting body-parts, *in vitro* fertilisation (conception in a test-tube) or the synthesis of biotechnology-based drugs to treat disease before the introduction of full gene therapy. Even so, the trend is clear: technological change is on the verge of creating a new world of health care.

This is true on several levels. Information networks, computer-assisted therapy, robotics and new drugs will increase efficiency and precision. Patients will be less damaged by the treatments they receive, which in turn should be more potent than their predecessors. Some robots and gene drugs will provide treatments where there was none before. The workload of doctors and surgeons should be significantly lighter as computers and robots take over many of their jobs and people become healthier.

Picture the new-age health-care consumer in 2010. In the 1990s an average person would visit a doctor four or five times a year. By 2010, or probably well before that, doctors will be on call via home personal computers, through electronic mail or teleconferencing. The consumer will anyway do a lot more of his own doctoring. By wearing a "healthwatch", he will keep a continuous medical check on his physical and mental state. The data will be fed direct to the computer. Individuals' medical records will be stored in two ways: in a database accessible to anybody with the right password, and on a smart card that is held by the individual.

The computer/doctor will diagnose whatever is wrong with the patient and determine the best treatment. By matching a personal medical profile to databases and services that are available globally, the computer/doctor will be able to tailor advice to patients' needs. If drugs are prescribed, these will be ordered electronically and mailed to the home; or by using a smart card they will be obtained from an automatic dispensing machine rather like bank cash machines. At home, on-line pharmacists or drug manufacturers will be able to advise about therapies.

If surgery is needed a patient will not need to go to hospital and stay there. The rapidity with which patients will recover from new surgical procedures will mean that most operations can be performed in a day. And if an overnight stay is necessary, a local "health-motel" will provide nursing and transport. A fleet of ambulances will also tour areas deprived of surgical facilities, doubling as mobile operating theatres. Instead of a patient travelling miles to the nearest hospital, the operating room will come to him. Many operations will be performed by robots assisted by nurses, although specialist surgeons will be called upon (via telemedicine) in emergencies or for tasks that robots can still not tackle alone.

What will happen to today's health-care infrastructure? Hospitals look likely to empty as traditional surgical wards become largely redundant. Many will close; others will tend only emergency patients or the chronically ill. Doctors' clinics will also be far less busy. The consumer will take far more responsibility for his own care. In return the availability and quality of medical help will improve, as those delivering health care will have a greater interest in ensuring that their treatments are successful.

As the health-care system switches to computers, and information begins to flow freely among doctors, nurses, drug makers and patients, the health-care market will become more transparent. The latest bulletins on the prices and the performance of health-care deliverers will be available on information networks for anybody to read, just as investors keep in touch with stockmarket prices. This will encourage more competitive buying not just by insurers and governments but also by patients themselves, making doctors and other health-care providers more accountable than ever before. Every patient will shop around for the health clinic that best suits his medical needs at fees that he can afford. Clinics will be linked to the health information network but will also belong to a larger managed-care conglomerate—call it Health Care Concern—that provides all medical services. Health Care Concern will keep a close track of all medical services, buying in only the most cost-effective in order to attract customers by offering them the best deal.

The patient moves into the driving seat

As for overall health-care costs, new investment in high technology may be largely offset by savings from hospital closures and fewer health-care staff—which currently account for the bulk of health-care spending. The balancing act between costs and savings may become harder, however, as demand for better medicine increases. When surgery is no more painful than visiting one's mother-in-law, many more will want quick treatment. However, if the net effect is to reduce the sickness in the population, governments and other health-care payers should end up profiting.

Such savings have often been promised before—for instance, with the introduction of health insurance in America, the establishment of Britain's National Health Service and almost every campaign for healthy living. Yet savings have rarely accrued. Indeed policy-makers have usually discovered that as life expectancy increases, new diseases or old-age complaints emerge that place huge extra demands on health-care systems. Hence the inexorable rise in spending in the past 50 years.

This time, though, things could be different. Most of humanity's serious diseases involve renegade genes—and so are curable through the right gene therapy. If new gene mutations or undiscovered infectious agents were to appear, as they certainly will, these too can be picked up by genetic screening and corrected by gene therapy. One worrisome exception is a group of diseases known as spongiform encephalopathies, which includes "mad cow" disease and its human equivalent, Creutzfeld-Jacob syndrome. Nobody knows what

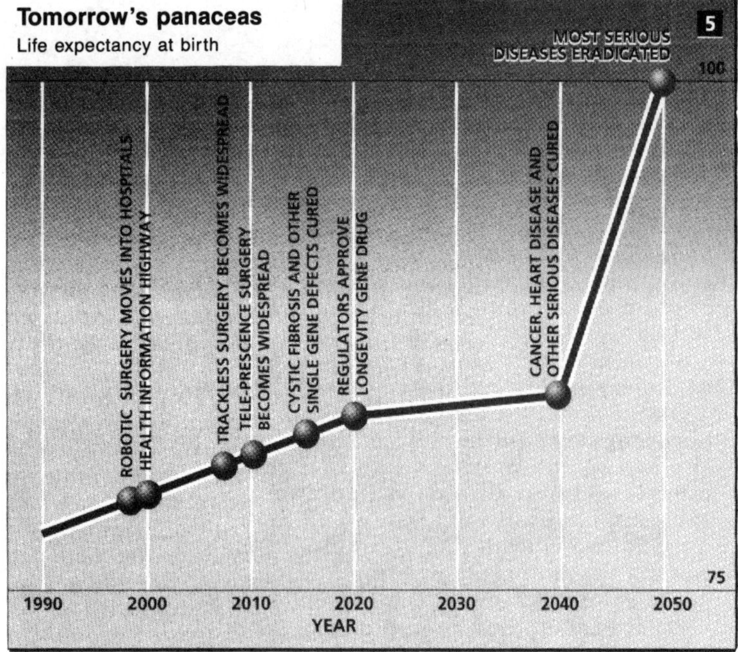

causes encephalopathies, but it does not seem to be genetic. There may be a risk that, with all other diseases cured, encephalopathies will run rampant. Even so, the elimination of other diseases should massively reduce health-care spending—as well as improving people's lives.

What's up doc?

The social consequences of the changes in health-care delivery will be equally significant. The implicit contract between doctor and patient will have to be rewritten. Patients, not doctors, will drive the system. Doctors will be relegated to mere members of a wider health-care team, which will include clever robots. For centuries doctors have claimed a monopoly on medical authority, based on their wide knowledge, training and experience—to which consumers had no access. According to Stephen Pauker, professor of medicine at Tufts University, medical information will now be out there for everybody. The difference between the skilled and the novice will lie less in the knowledge they already have than in knowing where to look for information. Nor will doctors be defined by their manipulative skills, as surgeons become those that control robots.

Computers will not dehumanise medicine any more than did the introduction of the stethoscope. There will still be a whole range of treatments that require flexible, human skills that cannot be replicated by computers. And doctors will anyway continue to have contact with patients through information networks. There is also something else that computers cannot replace: the placebo factor. Among patients with a migraine, the mere act of "seeing" a doctor induces recovery in nearly a third of cases.

Some of the medical practice for 2010 outlined above could be happening today—were it not for the dogged resistance of the medical profession, reluctant to take on board any new technology that threatens its position. However the introduction of managed-care systems first into America and then into Europe will give more power to those who pay for health care, forcing doctors to be more accountable to managers and patients. That will also provide more incentives for the spread of new technologies. Future arguments may indeed be more about their costs than about whether they usurp the role of doctors or hospitals.

And beyond 2010?

These new technologies, as this survey has stressed, are not just products in the vivid imaginations of a group of unhinged scientists. Many have already moved out of the laboratory to actual testing. The speed at which they will now come to the marketplace will depend on several things. The most important will be their performance in tests. According to Dr Anderson, if gene drugs prove to be as effective as antibiotics were in the 1940s in curing disease, the public demand to get them quickly will be too great for governments to resist. Antibiotics literally raised people from their death-beds. Similarly, the application of painless surgical procedures will be demanded by patients as they learn of the chances of cure by machines without bodily trauma.

Much will also depend on the speed of telecommunications advances—and especially how soon certain technological hiccups can be cured. For example, Masaaki Terada, director of the National Cancer Centre Research Institute in Tokyo, believes that image-guided therapy is still too insensitive to track cancers that have metastasized—the point when cancer cells spread from a primary tumour to other parts of the body. Such cells cannot be picked up by body scanners, but in 20 years, he believes, the electronic imagery should be good enough. But as a substitute for the surgical removal of solid tumours (which have not metastasized) image-guided therapy will still be used a lot more than invasive surgery. Only solid tumours are anyway operated on today.

All of this is about the immediate future: ie, the next decade or so. Look further ahead, say to 2050, and there is a distinct possibility that gene drugs will have dealt with most major serious diseases. By the middle of the next century, in other words, man could live a life free of illness, barring the odd accident—and he could be living a lot longer than he is now. Chart 5 offers a rough guide to what might happen when. There will be upheavals along the way; there may be resistance from medics or others with an interest in stopping change. But the concomitant health gains will be so great that such obstacles are bound to be overcome.

So is the future entirely rosy? Not to be disingenuous, there are several caveats, most of them ethical, to bear in mind before we can jump to that reassuringly comfortable conclusion.

(continued)

Hippocrates's dilemma

"I WILL prescribe regimen for the good of my patients according to my ability and my judgment and never do harm to anyone." So wrote Hippocrates, a Greek physician on Cos; hence doctors' Hippocratic oath. Though medicine is advancing towards potent therapies that produce better cures and less physical harm, talk of computer doctors and gene drugs will still frighten many into believing that we are heading towards Aldous Huxley's nightmare in "Brave New World". Most of these fears are baseless; but there are legitimate reasons for concern. That is the nature of medical innovation, which challenges traditional precepts. Even Hippocrates had to fight off critics of his day who argued that his empirical methods were worthless. "Desperate diseases require desperate remedies," he said.

The wholesale overhaul of health-care systems will produce an information network that puts more responsibility on consumers' shoulders. If doctors no longer act in patients' best interests and as general guardians of health, who will defend consumers against commercial interests? Or against prying governments? In tomorrow's medical world, highly personal information will swill around health information networks, from details about blood pressure to hidden genes predicting prospective states of health. This could be used by the unscrupulous. Last December China, which plans genetic screening of its population by 2000, announced that women carrying defective genes would be sterilised or prohibited from marrying. This sort of interference has prompted some opponents to argue that the information should not be collected in the first place.

But if health-care systems are to be made more efficient there must be some way of measuring their input (sick patients) and output (cured ones). To garner this sort of information a patient's welfare has to be tracked from medical records, data must be pooled and processed and the outcome of any treatments must be monitored. The more data there are, the greater the knowledge about what works and what does not. And there are ways to protect patients' privacy. Lawrence Fagan of Stanford University reckons that the level of security provided by electronics is now ten times better than that offered by hospital manual records today. The flow of medical data could be regulated. There may, for instance, be a case for restricting access to the results of genetic screening to the patient concerned, just as is now done for AIDS tests—unless and until treatments are found.

Human genetic engineering also has some opponents who believe that it is wrong in principle to interfere so blatantly with nature. Most people might think that the administration of genes to a sick person to cure a serious disease is welcome. But they might be less sure about extending gene therapy so that it changes people's offspring. After all, by genetically engineering individuals alone, many serious illnesses could be wiped off the face of the earth. But populations might then build up latent pools of "bad genes". Dr Anderson suggests that people could become fortgetful and not take gene drugs. Disease could then suddenly return to surprise all—as whooping cough has done today.

That is why Dr Anderson believes in genetically engineering germ cells (reproductive cells) to correct all "bad genes" in future generations and so eradicate disease once and for all. The only legitimate objection to this, he thinks, is the possibility of a genetic mishap causing apparently irrevocable damage to the unborn. But knowledge is progressing so fast that any conceivable mishap can easily be reversed by correcting the gene mix later.

What about life-enhancing, as opposed to disease-eliminating, gene therapy? Why should people not use gene therapy to improve their lot in life? Taking a growth gene might be compared to having a face-lift or other cosmetic surgery. Criticism of life-enhancing genes might be stilled if therapy were restricted to the individual. The newly-acquired traits would then not be passed on to children, who would be free to choose for themselves what characteristics they might like.

A word of warning

Not all life-enhancing traits should be considered in the same light, however. Widespread adoption of a longevity gene might cause social havoc as the proportion of the population aged 70 or more soars within a single generation. Isolation of behavioural genes—those associated with aggressiveness or athleticism, say—might raise concerns if everyone tried to choose the same types. At the moment, drugs have to demonstrate only safety and effectiveness to be approved. It is time for regulators to consider the social and ethical consequences of medicines, on a case-by-case basis.

A big remaining question will be who will pay for all this life enhancement. This is not just a matter of how much gene therapy itself might cost. It is more a question of broader costs if people start to live to 100-plus. Pension and other welfare arrangements will need to be changed. On the other hand, if a longer-lived population is also a healthier one, it could be economically a more productive one; assumptions about retirement ages must change.

Putting concerns about privacy and the ethics of human genetic engineering aside, the biggest worry may be "humanity's inescapable triumphalism". This, says John Maddox, editor of *Nature*, is what accompanies a rush of discoveries that leave the impression that scientists know much more than they really do. New technologies are adopted with wild enthusiasm, even when they need a lot of further work. This time, though, science is being cautious. New regulatory bodies have been set up to oversee genetic engineering. New medical products cannot come to market without undergoing rigorous testing—though there may be a case for broadening the tests' criteria.

What would Hippocrates have done? He would soon have found that, although many new technologies raise tricky medical, ethical and social problems, they can be managed with legislation and with the right regulatory constraints—just as society now decides how to deal with such controversial issues as *in vitro* fertilisation. Given this, it is hard to see why anyone should reject the opportunities that new medical technologies are likely to offer. The reward, after all, could be a guaranteed hale and hearty future for all.

HEAL THYSELF

Cancer, heart failure, kidney disease—serious problems, usually treated with surgery or powerful drugs. But new studies suggest that monitoring often is all that's needed

The best medicine for a surprising number of ills, including some forms of heart disease and cancer, may be: Watch and wait. While no one suggests that sick people should stay away from doctors' offices, evidence is growing that for a number of conditions, high-cost specialty care often makes no difference in the long run and may even hurt more than help. Hard data are slowly convincing doctors and insurance companies of the merits of nonmedical healing, such as diet and exercise. The most intriguing studies suggest that some worrisome medical problems often go away on their own when doctors simply monitor the conditions—a deliberate, seemingly hands-off approach that advocates dub "watchful waiting."

Such study findings mesh nicely with current efforts to control runaway health costs. The Clinton administration's proposed health care reforms would push medical consumers to health maintenance organizations and other managed-care plans that limit access to medical specialists and, thus, to the expensive tests and treatments that recent research increasingly calls into question. Among the latest reports:

- For most men with a slow-growing, "indolent" prostate tumor—one that hasn't spread beyond the gland—monitoring is sufficient.
- Most women with the kind of minimally abnormal Pap smears that are generally thought to signal precancerous cervical changes show clear improvement, often completely returning to normal, following nine months of careful monitoring.
- More than one third of heart transplant candidates at the University of California at Los Angeles who followed a personalized exercise program and took medication to reduce excess fluid and relax blood vessels improved so dramatically that they no longer needed new hearts.
- With membranous glomerulonephritis, an inflammation that's among the most common causes of kidney failure, the condition disappears or goes into remission within five years for 60 percent of patients who reject the standard treatment of steroids and immunity-suppressing drugs, if the protein in their urine stays within acceptable limits.

It is hardly surprising that doctors have not embraced this do-less approach. It bumps up against the search-and-destroy ethic drummed into generations of American physicians and reinforced by the abundant weaponry of medical technology. Besides, in today's medical world, physicians worry about malpractice suits if untreated patients get sicker. Moreover, patients tend to send a message to their doctors that they *expect* to be treated. For many sick people, waiting for a problem to disappear on its own would be unnerving.

"There's a great pressure to do *something,*" says Willett Whitmore, formerly an attending surgeon at Memorial Sloan-Kettering Cancer Center in New York. "If you don't do anything and things work out badly, you second-guess yourself and the patient's family second-guesses you." And if the patient dies after aggressive treatment, "You say, 'Well, I did all I can.' "

Of course, wait and see isn't an option for every condition. Chest pain should always trigger an immediate call to 911 or to a local emergency medical service. Less obvious hallmarks of heart attack, such as shortness of breath, restlessness and cold, clammy skin, likewise call for emergency measures. Similarly, no one should shrug off the earliest, somewhat vague symptoms of stroke, such as unexplained dizziness or sudden weakness or numbness of the face, arm or leg on one side of the body. People who are rushed to the closest large medical center as soon as such symptoms appear have the best chance for a successful recovery.

FRITZ HANSON, 62

CONDITION: *Early-stage prostate cancer*
■ Hanson passed up surgery because it is no sure cure and carries a risk of impotence or incontinence. Besides, prostate tumors generally grow slowly. Two years later, he doesn't regret his decision.

Nevertheless, Kylanne Green, director of managed care at the Health Insurance Association of America, a non-profit trade association, fully expects the wait-and-see option to become part of practice guidelines periodically issued by the federal government and by doctors' organization such as the American College of Obstetricians and Gynecologists for a variety of conditions.

Once physicians get on board, health insurers won't be far behind. After all, the notion that patients can do just as well minus the high cost and high technology—and can even heal themselves—has obvious appeal to those who foot the bills.

In July, for example, Mutual of Omaha became the first major insurer to announce plans to cover the costs of a program devised by California physician Dean Ornish that aims to reverse heart disease by combining a vegetarian diet, stress management, exercise and support-group sessions. Several studies show that the regimen can melt away artery-clogging plaque. Ornish's year-long program, which is starting up in six U.S. cities, consists of lengthy classes with health professionals to help patients change their lifestyles. (His *Eat More, Weigh Less*—from HarperCollins, $22.50—is a bestselling description of the program.) The course costs $5,000, while by-pass surgery—the most expensive of the standard treatments for coronary artery disease—can cost 10 times as

From *U.S. News & World Report,* November 22, 1993, pp. 64-66, 69-70, 72, 76.

much. Insurers say that many more such "alternative" treatment programs soon will win coverage.

Prostate cancer might not look like an obvious candidate for watchful waiting; the yearly death toll of 35,000 lags behind only lung cancer as the most lethal malignancy of American men. Yet it may be perfectly suited. Last May in the *Journal of the American Medical Association,* a team of researchers including medical epidemiologist John Wennberg of Dartmouth Medical School—who coined "watchful waiting" in 1988—pronounced a less aggressive approach a reasonable option for men 60 and older, who constitute the vast majority. After analyzing the medical literature and factoring in the impact of treatment on patients' quality of life, the team reported that surgery or radiation probably benefits only a small percentage of men ages 60 to 70 with tiny tumors confined to the prostate, and doctors can't predict which patients they will be. The team based its conclusion on the fact that prostate tumors typically grow very slowly, so most men older than 60 who are diagnosed with a tiny, localized tumor will die of other causes. (Only 16 percent of the men first diagnosed with prostate cancer are younger than 60.) For patients over 70, Wennberg's analysis shows that the possible complications from radiation or surgery—incontinence and impotence—could leave them *worse* off than before. And the risk of dying from prostate cancer surgery increases with age.

JOET RANKER, 69

CONDITION: *Congestive heart failure*

■ In 1989, Ranker was on the waiting list for a heart transplant because her own heart was failing. Fifteen months later, after a strict regimen of exercise and drugs, she was off the list and on the golf course.

"Given that treatment at best offers only limited benefits for most patients," says Wennberg, "some men over 60 may prefer to put the diagnosis of cancer out of their minds, if they can, and perhaps even consider forgoing monitoring." Bolstering that position, a 1992 Swedish study reported that only 19 out of 223 men with early, untreated prostate cancer died from the disease within 10 years of diagnosis.

Why treat? Both studies have their critics. Some doctors have noted that the average age of the Swedish patients was 72, probably too old to benefit from surgery. And Patrick Walsh, professor and director of urology at Johns Hopkins Medical Institutions in Baltimore, asserts that the Dartmouth team's analysis is based on an inadequate series of studies and unrealistic assumptions about the effectiveness of surgery and radiation. The American Urological Association will meet next month in Washington, D.C., to review the controversy.

Solid answers must likely await a pending study, directed by the National Cancer Institute and the Department of Veterans affairs, that is slated to begin next year. Researchers at 80 U.S. centers will randomly assign 2,000 men with early prostate cancer either to surgery or to observation (plus treatment, if necessary, to relieve symptoms). The condition and longevity of both groups of patients will be tracked for 15 years.

THELMA EDWARDS, 90

CONDITION: *Cataracts*

■ Neither cataracts nor a recent mild stroke has kept Edwards from her books, newspapers and magazines. She rejects cataract surgery. "I can see just about what I want to see," she says.

For now, men diagnosed with prostate cancer need a nothing-held-back conversation with their doctor about their condition and the options. A man who has a localized tumor but is otherwise in good health, for instance, may not care about the risk of impotence associated with surgery or radiation if he is not sexually active.

After Fritz Hanson, 62, was diagnosed with prostate cancer in 1991, he consulted three doctors and attended meetings of a prostate cancer support group. A Seattle resident retired from the Boeing Corp., Hanson weighed his risk of dying from the cancer against evidence that such cancers are generally slow growing and the risk of impotence or incontinence from the treatment. He will watch and wait—a decision that so far has stood him in good stead.

"I was upset." Like Hanson, Dana Fox, a 30-year-old gynecological nurse at the UCLA Medical Center, is going through a battle of nerves. In February 1991, a routine Pap smear showed cell changes that, while labeled "minimally abnormal," could indicate cancer. She took the standard next step: a colposcopy, or visual inspection of the cervix, which turned up nothing unusual. Her

When to watch and wait

Aggressive medicine isn't always necessary. Here are a few examples of less drastic alternatives that often work:

LOCALIZED PROSTATE CANCER

Conventional treatments: Surgical removal or radiation therapy, risking impotence and incontinence.

Alternatives: For men over 60 with tiny, localized tumors, do nothing, or simply monitor with PSA (prostate-specific antigen) test and rectal exam every six months. Additional options are less extensive surgery or hormonal therapy to shrink the prostate and relieve symptoms such as difficult urination.

CATARACTS

Conventional treatment: Surgically remove clouded lens.

Alternative: Progressively stronger eyeglasses.

GALLSTONES

Conventional treatments: Dissolve stones with drugs, pulverize them with sonic shock waves or remove gallbladder with laparoscopic surgery.

Alternative: Unless symptoms appear, do nothing. Often gallstones cause no symptoms and are discovered only during an unrelated medical evaluation.

CARDIOMYOPATHY

Conventional treatment: Drugs to treat symptoms of the failing heart, which generally continues to deteriorate. Without a transplant, death is inevitable.

Alternative: Exercise and medication to reduce excess fluid and relax blood vessels, thus easing the heart's load. This regimen eliminated the need for a transplant in 35 percent of the patients in one study at the University of California at Los Angeles.

UTERINE FIBROIDS

Conventional treatment: Hysterectomy (removal of uterus).

Alternative: Monitor if there's no excessive pain, bleeding or rapid growth of the fibroid. If symptoms are present, removing the fibroid may be feasible, sparing the uterus.

options included a $750 cone biopsy, in which a cone-shaped portion of the cervix thought to harbor the abnormal cells is removed for study, or burning or freezing the suspect tissue. Fox hesitated, well aware of the potential for future fertility problems: "I was very upset, very anxious."

Fox and her doctor finally decided that since the Pap smear changes were inconclusive, it would be safe to watch and wait for a while. They felt vindicated by a report last year in the journal *Obstetrics & Gynecology* that concluded that most "minimally abnormal" Pap smears improve or become completely normal within nine months and that close monitoring every three months is the only care indicated.

To reach that conclusion, a team headed by F. J. Montz, associate professor of gynecologic oncology at UCLA, had followed 294 women with minimally abnormal Pap smears, retesting them every three months with more smears and colposcopies for at least nine months. Any woman whose condition worsened received treatment. After nine months, about one fourth of the smears were abnormal but no worse than before—and smears for nearly the entire remaining three quarters of the women had returned to normal. (Seven other women had to be treated, but none suffered for waiting.) The Montz team's theory is that most Pap smears considered minimally abnormal are caused by active infections from two groups of human papilloma virus. The viruses are rarely linked to cancer and often subside on their own.

DANA FOX, 30

CONDITION: *Abnormal Pap smear*

■ Women with precancerous cervical changes often have the suspect tissue removed. Fox chose only to monitor her condition closely. "I don't have cancer," she says. "They're not taking anything of mine out until it gets to that point."

CLOCKS AND TAPE MEASURES

The latest in testing–take out the high technology

High technology gets the headlines, but some of the newest diagnostic tests are effective, cheap and bereft of digital readouts, computer chips and other conspicuous hallmarks of modern medicine.

A felt-tip pen, for instance, turns out to work nicely as an initial screening test for Alzheimer's disease. Asked to draw a clock with the hands at 11:10, someone who commits three or more errors, such as getting the numbers in the wrong order or leaving large gaps between them, should be given a complete work-up to see if Alzheimer's is to blame. By checking attention span, decision-making ability and comprehension of spatial relationships and numbers, the clock test is a window into the very factors that suffer in Alzheimer's patients, says Mario Mendez, associate professor of neurology at the University of Minnesota.

By permission of Mario F. Mendz, M.D., Ph.D., UCLA/West LA YAMC

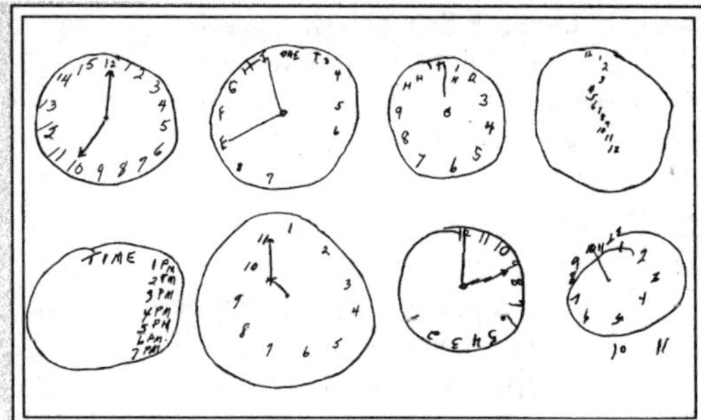

Dali-like. *Drawing an Alzheimer's connection*

Mendez's team tried out the one-minute test over six months with 46 patients previously diagnosed with Alzheimer's and 26 mentally alert people age 65 and over. As a check, each participant also took eight standard Alzheimer's screening tests, including mental-state exams. Test results were compared with the drawings, which were scored against a checklist of 20 items (for example: "all numbers 1-12 are indicated").

Even the non-Alzheimer's participants made mistakes, but rarely more than one or two, Mendez reported last year in the *Journal of the American Geriatrics Society*. The Alzheimer's patients averaged nine errors. Some rendered the time as "13" o'clock. Others drew one hand–or none. And over the six months, the Alzheimer's patients' clocks became increasingly Dali-like.

The results matched up well with conventional screening tests that take an hour or more to administer and cost several hundred dollars. Because many conditions can cause cognitive difficulties, however, only an autopsy can definitively diagnose Alzheimer's.

Mendez also stresses that his clock test is *not* a self-test. A doctor familiar with Mendez's checklist should review the results, and someone at risk should be tested for treatable causes of cognitive problems, such as drug side effects and brain lesions.

Clogging check. Other new no-tech tests, too, seem to work as well as their high-tech counterparts do. Two reports last July in the *Journal of the American Medical Association* showed that taking blood pressure readings in the ankle and the arm and comparing them can gauge the likelihood of clogged coronary arteries and the short-term risk of heart attack. Co-author Anne Newman, an assistant professor of medicine at Allegheny General Hospital in Pittsburgh, says that for people with an extremely low ankle-to-arm ratio, the simple check is as good at predicting risk as an echocardiogram–which must be done in a clinic, uses ultrasound equipment and costs hundreds of dollars. A *JAMA* editorial gave the screening test its blessing for use in doctors' offices.

And a study published in *Angiology*, a journal for heart specialists, shows that a tape measure can detect often painful blood clots in deep leg veins. A difference of more than 1 centimeter–about half an inch–between the thighs, the calves or the ankles indicates a significant clot in the larger leg. The technique is as accurate as the usual noninvasive test, which requires a device that measures the electrical resistance of the leg, takes about half an hour–and costs $200 or more.

DOUG PODOLSKY

The report takes on special significance in light of a federal campaign that began last June intended to motivate more women to get Pap smears. About 1 woman in 10 is likely to get a result other than normal—most of them "minimally abnormal." In all likelihood, these women need do nothing more than have their doctor keep a close eye on their condition.

Clearly, the most dramatic argument for medical minimalism would be it has the potential to make a $150,000 heart transplant unnecessary. In fact, that may be possible. Researchers at the Ahmanson-UCLA Cardiomyopathy Center in Los Angeles have shown that an individually tailored regimen of exercise and unexotic drugs can save many patients with failing hearts from the need for transplant surgery.

Originally, the investigators were simply looking for stopgap methods to keep patients alive while awaiting a scarce donor heart. But the scientists found that combining exercise—at first often as little as a daily half-block walk—with diuretics to flush out excess fluid and vasodilators to open up the blood vessels worked so well that 35 percent of the patients no longer needed a transplant.

Too busy to rest. Californian Joet Ranker, who was one of the fortunate, calls herself a "walking miracle." On a Hawaiian vacation in June 1989, Ranker, 69, found herself limp with exhaustion and suddenly gaining weight. After a week's hospitalization in Hawaii, Ranker was transferred to a hospital near her home and then admitted to UCLA. There she was diagnosed with cardiomyopathy, a condition in which the heart muscle is so weak that it cannot pump sufficiently. After giving her intensive treatment with diuretics and vasodilators, her doctors sent her home to bed to await a heart transplant.

But Ranker didn't stay in bed. The medication made her feel good enough to throw back the covers and start taking walks. "I just kept getting better," she recalls. Fifteen months later, she was doing well enough to be dropped from the transplant list. And now, still on medication, Ranker walks 2 to 3 miles a day, swims at least three times a week and plays nine holes of golf once or twice a week.

Doctors generally have not appreciated how well the body can cope with a heart working far below capacity, says Ranker's doctor, Lynne Warner Steven-

WHEN 'NEWER' ISN'T 'BETTER'

Taking a blunt look at cutting-edge treatments

In the 1930s, Japanese surgeons began treating nearsighted patients by making tiny cuts in the cornea. They had no idea that they were injuring 75 percent of the eyes or that this would often cause blindness and other problems 20 years later.

Radial keratotomy, as the procedure is called, is done far differently now; cuts are made at the front of the cornea rather than at the front and back, as before. It has improved the vision of millions since its 1978 introduction in America. For any given individual, however, the degree of improvement is still unpredictable and the long-term risk uncertain. In 1988, a study funded by the National Eye Institute of 435 patients five years after surgery found that 36 percent of them still wore glasses or contact lenses. Some people had to stop driving at night; cuts made too close to the pupil resulted in glare from oncoming headlights. And because health insurers consider the procedure unnecessary to health, they don't cover the $1,500 estimated cost.

Many other medical procedures become fashionable long before their effectiveness and safety are demonstrated. Surgeons no longer attempt to cure epilepsy, for example, by removing the healthy colons of epileptics. Still, no government agency bars surgeons from trying out new approaches. The current rage among some gynecologists is a new twist on vaginal hysterectomy. The way the procedure traditionally has been performed, the uterus and cervix are removed through a small incision in the vagina rather than through the abdomen; there's no unsightly scar and recovery is faster than with abdominal surgery.

Enter the laparoscope. Not all women are good candidates, however. Some doctors might reject women who have had pelvic surgery or disease that produced internal scarring, for example. The new version of the procedure enlists the aid of a laparoscope – a tube inserted through a small incision in the abdomen and connected to a video monitor to give the surgeon a close-up internal view. The uterus is cut free by instruments inserted through other small incisions, also in the abdomen. Proponents hail the new laparoscopic procedure as a breakthrough for women for whom vaginal hysterectomy otherwise would be ruled out because of scar tissue from previous surgery. But other doctors argue that many women are ruled out not because of their medical condition but because too many surgeons are inadequately trained in vaginal surgery. They fear that those surgeons are most likely to be enthusiastic about the procedure. Comparing the new technique with standard vaginal hysterectomy, a study in the December 1992 journal *Obstetrics and Gynecology* found that the laparoscopic procedure takes an hour longer, costs an average of $3,000 more and results in a more painful recovery.

A rule of thumb: Let a surgeon practice on someone else. Any new procedure has a learning curve, and hospitals set experience requirements, usually through quality-assurance or credentialing committees. Checking a surgeon's experience is crucial when a procedure is relatively untried. It might become tomorrow's standard treatment – or yesterday's unfortunate fad.

SUSAN BRINK

son, former director of the Ahmanson-UCLA Cardiomyopathy Center, who will assume a similar position next month at Boston's Brigham and Women's Hospital. "Before you think about a transplant," she observes, "this is certainly an easier route to try." Too often, she says, doctors focus on getting rid of a disease instead of improving the quality of life. "What's bothering the person is how he *feels* and what he can *do.*"

For instance, not all cataracts need to be removed, yet that surgery is the most common operation performed on Americans 65 and older. Surgery should not be performed if stronger glasses can compensate for a clouded lens well enough to allow daily activities to be carried out, a U.S. Public Health Service committee concluded last February. The health service's guidelines, which outline the diagnosis and suggest treatment for doctors and patients, emphasize that the need for cataract surgery should be literally in the eye of the patient, not of the doctor. "The whole question about vision really has to do with how you're able to function in your environment," says Denis O'Day, chairman of ophthalmology at Vanderbilt University School of Medicine in Tennessee, who led the federal panel. While dying from the surgery is only remotely possible, the operation can cause hemorrhaging or a detached retina.

As with other types of operations, patients must weigh the risks against the potential benefits, O'Day emphasizes. Someone who needs to drive at night might opt for surgery, while corrective glasses might be enough for an older person who is happy simply to be able to read. For instance, when O'Day asked 90-year-old Thelma Edwards, one of his patients, whether her small cataracts impaired her vision, she replied, "I can see just about what I want to see." Edwards quit driving two years ago but lives in her own home in Nashville, belongs to two bridge clubs and is an avid reader.

IRVING YAROSS, 70

CONDITION: *Membranous glomerulonephritis*

■ Doctors told Yaross in 1974 that he had kidney disease. He balked at potent drug therapy, preferring periodic monitoring instead. "Lo and behold, over a period of years it just went away," he marvels.

Finding a happy medium. Some research raises the specter that aggressively treating a disease sometimes not only diminishes the quality of life but might even shorten it. In analyzing the records of nearly 31,000 white and black heart attack patients in veteran's hospitals nationwide, cardiologist Eric Peterson and colleagues at the Brockton/West Roxbury Veterans Affairs Medical Center in Massachusetts found that white patients were twice as likely to undergo bypass surgery and 1½ times as likely to have a cardiac catheterization as were black patients. But blacks were 16 percent more likely to be alive 30 days later and 10 percent more likely to survive a year after their heart attack. "One potential explanation is that blacks are less sick than whites," says Peterson, but he notes that numerous studies have found that blacks have higher rates of hypertension and diabetes, which exacerbate heart disease. "Just because the blacks got fewer procedures doesn't mean they got worse care," says Peterson, now a cardiology fellow at the Duke University School of Medicine in North Carolina. "There is a lot of evidence out there that aggressive care may not always be better."

Even when watching and waiting is one of the options, it imposes its own set of demands. Nail-biters may find the prospect of years of uncertainty too unsettling to contemplate. An I'll-get-through-this attitude is a necessity—as is, obviously, a cooperative physician. Chicagoan Irving Yaross, 70, had both. He and his doctor decided to wait rather than resort to potent and sometimes toxic drugs when membranous glomerulonephritis, a kidney disease that often leads to renal failure, was diagnosed in 1974. By the early 1980s his problem had disappeared, as happens in about 3 in 5 patients. "I'm glad it's behind me," Yaross says today of his years of watchfulness. "It was like being the guy who falls from a 30-story building. As he passes the 15th floor, he says: 'So far, so good.' "

DOUG PODOLSKY AND RITA RUBIN

WHEN DOCTORS JUMP THE GUN

In 1962, physicians developed a dramatic new treatment designed to cure bleeding ulcers by freezing them. But the first controlled clinical trial of the treatment didn't come until seven years later. It conclusively demonstrated that freezing worked no better than a placebo, or sham procedure. Meanwhile, a number of patients had died from intestinal gangrene caused by the freezing.

The authors of the study sternly called for stricter scientific evaluation of new procedures. But little has changed since then; if anything, new but unproved medical techniques proliferate.

The U.S. Food and Drug Administration approves the vast majority of medical devices without rigorous evaluation. Into that regulatory vacuum rush the marketers, who dominate medical conferences with extravagant displays of new techniques and flood doctors' offices with glossy come-ons. Even without that prodding, some doctors would be seduced by the sheer technological wizardry of devices like the surgical laser; by the status, power, and higher fees that new techniques command; or by the demands of patients exposed to news reports often inspired by public-relations specialists.

This report discusses several of the most frequently used procedures in which the widespread use of technology appears to have jumped ahead of the scientific evidence of its value.

Keyhole surgery

In 1988, a Tennessee surgeon introduced a new way to remove a gallbladder, a type of surgery sometimes necessary when the gallbladder is forming stones that cause painful attacks. The new method, known as laparoscopic cholecystectomy, requires only four small incisions, each roughly half an inch long, compared with a typically six-inch incision required by the traditional operation. Through those incisions the surgeon inserts the surgical instruments and a laparoscope—a lighted tube equipped with a miniature camera—and operates with the aid of a video monitor. A properly performed laparoscopic cholecystectomy reduces postsurgical pain, decreases the hospital stay from seven days to two or three days, and cuts recovery time from up to six weeks to less than two.

The rush to use the latest medical 'advance' often has only the flimsiest scientific support.

Surgeons have switched to laparoscopic cholecystectomy in droves; it now accounts for at least 85 percent of the roughly 600,000 gallstone operations performed each year. That revolution took place before researchers had completed any clinical trials comparing the two procedures.

The scanty available evidence suggests that the new procedure may be reasonably safe when it's done by a properly trained surgeon. (Other "keyhole" techniques used to treat orthopedic and gynecological disorders do seem to be safe enough.) But some doctors are doing laparoscopic cholecystectomy without proper training. Reports of serious complications from the operation have forced New York State to establish minimum standards of training for laparoscopy—the only surgical procedure the state has ever regulated in that way. A key requirement: A surgeon must train by performing at least 10 procedures under the supervision of an experienced surgeon.

Enthusiasm for the new procedure has gotten out of hand in another, equally troubling, way. Studies in two states and in one nationwide health maintenance organization suggest that the total number of gallbladder operations has jumped sharply, by at least 30 percent, since the introduction of laparoscopy, while the number of other abdominal surgeries has not increased. Presumably, some doctors have decided without any scientific justification to expand the standard indication for gallbladder surgery—stones plus severe pain or moderate recurrent pain—to include stones that cause little or no pain. Studies have already indicated that removing the gallbladder does not prolong the lives of patients without severe symptoms. A recent consensus conference sponsored by the National Institutes of Health concluded that surgeons should not perform a major operation like laparoscopy just to relieve mild gallbladder symp-

Reprinted with permission from *Consumer Reports on Health*, September 1994, pp. 97-100.

toms or to prevent possible problems in the future.

Now laparoscopic surgery has started spreading to the treatment of other abdominal ailments. Two of those new applications are particularly troubling, and should generally be avoided until further studies show that they're safe and effective:

■ **Hernia repair.** An estimated 10 to 20 percent of all operations to fix a hernia—protrusion of an abdominal organ through a rupture in the groin muscles—are now done laparoscopically. That approach does minimize discomfort and shorten recovery time. However, the best traditional procedure, known as the Canadian method, requires no hospitalization, needs only local anesthesia, and is exceptionally safe and effective. In contrast, laparoscopy usually requires general anesthesia, sometimes necessitates an overnight stay in the hospital, and poses a greater risk to the abdominal organs. Moreover, laparoscopy necessitates a new, experimental method, using staples and plastic mesh, to close the rupture. No one knows whether stapling will keep the rupture permanently closed. Concern about those drawbacks recently led all the participating surgeons at a prominent Boston hospital to withdraw from a multi-center study of laparoscopic repair.

■ **Colon surgery.** A standard treatment for colon cancer and several other diseases of the colon is removal of the affected segment of the bowel. That's a particularly formidable job when done with a laparoscope. Without viewing the colon directly, the surgeon must meticulously cut a large segment of the bowel away from the surrounding tissues, remove that segment, and rejoin the cut ends of the bowel with a watertight seal. In the few studies done so far, laparoscopic colon surgery has caused many complications. Treating colon cancer with the laparoscope is particularly difficult, since the surgeon also has to remove the nearby lymph nodes. Some reports suggest that cancer cells may spread when surgeons try to squeeze a large, cancerous segment of the bowel through one of the tiny incisions.

The magnetic allure of MRI

Getting a clear look at anything inside the body except the bones requires special imaging techniques, such as ultrasound and computerized X-rays, or CT scans. But physicians generally get the clearest views from magnetic resonance imaging (MRI). That technique uses powerful magnets to stimulate the body's tissues to emit their own electromagnetic signals, which a computer transforms into detailed pictures.

Most large hospitals and many physicians in private practice have now invested the one to two million dollars needed to obtain this seductive new technology. The combination of impressive pictures and a huge investment to recoup creates a seemingly irresistible incentive to use the device at every opportunity—at an average cost to patients of about $1300 per scan, nearly twice the average cost of a CT scan. According to the latest available figures, the number of MRI scans done in hospitals increased nearly 15-fold between 1986—shortly after Medicare started paying for the scans—and 1992. And a Government report published in June showed that doctors who have invested in an MRI machine order the scans three times more often than other doctors do.

But improved pictures are not themselves a clinical advantage if the images from a CT scanner or other device provide enough information, or if the results of the scan will not affect treatment. And sharper pictures are more likely to reveal potentially misleading information, such as a harmless anatomical deformity, that leads to further testing or even unnecessary treatment.

Indeed, there's surprisingly little evidence to demonstrate that MRI scans are worth the extra cost in most cases. A comprehensive review published in May in the Annals of Internal Medicine found few reliable studies on whether MRI actually changes treatment decisions or improves the patient's final outcome. The limited evidence the authors did find suggests that MRI's are seldom warranted, but frequently ordered, to aid in the diagnosis of a number of common conditions.

■ **Stroke.** Most strokes are caused by a clot in an artery feeding the brain, so doctors generally treat them with anticlotting drugs. But first they have to rule out two other possible causes of stroke or strokelike symptoms, a hemorrhaging blood vessel or a tumor. A CT scan of the brain is generally sufficient for that purpose, since it will accurately detect bleeding and nearly all tumors in stroke patients. Only when unexplained symptoms persist after a CT scan might an MRI be warranted.

■ **Alzheimer's disease.** Doctors can almost always diagnose Alzheimer's from the patient's symptoms and medical history alone. Confirming the diagnosis with a brain scan rarely has any practical payoff, since there's no effective treatment for Alzheimer's disease. Dementia that worsens unusually rapidly might be caused by some other, treatable disorder; but blood tests will usually identify the problem. Only if those tests are negative might the patient need a brain scan, to rule out a potential tumor. Even then, a CT scan will rarely miss a growth that an MRI would have caught:

■ **Low back pain.** This common problem is usually caused by a muscle or ligament strain, something doctors can confirm simply by questioning the patient. Even back pain that radiates down the rear of the legs, a sign of pressure on a spinal nerve, initially requires no special tests, since the pain usually clears up as inflammation around the nerve subsides. Only when the pain is particularly severe or persists for more than a month or two would an imaging test be needed to search for a protruding vertebral disk or other abnormality that might require surgery. In that case, MRI would be preferable, since the tissues pressing on a nerve may be difficult to identify with other tests.

■ **Headaches and dizziness.** These common complaints are so rarely caused by a tumor or other physical abnormality in the brain that imaging tests are not worth doing unless the person has some other, more serious neurological symptom. Even then, MRI should be reserved for problems that persist after a CT scan has failed to pinpoint the cause.

If a physician recommends that you undergo an MRI, you may be able to avoid unnecessary trouble and expense by asking these key questions: What is the chance that the test will find something wrong? Is the test more likely than a CT scan to detect a significant problem? And, most important, will the results have any effect on treatment?

Lasers: Magic ray or flash in the pan?

Doctors have started using this technological marvel to treat everything from snoring and droopy eyelids to coronary heart disease. For certain types of surgery, lasers do indeed have potential advantages over scalpels and other mechanical cutters. For example, lasers can be focused precisely, allowing physicians to remove certain birthmarks with less scarring of the surrounding tissue than other methods cause. Lasers can reduce bleeding during surgery by sealing off the severed capillaries. And they can pass harmlessly through the transparent front of the eye, while destroying unwanted tissue inside the eye, such as proliferating blood vessels in the retina of people with diabetes.

But in many cases, conventional instruments work at least as well as lasers do, and cost considerably less. Here are three important examples:

■ **Cutting down the prostate.** The prostate gland tends to get larger as a man gets older, often making urination more difficult and more frequent. When symptoms keep getting worse and drugs don't help, surgery may. In the traditional operation, surgeons remove part of the prostate, usually by threading a tiny electric cutter through the penis and into the gland.

Now, an increasing number of prostate surgeries are being performed by inserting a flexible laser device into the prostate, where the beam destroys the excess tissue. The new approach causes less blood loss than the traditional procedure. But the laser does not ease the original urinary problem as effectively as the standard operation. Further, it causes more postoperative pain during urination and requires more prolonged use of a catheter for urination. Most important, no one knows what long-term complications may develop and how soon the operation may have to be repeated.

■ **Clearing clogged arteries.** In standard angioplasty, designed to open a constricted artery feeding a leg or the heart, surgeons inflate a tiny balloon inside the artery to flatten the obstructing plaque deposit against the artery wall. But the flattened plaque tends to attract new deposits, which reclog the artery in about one-fourth of cases within six months. When the FDA approved lasers for angioplasty in 1987, proponents hoped that vaporizing the plaque would keep the arteries open permanently. Surgeons were soon performing some 10,000 laser angioplasties per year.

At first, surgeons used the laser to heat a metal-tipped probe that they threaded through the artery and into the plaque. Unfortunately, the heat not only melted the plaque deposit but also burned the artery walls, leaving a roughened surface that attracted new deposits even faster than the plaque flattened by a balloon.

Undaunted, the manufacturers introduced a "cold" laser, which destroys the plaque's chemical bonds. Although the new method works better than its predecessor, it too damages the artery; it has led to at least as much reclogging as the balloon does. That hasn't stopped some hospitals from aggressively encouraging patients to have their clogged arteries treated with the cold laser.

■ **Hemorrhoids.** According to a half-page ad in the Manhattan yellow pages, lasers "enable doctors to successfully treat hemorrhoids painlessly without surgery . . . [or] risky anesthesia. Most patients . . . return to normal activities immediately." Actually, lasers seem to offer no advantage over traditional hemorrhoid surgery, a relatively simple outpatient procedure that usually requires only local anesthesia. In fact, the lone clinical trial that compared the two procedures found only one significant difference: Lasers left patients with more postoperative inflammation. And laser treatment typically costs about $2300, some $500 more than the standard procedure. Fortunately, hemorrhoid patients rarely need surgery at all, since self-help measures or treatment such as injections or rubber banding will usually relieve the problem (see CRH, 2/94).

Timing Is Everything

In sickness, as in health, rhythm is a critical factor. Effective treatments must work with the body's clocks, not against them.

WILLIAM J. M. HRUSHESKY

William J. M. Hrushesky is professor of medicine at Albany Medical College in New York, and an oncologist at the Samuel S. Stratton Medical Center, Department of Veterans Affairs. This article is adapted from "Chaos, Clocks, and Cancer," a lecture he gave to the Biomedical Section of the New York Academy of Sciences on May 4, 1994.

Each thing is of like form from everlasting and comes round again in its cycle.
—Marcus Aurelius, second century A.D.

In 1729 the French astronomer Jean-Jacques de Mairan tested a phenomenon that had intrigued observers since ancient times: the leaves of certain plants regularly open in the daytime and then close at night. It had long been assumed that such activity was cued by the alternating sunlight and darkness. But de Mairan, using *Kalanchoë blossfeldiana,* a plant with small red flowers, made a startling discovery: the leaves and petals adhered faithfully to their routine even when kept in the dark. The implication was clear: something other than the fluctuations of light was causing *Kalanchoë* to open and close on a daily basis.

De Mairan's experiment was the earliest recorded exercise in what is now known as chronobiology (from the Greek *chronos,* meaning time), the study of rhythmic temporal patterns in biological phenomena. Like the movements of *Kalanchoë,* many such patterns follow roughly a twenty-four-hour schedule; hence they are referred to as circadian (Latin for about a day) rhythms. As de Mairan's work was the first to suggest, circadian rhythms are widely held to be endogenous, or innate, to living systems, governed by shadowy physiological mechanisms known as biological clocks. Indeed, in the past two and a half centuries endogenous timekeeping rhythms have been demonstrated in yeasts and nucleated unicells and at all levels of biological organization—cell, tissue and organ—as well as in the human body as a whole.

Ponder for a moment a few of the ways the time of day has been observed to govern people's lives: In the morning, on awakening, one's pulse rate and blood pressure rise sharply, a trend that may be linked to the high frequency of heart attack and stroke at that time of day. Body temperatures also rise during the day and, with the pulse and blood pressure, fall off sharply at night. One's tolerance for alcohol peaks at around five o'clock in the afternoon. The secretion of countless hormones, essential for the control of life's processes, ebbs and flows with faithful circadian regularity. The number of white blood cells in the immune system also fluctuates widely and regularly, with a normal variation of as much as 50 percent in a day. The daily pattern of sleep and activity is so much a part of what it means to be human that it is scarcely noticed, except perhaps by insomniacs and narcoleptics. The time the Swedish filmmaker Ingmar Bergman called the *Hour of the Wolf*—the gloomy hour "between night and dawn"—is the most likely time to be born or to die.

Why do all living organisms do virtually everything cyclically? Daily cycles of life, as well as seasonal and monthly ones, arose, quite simply, because life evolved on this planet. The waxing and waning of light, heat and electromagnetic and gravitational forces caused rhythmic changes both in the availability of energy and in the physical medium in which evolution was unfolding. But even more basic than the happenstance of geophysical location to evolution, the rhythmic organization of temporal processes maximizes the stability of living things and ensures that they not waste precious energy.

Life's absolute need for stability requires continuous readjustment to external and internal dynamic requirements. The adjustment can be pictured as cyclical: a phase of activation or production; then an assessment of stability; a "midcourse correction," based on feedback from the outcome of the activity in the first phase of the cycle; and a return to the beginning of the cycle. A second cycle of activity then begins at the optimum time if it would promote stability. If stability is already optimum, the first phase of the new cycle begins with minimal or nonexistent productive activity. The breakdown of such cyclical temporal ordering has lethal consequences for the organism.

One of the most important and practical applications of the emerging understanding of the role of cycles in biology is the treatment of disease. The abnormalities associated with virtually every disease—from allergy, arthritis and asthma to cardiovascular disease and cancer—are themselves organized cyclically and, in particular, along circadian lines. The treatment of such illnesses according to daily rhythms is commonly referred to as chronotherapy. Only recently has the medical community integrated chronotherapy into the development and delivery of pharmaceuticals. Circadian variations in symptoms and in the ability of certain tissues to absorb certain drugs help determine whether a given treatment will be successful or dangerously toxic. A growing body of evidence suggests that therapy could be improved and toxicity reduced by administering drugs at carefully selected times of day. A brief survey of the cases in which chronotherapy is most effective will suggest how much has been learned, and how much remains to be done.

THE DRUGS USED TO CONTROL ALLERGY SYMPtoms—among them, antihistamines and decongestants—represent one of the largest and most profitable pharmaceutical markets in the world. A great deal of effort, time and money has been spent developing such drugs, with an eye toward diminishing their sedative or stimulatory side effects. It does not take a genius, however, to realize that antihistamines, which generally act as sedatives, are better taken in the evening, and that decongestants, which exert a stimulatory effect, should be used during the day and be avoided at night. Aside from that kind of logical treatment, other, less obvious and even surprising circadian differences in drug absorption, excretion, metabolism and effectiveness have recently become clear.

Allergic reactions are cued by the overzealous response of the body's primordial defense against invasion, the inflammatory reaction. When a person is exposed to an allergen, be it dust, pollen or a particular food, the bloodstream sends a crowd of circulating white blood cells to the site of contact. There they proceed to react with and engulf the foreign agent. Some of those white cells, the basophils, release histamines, chemicals that increase local blood flow; cause leaks in small blood vessels; and spark a flood of more white cells. The result is swelling, pain and itchiness, burning and redness. That response can serve as the takeoff point for either allergy or exaggerated inflammation. Inflammation can also trigger an aberrant immune response against normal tissues.

Both the immune system and the inflammatory response are orchestrated primarily by circadian rhythms in the release and action of glucocorticoids, steroid hormones made in the adrenal gland. Glucocorticoids, cortisol above all, promote the manufacture of glucose out of protein and fat stored in the body. Their intense release, along with the release of adrenaline, is part of the flight-or-fight response to times of heightened, short-term stress (a mugging, say, or a job interview). Glucocorticoids also regulate and, if present in excess, depress the immune system, which may explain why people are more susceptible to illness when they are under stress—and why the hormones, cortisol especially, turn out to be valuable in reducing the redness, pain and burning of inflammation.

Cortisol concentration in the blood is highest in the morning, around five or six o'clock; as expected, the inflammatory reaction is weakest at that time. But in the evening, when the blood concentration of cortisol is lowest, inflammatory activity is at its strongest. The daily waxing and waning of cortisol concentration has broad implications for the timing of virtually any anti-inflammatory agent. That profoundly stable rhythm may also be responsible, at least in part, for the circadian coordination of all the body's defense networks and even the daily pattern of cell division—in other words, for the renewal of almost all bodily tissues.

ARTHRITIS, AN ALL TOO COMMON INFLAMMAtory disease of the joints, also runs on a biological clock. The condition comes in two major varieties. In rheumatoid arthritis a disordered immune system attacks components of the joint. Nonrheumatic arthritis includes a wide range of degenerative diseases. Some of them are associated with the formation of crystal deposits in the joints; others are set off by wear and tear, trauma or infection. Various forms of rheumatoid arthritis affect millions of people, whereas nonrheumatic arthritis to some extent affects most people who live past the age of forty.

For generations physicians have differentiated between the two kinds of arthritis according to the circadian patterns of their symptoms. In rheumatoid arthritis the joints are most stiff, swollen, hot and painful when one arises; they "work themselves out" as the day progresses. In contrast, in nonrheumatic arthritis, such as osteoarthritis, the redness, pain and swelling build throughout the day and get relieved only by a good night's rest. By timing the medication and optimizing the relation between dose and time of day, one can better control the symptoms and reduce the side effects of drugs.

Arthritis is often treated with NSAIDs (nonsteroidal anti-inflammatory drugs), among which are aspirin and ibuprofen. Depending on the release characteristics of the specific preparation, NSAIDs can best be taken at one time of day or another. An NSAID taken in the evening that hits its peak of release within four to ten hours after ingestion would best treat rheumatic diseases. A once-a-day preparation taken at bedtime for osteoarthritis, however, should peak the following afternoon, between fourteen and twenty hours later.

In addition to symptom patterns, many other considerations relate to the construction of an optimized pill—one that, taken at a certain time of day, provides the highest levels of its active ingredient when it is needed and the lowest levels when it is least needed and most damaging. The absorption of a standard drug preparation in the gut also depends on when the drug is taken. Sodium salicylate, for instance, which is prescribed for osteoarthritis, is absorbed relatively slowly in the morning; ketoprofen, prescribed for the same condition, is absorbed quickly in the morning.

Sometimes NSAIDs are not enough. For the most severe cases of rheumatoid arthritis, physicians typically prescribe steroids. Because steroids are hormones that occur naturally in the body, their side effects—including weight gain, thinning bones, diabetes, mania, high blood pressure, suppression of the adrenal gland and increased risk of infection—can be diminished if the hormones' usual circadian rhythms are mimicked, taking advantage of the body's capacity to neutralize their toxic effects. The patient takes most of each day's dose on arising or takes a larger morning dose every other day.

PERHAPS THE MOST PROMINENTLY CIRCADIAN of all diseases is asthma, which affects one of every twenty people worldwide. Asthma is a contraction of the smooth muscle surrounding the airways that makes it excruciatingly difficult to breathe. The great majority of asthma attacks take place between two and six o'clock in the morning. That circadian pattern is caused by the co-occurrence of many normal physiological processes.

Airway size and breathing patterns change rhythmically throughout the day in healthy people as well as in asthmatics. Generally the airways are open widest during the day. There is a rhythmic reduction in the airflow after midnight, and particularly between the critical hours of two and six in the morning. Those normal fluctuations can become extreme in response to both internal and external stimuli: allergens in the sleeping room, the supine posture and mucus retention during sleep, the cooling of the airway caused by breathing through the mouth, and circadian patterns in muscle and sympathetic nervous tone and in the circulation of cortisol, histamine and the hormone epinephrine.

The so-called chronopathology of asthma suggests that drug treatments should be designed to anticipate the temporal onset of an attack. One of the most successful kinds of chronotherapy yet developed is the bronchodilator preparation for nocturnal asthma. Many such drugs are on the market, each one absorbed, metabolized and excreted differently, depending on when it is ingested. The optimal once-a-day bronchodilator must make its active ingredient most available between the critical hours of two and six in the morning. Thus an evening dose should delay delivery for between four and six hours, and a morning dose should do so for between sixteen and eighteen hours.

ONLY RECENTLY HAS IT COME TO BE UNDERstood that cardiovascular disease, the number-one killer of adults, is heavily influenced by circadian rhythms in pulse rate, blood pressure, the tendency of blood to clot, the interactions between blood cells and the walls of the blood vessels, and important interactions in the part of the nervous system that controls involuntary functions.

Consider angina pectoris, a chest pain caused when the heart muscle does not get enough oxygen. Oxygen is carried to the heart by the blood through the coronary arteries. A partial blockage of those arteries may prevent some area of the heart muscle from getting enough blood, an ongoing condition known as myocardial ischemia; ischemia can be silent or it can manifest itself as angina. The timing of ischemia during the day makes it clear that getting oxygen to the heart muscle is quite sensitive to circadian rhythms, and so those rhythms are potentially highly relevant to coronary artery disease. Several large studies have shown that ischemia is much more frequent and severe in the four to six hours after people arise in the morning than it is at other times of day. Whatever its precise cause, that finding has obvious implications for the development of anti-anginal-drug delivery systems.

Several large studies have demonstrated that myocardial infarctions—heart attacks—strike twice as often in the morning as they do during the rest of the day. Like angina, heart attacks result from a lack of blood, and hence of oxygen, in the heart muscle. The condition can arise from a variety of problems inside the blood vessels, and one of the most significant of those problems is high blood pressure, or hypertension.

Blood pressure, as I noted earlier, is strongly circadian; thus transient hypertension in response to daily stresses may not be as ominous as blood pressure that is abnormally elevated at a time of day when it is usually much lower. The main problem with hypertension is that it gives an unhealthy battering to the walls of the blood vessels. That raises the odds that the vessels will be damaged, giving rise to a blood clot and causing a heart attack or a stroke.

Another threat to the blood vessels is intensified shear stress—the pulling or tearing force exerted on the vessel wall by the flow of blood cells. Shear stress relates in complicated ways to blood pressure, to the rate of blood flow and to the diameter of the blood vessel. The most prominent increase in shear stress takes place, again, when one gets up in the morning: when one stands upright after lying down for a long while, the nervous system cues an increase in blood pressure and a change in blood flow, as well as a constriction of the blood vessels. The shear stress and change in blood pressure ultimately damage the vessel walls.

A THIRD IMPORTANT factor in the evolution of heart disease is an unfortunate side effect of the body's mechanisms for controlling bleeding. When a small wound opens in the skin, the blood cells known as platelets clump together at the site of the injury. But blood vessels damaged by hypertension or shear stress also appear wounded to the platelets, and so large numbers of platelets can aggregate inside the blood vessels and eventually set off a chain reaction that can block the passage of the blood. Platelets tend to be stickier in the morning than they are at other times of day; hence it is safer to shave in the morning than it is at night. The tendency is associated with increased levels of catecholamines, stress hormones released when a person assumes an upright posture. Any drug that might suppress the morning surge in stress hormones should reduce the tendency of arterial platelets to clump together. Also, drugs that directly interfere with platelet function should be given in such a way that most of their activity takes place in the morning.

Another important factor in the control of bleeding is fibrinogen, the main clotting protein in the blood. The concentrations of fibrinogen in blood plasma peak in the morning and then plunge into an evening trough. In normal circumstances blood clots are constantly dissolved by fibrinolysis, a process whereby the crucial clotting proteins are absorbed by the body. Fibrinolytic activity has a prominent circadian rhythm, with a morning trough and a nocturnal peak—which helps account for the inverse pattern of fibrinogen concentration.

Any strategy for interrupting the cascade of events leading to a heart attack would do well to account for all the foregoing circadian dynamics. In the morning the heart's need for oxygen should be decreased; small doses of anticoagulants should be prescribed; blockers of the effects of stress hormones must be administered to counteract the tendency of damaged blood vessels feeding the heart muscle to contract and thereby decrease the flow of oxygen; and blood pressure, which tends to leap after one awakens, must be modulated.

CANCER, IN ITS VARIOUS FORMS, WILL BE REsponsible for 600,000 deaths this year in the United States alone, making it second only to heart disease in frequency and lethality. A number of natural cycles govern the delicate balance between a person and an incipient or established cancer—seasonal cycles, fertility cycles and circadian cycles. Breast cancer tumors grow more rapidly, and are most likely to be discovered, in spring; the opposite is true in fall, and growth in winter and summer lies somewhere in between. In men the discovery of two main kinds of testicular cancer peaks at different times, one in early winter and the other in late summer. As for fertility cycles, recent studies have confirmed that the cure of a breast tumor by surgery is dramatically more likely between two and three weeks from the first day of the patient's menstrual period than it is at other times in the menstrual cycle.

The effects of circadian rhythms in cancer are somewhat less obvious than they are for arthritis or asthma. But they bear enormously on treatment, especially because the stakes are so high: cancer is life-threatening, and the cure often involves chemotherapy, the use of drugs with frequently serious side effects.

Chemotherapeutic drugs generally kill human cells by exploiting their relative vulnerability during cell division: they damage actively reproducing cells far more severely than they damage cells that are not dividing. Thus the drugs kill cancer cells preferentially, because such cells, by definition, grow and proliferate at an abnormally high rate. The catch is that anticancer drugs also sometimes damage and destroy noncancerous cells, usually including the white blood cells of the immune system, the precursor immune cells in the bone marrow and the cells that line the gut.

Most oncologists give little thought to the time of day when a drug is given: generally the deciding factor is convenience for the medical staff. But a growing body of data suggests that the patient can gain an optimal therapeutic effect with minimal toxicity if the drugs are dispensed at carefully selected times. Regular circadian rhythms in the division of cells in the bone marrow and in the gut may partly explain why chemotherapy is more toxic to those normal cells at certain times of day. There is also evidence that suggests the division of human tumor cells follows a synchronized circadian pattern. An understanding of that pattern could reap extraordinary benefits. For example, if the daily periods of cell division in healthy and cancerous cells are not identical, chemotherapy could be tailored to work when only the cancerous cells are dividing.

Although much work remains to be done, the benefits of timing have so far been demonstrated for a diverse class of anticancer drugs. Consider doxorubicin, a complex fungal derivative that attacks the DNA of all kinds of cell, cancerous as well as benign. Often taken in conjunction with a platinum-based drug called cisplatin, doxorubicin significantly depresses the body's concentration of white blood cells. Although the effect is not understood, when doxorubicin is given in the morning, the dip in white blood cells is much less profound, and recovery to normal levels is complete within twenty-one days. In contrast, when doxorubicin is administered in the late afternoon or early evening, full recovery does not take place even after twenty-eight days. Women with ovarian cancer who receive optimally timed doses of doxorubicin and cisplatin are four times more likely to survive for five years than are women who receive the same drugs in ill-timed doses.

MOST ONCOLOGISTS GIVE LITTLE THOUGHT TO THE TIME OF DAY *when a drug is given: generally the deciding factor is convenience for the staff.*

Recent multicenter studies by workers in Canada, France and the U.S. suggest that for certain cancers drugs in the fluoropyrimidine family—widely used in chemotherapy—are safest when most of the daily dose is given at night. Moreover, the French trial found that nighttime doses of fluoropyrimidines given with daytime platinum-based drugs are safer and dramatically more effective against colon cancer than the same drugs given at a constant rate in daytime hours. Other data suggest that circadian timing is even more crucial for certain cancer therapies involving growth factors and peptides that stimulate infection-fighting white cells.

ANTICANCER DRUG DEVELOPMENT IS A COMplex, protracted and expensive high-risk venture. The few agents that graduate from in vitro screening to trials in whole animals or in humans have high rates of failure. And so it is ironic that the results of such trials may themselves depend on time of day.

Consider the development of a new, so-called S-phase (for synthesis phase) active agent: a drug that damages only cells engaged in making DNA for self-replication. Suppose the S-phase agent targets an enzyme in the cell required for the synthesis of a nucleic acid necessary to replicate DNA. If the agent is evaluated for toxicity at the time of day when little DNA tends to be synthesized in the gut or bone marrow, the agent will be classed as highly therapeutic and scarcely toxic.

As it turns out, drug trials are usually run in the first half of the working day. That happens to coincide with the first half of the daily sleep cycle of the laboratory mouse, when relatively low levels of DNA are synthesized in the gut and bone marrow. When the drug passes the mouse test, it generally goes on to a clinical trial with real cancer patients. Those initial trials are also carried out in the first half of the working day—and therein lies a rub. At that time of day the level of DNA synthesis in people is at its highest—the reverse of its level in mice. Thus a potentially useful drug that works well in mice may well be prematurely discarded as too toxic.

The outcome could be quite different if laboratory studies were focused on finding the optimum circadian time for therapy and then, as a result, setting up the clinical trials at the appropriate time of day. Here, as in much else in life, timing is everything. In some instances, proper circadian timing may enable effective drugs to be distinguished from the ones that have no effect. That knowledge, in turn, can make the difference between tumor control and tumor enhancement growth: between life and death.

Do HEALTH CARE COSTS MATTER?

William J. Baumol

WILLIAM J. BAUMOL is director of the C.V. Starr Center for Applied Economics at New York University. This article is based on a longer paper to be published by the American Philosophical Society.

The exploding cost of health care is clearly a matter of concern across the industrialized world. In the United States the president has stressed this issue as one of the most critical facing us, arguing that soaring health care costs not only drain the economy, but price good health out of the reach of many Americans. The issue, it is important to note, is not just absolute levels of health care costs, but the *rate* at which they're rising and the growing share of the national economy they occupy. The reasons cited for this are many—from the greed of drug and insurance companies to an increasingly aged population. But there's also something else at work here: a deep economic force that suggests the relative increase in health care costs compared with the rest of the economy is an inevitable and ineradicable part of a developed economy. The attempt to do anything about it may be as foolhardy as it is impossible.

But first some facts. The relative rate of growth of health care costs is indisputable. From 1948 to 1992 the price of a doctor's services increased more than 5.5 percent a year, compared with an average annual increase of 4 percent in the Consumer Price Index. This gap may not seem very large for any one year, but over the forty-four years in question it means that the price of a doctor's services increased by more than 100 percent in real terms. In the same period, the price of a hospital room grew even more rapidly: by 700 percent in real terms.

In America the phenomenon has been worse than in other countries, but there is no other advanced country in which complaints about rates of cost increase are not heard. According to the latest Organization for Economic Cooperation and Development medical-consumption price index, in fourteen of eighteen countries in the years 1960 through 1990, health care prices rose more rapidly than prices in general. The U.S. rate of increase was exceeded by that in seven countries—Australia, Austria, Canada, the Netherlands, New Zealand, Norway and Switzerland. Although in recent years the growth rate of U.S. costs has accelerated relative to that of the other leading economies (and the proportion of health spending here is still higher than in other countries), the universality and persistence of the problem suggest it lies deeper than the particular administrative or institutional arrangements adopted in any single country.

What, then, can its source be? There are many influences, actual or alleged. Lawsuits against doctors, lack of competitiveness in the profession and high earnings of physicians clearly help explain the *levels* of those costs. But I am aware of no source besides the one about to be described that seems to account for the many countries in which *growth* in health costs persistently outpaces the rate of inflation.

If litigation could explain the rise in medical costs, it, and the size of jury awards, would have to have been increasing throughout the last few decades. I know of no evidence that this was so, or that it was so in the other countries in which costs have been rising faster than ours. Recent evidence even seems to suggest that the pertinent litigation in the United States has been leveling off or declining. There has been no discernible trend in the size of jury awards, but the frequency of plaintiff victories has been declining, meaning that the total cost of malpractice awards has also probably been falling.

Similarly, if lack of competitiveness were the problem, the degree of competitiveness would have to have been falling over the years. The evidence, however, is to the contrary. The rapid growth in the number and membership of HMOs has added to the forces of competition. The number of physicians per capita has been expanding since 1960 and, with that, the pressures for doctors to compete for patients. Moreover, the proportion of applicants to medical school who are granted admission and the proportion of medical students who graduate have also grown. The other alleged cause of the relative rise of health care costs—doctors' incomes—also doesn't seem to explain much. Over the past fifteen years, the real earnings of doctors in the United States have been virtually constant. The 1991 *U.S. Statistical Abstract* reports the trends in median net physician incomes for the period 1975-1988. In 1988 real average physician income was somewhat less than where it had begun, at $53,600 in 1975 dollars.

Where, then, does that leave us? It is almost exactly a quarter-century since William Bowen and I first reported our analysis of what is now called "the cost disease of the personal services," including health care, education and a number of other services. A major source of the cost disease, we argued, was the different productivity growth rates of the various parts of a developed economy. Put simply, we noted that some parts of the economy—what we called the "stagnant services"—experienced consistently lower productivity growth rates than other sectors did. These services—notably health care, education, law, welfare programs, mail, police, sanitation, repairs, the performing arts and restaurant services—all had in common the handicraft attribute of their supply processes. None of them had been fully liberated from the requirement of a large residue of personal attention by their producers. Not that the growth rate of their labor productivity had been zero. In almost every case there was some productivity gain with the passage of time; but in the long run, it was far slower than the rate of productivity increase in the economy as a whole.

There are at least two reasons why this is so. First, these services are inherently resistant to automation. The manufacture of thousands of identical cars can be carried out on an assembly line, but the repair of a car just hauled to a garage from the site of an accident can not be entrusted completely to automated processes. Second, in many of these services, quality is, or is at least believed to be, inescapably correlated with the amount of labor expended on their production. Doctors who speed up the examination of their patients, or police forces that spend less time on the beat, are held to be shortchanging those they serve. This has a real effect on the relative share of GNP and relative sector labor costs that exist in an advanced economy.

To see why, imagine an economy divided into two sectors: one, the progressive sector, in which productivity is rising, and another, the stagnant sector, in which productivity is constant. Suppose the first economic sector produces cars, and the second, performances of Mozart quartets. Assume that in car production, where technological improvements are possible, output per work-hour is increasing at an annual rate of 4 percent, while the productivity of quartet players remains unchanged year after year. Imagine now that the workers in the car industry recognize the growth in their own productivity and persuade management to agree to a matching rise in wages. The effect on the auto industry is easy to trace. Each year the average worker's wages go up by 4 percent, but her output increases by exactly the same percentage. Then the one effect on cost is exactly offset by the other—total cost and output both rise 4 percent. So labor cost *per unit* (the ratio between total labor cost and total output) remains absolutely unchanged. This process can continue indefinitely in our imaginary world, with auto workers earning more and more each year, with cost per car remaining stationary, and with no rise in car prices necessary to maintain company profits.

But what of the other industry in our little economy? How is quartet performance faring in this society of growing abundance? Suppose that the quartet players somehow succeed in getting their wages raised, and that their standard of living, though below that of the auto workers, maintains its relative position, also increasing 4 percent per year. What does this situation imply for the costs of quartet performance? If the earnings of string players increase by 4 percent per year while their productivity remains unchanged, it follows that the direct labor cost per unit of their output must also rise at 4 percent, since cost per unit is equal to total cost divided by the number of units of output. If in a forty-hour week the string player provides just as many performances as he did the previous year but his wage is 4 percent higher, then the cost per performance must have risen correspondingly. Moreover, there is nothing in the nature of this situation to prevent the cost of performance from rising indefinitely and at a compounded rate. So long as the musicians are successful in resisting erosion of their relative incomes, the cost per performance must continue to increase along with the performers' income. Cumulatively rising costs will beset the performing arts with absolute inevitability.

It is important to recognize that ordinary price inflation plays no role in the logic of our analysis. That is, as long as the wages of musicians in this two-sector economy continue to increase at all, the cost of a live performance will rise, cumulatively and persistently, relative to the cost of a car, whether or not the general price level in the economy is changing; the extent of the increase in the relative cost of the performance will depend directly on the relative rate of growth of productivity in the car industry. Moreover, though it is always tempting to seek some villain to explain such a run of real price increases, there is no guilty party here. Neither wasteful expenditure nor greed plays any role. It is the relatively stagnant technology of live musical performance—its inherent resistance to productivity improvements—that accounts for the compounding rise in the cost of performance of quartets.

It's clear how this analysis applies to the relatively increasing cost of health care. Clearly, health care has taken giant steps in quality improvement over the decades, but while the amount of physician time spent per patient visit or per illness may have declined somewhat, it has done so only marginally. Even the most elaborate technology needs to be applied patient-by-patient in a painstakingly labor-intensive fashion. The upshot is that this service must suffer from a rise in its cost that is terrifyingly rapid and frighteningly persistent. It threatens the strained budgets of individual families, as well as of central governments.

Is there a way out of this morass? The bad news is: unfortunately not. The good news is: on closer inspection, the morass is not as depressing as it first looks. In truth, the very structure of the problem is such as to offer society all the resources for its solution. We can afford ever more ample medical care, ever more abundant education, ever more adequate support of the indigent, and all this along with a growing abundance of private comforts and luxuries. This conclusion may sound implausible in light of all that has been said. But it's inescapable, if only our future productivity record bears any resemblance to that of decades past, which brought us ever better health care, despite rising costs. There are two fundamental reasons why this must be so.

The small, but positive, productivity growth rate in the stagnant services. In *A Connecticut Yankee in King Arthur's Court,* Mark Twain devotes an entire chapter to Sir Boss's unsuccessful bid to explain the concept of real wages to his primitive hosts. He argues passionately that the monetary magnitudes of wages are irrelevant; that, regardless of their value as expressed in terms of money, wages are really higher only when it takes fewer hours of labor to earn the wages needed to purchase a given set of goods. Yet, precisely that is true of stagnant services. Their money prices are indeed rising ever higher, their exchange rate against manufactured goods constantly increasing. But in terms of the number of labor hours it takes to acquire them, over the longer run, their cost is decreasing steadily, if slowly. It is immediately obvious that the claim that we cannot afford them is simply a manifestation of what economists call "money illusion."

But how can that be? The answer is that even the most stagnant of services is undergoing some, albeit modest, productivity growth. The cost disease analysis does not claim otherwise; its workings merely require productivity in the stagnant services to grow much more slowly than that of the economy overall. To illustrate the point, let me return to my favorite example. If the hypothetical Mozart string quartet had been scored for a half-hour performance, then its performance in 1990 required two person-hours of labor, just as it did in 1790, when it might have been written. Thus, there is apparently no scope for the slightest increase in labor productivity. Yet that is only an illusion. Assume that the more recent performance was by a Viennese group of musicians, and that it was played in Frankfurt. A 1990 trip from their Austrian home base to the German auditorium surely would normally have taken no more than several hours. But when Mozart made the trip in 1790 it required six days of extreme discomfort. Certainly, technical progress has reduced the number of hours of labor required to provide a unit of the output in question, thus raising the labor productivity of every itinerant performer, even in live performance (and we know that performers are virtually all itinerant).

There is in fact no service whose productivity is untouched by technical progress to some degree. This rise in labor productivity means, by definition, that it requires ever less labor time to produce a unit of such a service. And every resulting reduction in labor time spent in producing the service means that those purchasing the service must expend that much less labor time to acquire the wherewithal needed to purchase it. That is the sense in which even education and medical care have really grown steadily cheaper (albeit at a snail's pace, compared to other outputs), even as they appear to become steadily more unaffordable. However, this, at best, can only make a minor contribution toward solving the politico-budgetary problems that stem from the cost disease. More powerful aid must come from a second source.

Productivity growth in the entire economy means we can afford more of everything. In an economy in which productivity is growing in almost every sector and declining in none, it is a tautology that consumers can have more of every good and service: they simply have to transfer some of the gains from the sector that's becoming much more productive into the sector that's becoming only a little more productive. Impossible? Imagine that the real price of health care continues to grow at its current rate for fifty years, and that overall U.S. productivity rises for that period at its historic rate of around 2 percent. In fifty years, the output of every good and service, including education and health care, can increase to more than 3.5 times its 1990 magnitude: an enormous increase in wealth for everyone. But the catch is: the relative composition of the sectors will be drastically different. Medical outlays, instead of constituting 12 percent of the total, as they did in 1990, must rise to more than 35 percent in 2040! And Bill Clinton thought he had a problem.

An analogy can perhaps make this clearer. Suppose we think of the public's consumption of goods and services as the purchase of a bundle containing many components, just as the purchase of a car includes the acquisition of seats, tire, steering wheel, etc. Imagine that the price of steering wheels is increasing at an impressive rate, but that because of the decline in the costs of the other components, cars (equipped with steering wheels) grow less expensive every year. Would one really conclude that steering wheels are growing unaffordable, even when their price grows to 65 percent of the price of the car?

Yes, this happy conclusion is just a bit simplistic. Making the stagnant services affordable for the poor will still be necessary. Managing a service sector of more than 50 percent of the economy will be a massive headache. So, too, will educating the public to understand the difference between the reality and the illusion in the behavior of costs. It will not be easy to convince the layperson that, even though prices of personal services appear to be rising at a phenomenal rate, in fact the costs of those services (in terms of their labor time equivalent) are really declining, because of increases in their labor productivity. But these are the real problems of our future economy. The share of GNP devoted to health care costs isn't one of them.

Contemporary Health Hazards

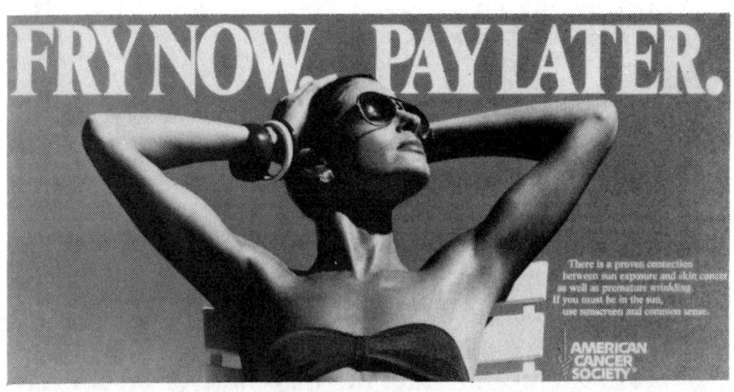

During the past few years, we have been inundated with health warnings about toxic substances in our air, water, and even in the food we eat. Unfortunately, the American public has come to believe that these reports are simply warnings and need not be taken too seriously. Reports of poisonous chemicals polluting our waters, seeping from the earth, and spewing into our skies are indeed overwhelming. Although awareness of the problems has increased, we have yet to make significant strides in our move to clean up our environment. Clearly, the major obstacle to such an effort is the complex economic aspects involved. If we as a people demanded that all offenders stop polluting our environment today, all of us would have to permanently park our cars, risk having our heat turned off, and face losing our jobs. The results would probably be more detrimental to our health than the toxins themselves. Certainly this is not the answer to our environmental problems.

While some improvement has been observed in the areas of air and water pollution, much remains to be done, and new areas of concern continue to surface. Of all the environmental health issues, atmospheric pollution by chlorofluorocarbon compounds (CFCs) and carbon dioxide seems to have generated the most concern worldwide. CFCs are synthetic products that have achieved worldwide acceptance as components of refrigerants, propellants, and solvents. Unfortunately, when these compounds are released into the atmosphere they destroy the ozone layer that shields the earth from ultraviolet (UV) radiation. This protective layer is undergoing a rapid depletion. Consequently, there has been a steady rise in the amount of UV radiation to which we are exposed. Most experts agree that we will witness significant increases in the incidence of skin cancer because of this depletion. To protect ourselves against the damaging effects of this form of radiation, medical authorities have encouraged us to apply liberal amounts of sunscreen to our skin. According to some researchers, adherence to this advice may prove to be deadly. While sunscreens appear to be effective in blocking the shorter ultraviolet (UVB) rays that cause sunburns, they provide little protection against the longer ultraviolet wavelengths (UVA radiation), which constitute 95 percent of the UV radiation and is associated with malignant melanoma, the most deadly form of skin cancer. Opponents of sunscreens argue that they disable our bodies natural alarm system (sunburn response) and expose us to very high doses of the more dangerous UVA radiation. Michael Castleman's article "Beach Bummer" discusses the controversy concerning the use of sunscreens and the prevention of cancer. (See also in unit 9, "Sunscreens: Everything New under the Sun.")

In addition to man-made pollutants, there are numerous naturally occurring substances that pollute the air we breathe. While substances such as pollen, dust, cat dander, and mold spores are not normally classified as environmental toxins, they are capable of triggering physiological reactions in some individuals that range from minor irritations to death. Scientists have termed this class of substances allergens, and while allergens normally contain no specific toxic substances, they affect as many as 50 million people in the United States alone. Allergic reactions to airborne pollen is the most common type of allergy, and the symptoms that accompany this particular allergen include sneezing, wheezing, watery eyes, and headaches. The symptoms just described constitute what is commonly termed allergic rhinitis or "hay fever." This particular allergic condition affects an estimated 22 million Americans. Most allergic reactions produce only mild to moderate discomfort, but for certain individuals allergens can trigger physiological responses that can be deadly. Anaphylactic shock and asthma (a chronic breathing disorder) are deadly forms of allergic reactions, and together they account for more than 6,000 American deaths annually. While the airborne allergens are the most common, foods, medications, and insect bites are also capable of triggering allergic responses. Because most allergic reactions produce only minor discomfort, they may be overlooked as a health hazard. However, they account for one out of every nine visits to the doctor among adults, and for children the rate jumps to one in five. Larry Katzenstein's article "Allergies: Nothing to Sneeze At" examines why allergic reactions occur and discusses the nature and scope of this health problem.

Another example of an exogenous health hazard is the presence of hazardous substances in our food. Despite the numerous safety precautions taken by the food industry, there may be as many as 80 million cases of "food poisoning" annually in the United States. The exact number is difficult to track because most of the cases are

Unit 2

never reported. According to the Centers for Disease Control (CDC), the number of cases of food poisoning attributable to botulism and trichinosis are declining, but food-borne illnesses such as salmonella have increased over 200 percent in the last 25 years. What is most alarming is that another food-borne pathogen named campylobacter may be even more common than salmonella. Recent studies have confirmed the threat that these pathogens pose by finding evidence of their presence in over 65 percent of all raw meat and poultry sold for human consumption in the United States. Because the level of contamination is so widespread, the CDC recommends that consumers view every product of animal origin as if it were contaminated and treat it accordingly. "Uninvited Guests" by Winifred Conkling examines specific types of food poisoning, including symptoms, food sources, and preventative measures.

Over the past 20 years, many Americans have come to believe that we have won the war against infectious bacteria. However, within the last two years there have been numerous reports suggesting that we are currently in the midst of a microbial resurgence of frightening proportions. Clearly, the most frightening of all the microbes that have surfaced is Streptococcus pyogenes, also know as the "flesh-eating bacteria." Given the tendency of the mass media to hype stories of a bizarre nature, one may question the authenticity of this so-called microbial invasion. According to the CDC, we have entered an era in which the spectrum of infectious diseases is growing, and many infectious diseases once thought to be controlled are increasing. Just as frightening as the emergence of new infections is the fact that the antibiotics we use to combat these illnesses are losing their effectiveness. Ironically, many of the antibiotic-resistant bacteria found today probably had their origins in our hospitals where massive amounts of antibiotics are used. "Return of the Germ" by Richard Saltus examines this new wave of infectious illness and discusses why bacterial infections appear to be on the rise. He also presents some useful suggestions on steps that can be taken to guard against these infections.

While AIDS has clearly dominated the press coverage of sexually transmitted diseases (STDs), other STDs such as human papilloma virus (HPV) and genital herpes infect hundreds of thousands of individuals each year. HPV, also known as genital warts, is a viral disease for which there is no vaccination or cure. The symptoms of this disease can range from cauliflower-like warts that appear on the genitals to cancer of the genitals, especially cancer of the cervix. Experts estimate that as many as 750,000 people a year are infected with this disease. "Sleeping with the Enemy" provides a short discussion of the eight most common STDs, including information regarding their incidence, symptomatology, and medical complications.

Another health hazard that warrants inclusion in a unit such as this is rape. Rape is an act of violence against another human being and, as such, should be considered a health hazard. Date rape or acquaintance rape has recently emerged as a major security issue at numerous colleges and universities throughout the United States. At this time, it is difficult to determine whether this form of sexual violence is relatively new, or has been going on for years, undetected, like wife beating or sexual harassment. We do know that date rape is widespread, with the number of reported cases growing rapidly. In 1989 it was estimated that between 13 and 25 percent of all coeds attending American universities were victims of date rape. Statistics also indicated that in most cases the victims knew their assailants. Sexual violence has become so common on college campuses that it frequently surpasses theft as the foremost security issue. "What Every Woman Needs to Know about Personal Safety" discusses the safety measures women can take to reduce their risk of becoming victims of rape or some other violent crime.

While this unit focused on exogenous factors that influence our state of health, it is important to remember that health is the dynamic state representing the degree of harmony or balance that exists between internal and external factors. This concept of balance applies to the environment as well.

Looking Ahead: Challenge Questions

What do you consider to be our greatest environmental health hazard today?

Are you concerned about the damaging effect of UV radiation on your skin? What steps are you taking to prevent such damage?

What steps can one take to reduce the risk of contracting food poisoning?

How has our use of antibiotics contributed to the resurgence of infectious illnesses?

What could the government do to help cut the spread of STDs? What are you personally doing to reduce your risk of contracting them?

What steps can a person take to reduce the likelihood of experiencing an allergic reaction?

What safety measures could a woman take to reduce her chance of being a victim of date rape or some other form of violent crime?

Beach bummer

New evidence suggests that sunscreens don't prevent skin cancer and may even promote some forms of it. The manufacturers know it. Some researchers know it. Why don't consumers?

Michael Castleman

Medical journalist Michael Castleman writes for national magazines and has authored six books, most recently An Aspirin A Day *(Hyperion). Kerry Lauerman of* Mother Jones *contributed additional reporting to this story.*

Anyone who's ever heard a smoke alarm go off knows how horrid its whine can be. Why keep it around? Because a little unpleasantness can prevent injury or death in a fire. But in the last few decades, millions of people who cherish smoke detectors may have disabled one of nature's equally protective, if annoying, alarms. They've rubbed on sunscreen, never thinking that sunburns, like smoke alarms, might prevent a greater harm.

As experts persuaded more and more Americans to use sunscreens, melanoma became an epidemic, with new diagnoses roughly paralleling sunscreen sales.

Ironically, sunscreen devotees have turned off their dermatological smoke detectors in the name of preventive medicine. Sunburn, experts say, is a key risk factor for malignant melanoma, the potentially fatal skin cancer that's become a headline-grabbing epidemic since 1980. Forget what used to be called a "healthy tan." Today, experts insist, we're paying for decades of naïve, post–World War II, beach-blanket sun worship with an unprecedented melanoma rate. But there's hope, they tell us. If you can't avoid the midday sun, pour on the sunscreen.

Unfortunately, the public health authorities who urge routine, liberal use of sunscreen (especially on children) fail to mention that *sunscreens have never been shown to prevent melanoma.* The medical research community knows this. The Food and Drug Administration knows it. And sunscreen makers know it. Yet, as a result of scientific myopia, bureaucratic inertia, and the almighty bottom line, they've essentially told us to use sunscreen and not to worry.

But two San Diego epidemiologists, Cedric and Frank Garland, *are* worried. Best known for their work linking sunshine with the prevention of breast and colon cancer, the Garland brothers (with research associate Edward Gorham) have compiled a body of evidence suggesting that sunscreens dupe the public into believing they're covered by state-of-the-art melanoma protection, when, in fact, they may be highly vulnerable to the disease. Even worse, the Garlands' research suggests that sunscreen use just might *promote* melanoma.

Unfortunately for the public health, the Garlands refuse to discuss their theory for fear of professional ostracism. After they presented their case against sunscreens at a 1990 epidemiological meeting in Los Angeles, both the *New York Times* and the *Washington Post* ran articles explaining their theory. Epidemiologists accused the Garlands of grandstanding for speaking to the press before publishing their analysis in a scientific journal. Stung by this criticism (which could threaten funding of their other work), the brothers have since avoided journalists. But anyone who examines the Garlands' claims might feel, well, burned by sunscreens.

Meanwhile, most dermatologists, epidemiologists, and sunscreen makers continue to suggest that sunscreens prevent melanoma. With a $380 million market at stake, the sunscreen industry in particular has an interest in keeping the Garlands' argument out of the public eye. Perhaps, as the industry claims, sunscreens prevent melanoma; perhaps they promote it. No one knows for certain, but worse, almost no one is trying to find out. So before you rub on another drop of sunscreen, consider the evidence. Because sunscreen makers are watching out for everything except your health.

Malignant melanoma's dark, mole-derived tumors are the fastest-rising cancer under the sun. From 1975 to 1992, the number of melanoma cases reported annually in the U.S. tripled, increasing more than any other cancer. Since the 1950s, melanoma rates have also risen dramatically among fair-skinned Australians, Brits, Canadians, and Scandinavians (it is extremely unusual for dark-skinned people to get skin cancer).

Melanoma now strikes thirty-two thousand Americans each year and kills sixty-eight hundred. But before 1950 it was quite rare. Two other skin cancers, basal and squamous cell skin tumors, were dermatologists' major concern. These slow-spreading cancers usually occur in white men over forty-five who work outdoors or live near the equator. They are by far the nation's most prevalent cancers, with 600,000 new diagnoses each year, but they rarely prove fatal, with successful treatment in 99 percent of cases.

Around the turn of the century, doctors linked risk of basal and squamous cell tumors with lifetime sun exposure—the more sun, the more risk. They also discovered a far rarer—and more fatal—skin cancer, later dubbed malignant melanoma, which they believed had nothing to do with sunlight because it usually appeared in people who spent little time in the sun. Victims of the fatal cancer had only two things in common—fair skin and red or blonde hair. Doctors concluded that the cancer was a consequence of being fair-skinned and light-haired.

But by the late 1960s, numerous studies showed a connection between melanoma and the ultraviolet radiation in sunlight, demonstrating, for example, that whites who live near the equator have higher melanoma rates than those in temperate climes.

The fact that outdoor workers rarely develop melanoma was apparently explained when researchers shifted their attention from sun*light* to sun*burn*. They hypothesized that deeply tanned skin protects against melanoma, even though it increases the risk of basal and squamous cell cancers. Indoor office workers have brief, intense exposures to the sun—the kind that cause sunburn, which in turn could lead to melanoma.

During the 1970s, scientists used the sunburn theory to explain the dramatic rise in the melanoma rate in the second half of this century. After World War II, they argued, record numbers of Americans became white-collar workers, which limited their sun exposure and, as a result, increased their risk of weekend sunburns. In addition, sunbathing became a national pastime, and women's swimsuits became more revealing.

Because melanoma has been associated with teenage sunburns, but the median age for diagnosis is in the forties, researchers concluded that melanoma, like many cancers, takes decades to develop. Estimating a twenty-five- to thirty-year lag time, proponents of the sunburn theory claim that postwar sunbathing resulted in the melanoma epidemic of the 1980s.

There is no animal model for melanoma (as there is for squamous cell skin cancer, which mice can contract), so it is impossible to conduct laboratory experiments to discover exactly what causes the disease. And, although the sunburn theory is an advance over the "fate of the fair-skinned" theory, it fails to explain a few things.

For instance, sunburn was a common medical problem long before people started wearing bikinis. Turn-of-the-century medical texts dealt with it as a fact of life, and folk medicine abounds with remedies. Yet melanoma was extremely rare before 1950.

Many of the social changes sunburn-theory supporters attribute to the 1950s actually occurred about thirty years earlier. Sunbathing first became popular during the 1920s, thanks to fashion designer Coco Chanel, who launched a tanning chic after returning from a yachting vacation with a golden tan. Assuming a lag time of twenty-five to thirty years, the melanoma rate should have risen considerably starting in the mid-1940s. It didn't.

Furthermore, several studies suggest that melanoma actually may have a short lag time. Sunspots, which cause complex

New kid on the (sun)block

When the Garland brothers took aim at sunscreens that protect skin only from UVB rays, many sunscreen makers referred media calls to the Academy of American Dermatology, which issued a rebuttal stating, "No studies have suggested direct relationships between melanoma and ultraviolet A."

Less than three years later, the AAD is recommending UVA protection and it is the major focus of sunscreen marketing efforts. Part of the reason is the FDA's approval of the UVA-screening chemical Parsol 1789 (until recently available only in Herbert Laboratories' Photoplex). Although previous sunscreens had claimed to block UVA, they blocked only about one-third of the UVA spectrum. In fact, in 1990 the FDA warned Schering-Plough, makers of Coppertone, that adopting its own proposed UVA rating system would constitute "false and misleading" labeling.

If the Garlands are right about the dangers of sunscreen, then UVA-blockers might go a long way toward solving the problem. Of course, that's what everyone thought twenty years ago about blocking UVB. . . . So before you rush out to buy Photoplex or any other broad-spectrum sunscreen, remember: scientists still don't know what causes or prevents melanoma. Assertions that UVA blockage protects against melanoma are purely speculative.

Hot tip

"Sun Protection Factor" (SPF) numbers may not be as useful as you think. A sunscreen's protection depends not only on the SPF, but also on the thickness and uniformity of the application and the product's chemical stability. The SPF standard assumes liberal application. A thin coat might provide only half the SPF on the product label.

—M. C.

effects in the upper atmosphere, appear cyclically on the sun's surface about every eleven years. A study of sunspot activity between 1935 and 1975 showed that every sunspot cycle was followed a few years later by a small but significant increase in the melanoma rate.

A Scottish study corroborated the idea of a short lag time by finding a "highly significant" correlation between melanoma diagnoses and severe sunburns occurring just five years earlier. Melanoma diagnoses in fifteen- to twenty-four-year-olds have increased noticeably since 1973. And studies in Sweden, Hawaii, and the continental U.S. have shown consistent seasonal patterns in melanoma diagnoses, another hallmark of biological events with short lag times.

But if melanoma has a lag time of only a few years, then the explosive increases of the 1960s, 1970s, and 1980s can't be blamed on changes in beach attire of the 1920s *or* the 1940s. The factor that accounts for these changes must have appeared in the middle or late 1950s and become gradually more significant as time has progressed.

No one knows what this factor is. But Cedric and Frank Garland are afraid that it may be sunscreen use.

What about the ozone?

The melanoma epidemic became a major news story six years ago when the ozone "hole" (thinning is a more accurate description) opened up over Antarctica. However, what's been happening over the bottom of the world has nothing to do with the melanoma rate in the U.S.

In a 1991 report, the Environmental Protection Agency estimated a 5 percent ozone loss over the U.S. during the last decade. But the amount of UV radiation striking the country actually decreased a bit, according to the National Cancer Institute, because of another UV filter—air pollution. If ozone loss on the order of Antarctica's happens over the U.S., our melanoma rate might well soar in the future. But melanoma epidemiologists agree that, to date, Antarctic ozone loss has played no role in our Melanoma epidemic.

—M.C.

Most sunscreens block about 5 percent of ultraviolet radiation—the UVB rays that cause burning. The other 95 percent of the UV spectrum, UVA, has long been thought to play a minor role in sunburn, so sunscreens block only a small portion of it (see box on preceding page). But studies have shown that UVA may play an important role in skin cancer. UVA radiation penetrates more deeply into the skin than UVB, down to the melanocytes, the cells that turn cancerous in melanoma.

Scientists have yet to identify exactly what corrupts healthy melanocytes, largely because there is no animal model for melanoma. But mice develop *non*melanoma skin cancers under UV light.

The sunscreen-melanoma link might also explain why professionals are at greater risk than clerical workers.

Proponents of the sunburn theory are quick to point to a Danish study in which sunscreen was shown to delay (but not completely prevent) the development of squamous cell tumors in mice exposed to artificial sunlight. The higher the sunscreen's sun protection factor, the longer it took the mice to develop tumors. To date, this is the closest scientists have come to establishing the preventive value of sunscreens.

However, another study at the same lab should give sunscreen advocates pause. In this experiment, mice exposed to artificial sunlight developed a small number of squamous cell tumors. But ones exposed to artificial sunlight followed by additional UVA developed more than twice as many tumors.

Not only does this study suggest that UVA may play a role in skin cancer, it also points to the particular danger of sunlight followed by UVA alone—a cycle similar to that which occurs when people use sunscreen. They hit the beach, playground, or ballfield and remove some clothing, exposing themselves to full-spectrum sunlight. Then they apply sunscreen, blocking UVB, but continuing their exposure to UVA. As the sunscreen wears off, they're again exposed to full sun. After reapplying sunscreen, they get additional UVA—and possibly cancer.

Of course, mice are not human beings, and squamous cell cancers are not melanoma, so either study (or both) may mean nothing. But melanoma experts trumpet the implications of the first study, that sunscreens help prevent skin cancer, while ignoring those of the second, that sunscreen use fosters a cancer-promoting pattern of UV exposure.

The Garlands have more disturbing news about sunscreen: by impairing the body's production of vitamin D, it may also remove a defense against cancer. According to studies, vitamin D has a hormone-like effect that interferes with the growth of several tumors, including those associated with melanoma and colon and breast cancers. Although we get small amounts of the vitamin from milk and cold-water fish, most of our bodies' supply is produced when skin is exposed to UVB. By blocking UVB, sunscreens interfere with vitamin D synthesis. A recent study shows that habitual sunscreen users have unusually low vitamin D levels—sometimes low enough that researchers call them "deficient."

A sunscreen-melanoma link might also illuminate a peculiar fact unexplained by the sunburn theory: melanoma risk rises with income. Although both professionals and clerical workers work indoors, the former have a significantly higher melanoma rate. Because health consciousness is generally an upper-income phenomenon, sunscreens presumably appeal to the more affluent.

Even if sunscreen is one day shown to protect against melanoma, the Garlands worry that it may give users a dangerously false sense of security. No one knows how large doses of

UVA might affect the body. Historically, whites would have been dangerously sunburned long before they received the levels of UVA radiation that they may now get in one sunscreen-wearing day at the beach. Whatever UVA's role in causing melanoma, the Garlands strongly recommend that you not make yourself a guinea pig.

Remember those old Coppertone ads with the puppy pulling down the little girl's bathing suit? Suntan lotions, introduced in the mid-1950s for cosmetic purposes, were the first commercial use of sunscreens. As sales increased throughout the 1950s and 1960s, so did the melanoma rate.

During the 1970s and 1980s, suntan lotions were repositioned as sunscreens, which, experts said, prevented skin cancer by preventing sunburn. Sales in 1991 were $380 million, more than twice as much as a decade earlier. But as experts persuaded more and more Americans to use sunscreens, melanoma became an epidemic, with new diagnoses roughly paralleling sunscreen sales.

This epidemic has been a godsend for sunscreen makers. According to the journal *Drug and Cosmetic Industry,* "Every indicator that skin cancer is on the rise, every utterance by a dermatologist . . . seems to reinforce the need for consumers to use more of these products. The missionary work required to double the market [by 1995] has already been done, and not just by the industry."

Sunscreen makers frankly admit that their products have never been shown to prevent human skin cancers. "The studies show that sunscreens prevent squamous cell cancers in animals," says Patricia Agin, sunscreen product manager for Schering-Plough, whose brands, including Coppertone, account for one-third of the market. "I think they do the same in humans. But . . . we don't know for certain. Because there's no animal model for [melanoma], we don't know if sunscreens prevent it. I see no reason to think that they wouldn't, but we have no proof that they do."

Jack Surrette, marketing vice-president of Tanning Research Laboratories (makers of Hawaiian Tropic sunscreens), goes further. "To some extent, when you protect only for UVB, it would seem to run a risk for potential skin cancer," he says. "UVA is a more damaging ray. We may be hurting ourselves by protecting ourselves too well on the UVB side."

Unfortunately, sunscreen labels do not reflect Agin or Surrette's understanding of the research. They echo the claims of dermatologists and cancer-education organizations: "Regular use may prevent skin cancer." Of course, when a label says "skin cancer," sunscreen makers insist that it means nonfatal squamous cell skin cancer. But if the label doesn't distinguish between melanoma and other skin cancers, then how can consumers be expected to?

Further confusing consumers, most sunscreens carry a seal of approval from the nonprofit Skin Cancer Foundation, which claims to alert people to safe products. More than 130 different suncare products have earned the right to display this seal—for a price. In addition to submitting their products for testing and review, corporations also dole out ten thousand dollars to use

What you can do

To prevent malignant melanoma, start by using common sense instead of just sunscreens. First, assess your risk. Risk factors include: fair skin; blonde, red, or light brown hair; blue or green eyes; a family history of melanoma; an indoor occupation; outdoor leisure activities; numerous moles; freckling on the upper back; a tendency to sunburn easily and tan poorly; and actinic keratoses, rough, red, sun-induced bumps which sometimes develop on fair skin. The more risk factors you have, the more concerned you need to be. Anyone, even a black person, can develop melanoma, but for those without risk factors the danger is slight.

Dermatologists, the Skin Cancer Foundation, and the American Cancer Society all agree that the best way to prevent harm from sunlight—burning, wrinkling, and all forms of skin cancer—is to avoid direct sun between 10 a.m. and 3 p.m. Just take reasonable precautions: Don't sunbathe. If you love the beach, invest in an umbrella. Don't patronize tanning salons. In summer, adjust your schedule to engage in outdoor activities in the early morning or late afternoon. When out on summer days, wear a hat, sunglasses, and lightweight, long-limbed clothing. In winter, particularly if skiing, cover up with clothing.

There's no such thing as a "healthy tan," so don't go looking for one. Even if you take all the precautions listed above, you'll still acquire some color in the summer without significantly raising your melanoma risk.

How to spot it

Few people understand how life-saving early melanoma detection can be. Seventy percent of melanoma tumors develop from pre-existing moles. So examine your moles regularly—or have someone else do it—and know the ABCD's of melanoma detection:

- Asymmetry. Most normal moles are round and symmetrical. Melanomas are oddly shaped and asymmetrical.
- Border. Most normal moles have smooth edges. Melanomas often have notched or scalloped edges.
- Color. Most normal moles are a single shade of brown. Melanomas are black, blue, pink, and multicolored.
- Diameter. Most normal moles are less than one-quarter inch in diameter. Early melanomas grow outward and become larger.

Even before melanoma moles undergo visual changes, they often itch. If one of your moles starts to itch, or if you become nervous about a mole for any reason, ask you doctor for a referral to a dermatologist. If you have significant melanoma risk factors, see a dermatologist annually.

—M. C.

the seal. John Epstein, who sits on the Skin Cancer Foundation's four-member seal review committee, says he can't recall anyone ever being denied the seal, but companies that file inadequate paperwork must resubmit their requests. (A foundation spokesperson claimed that some companies have withdrawn rather than resubmit their applications.)

The foundation, which boasts celebrity backers such as Tom Selleck, Lauren Bacall, Dick Cavett, Paul Newman, and Joanne Woodward, earns about one-fourth of its $1.7 million budget from corporate donations. Recently the foundation sent sixty thousand elementary schools posters that urge students: "Always use sunscreen when you go outdoors, no matter the season or the color of your skin."

The Skin Cancer Foundation isn't the only case of corporate funding blurring the boundary between public health and the bottom line. The Skin Phototrauma Foundation (acronym: SPF) was founded by Ortho Pharmaceuticals (whose parent company, Johnson & Johnson, makes Sundown sunscreens), Procter & Gamble (Bain de Soleil), and Mary Kay Cosmetics (Sun Essentials). Even the Academy of American Dermatology, a medical association that counts 98 percent of dermatologists in the United States and Canada among its members, uses corporate donations to fund its public-education efforts.

So who should consumers turn to for an untainted view of sunscreens? The likely choice would be the Food and Drug Administration. Sometime this year, the FDA plans to release new labeling regulations for the first time since 1978. One proposal would require all sunscreen labels to carry "sun alerts," warning consumers that preventing sunburn may not protect them against wrinkling and skin cancer. But even after new regulations are released, the public and sunscreen makers will have eighteen months to comment before the FDA issues its final regulations, probably in 1995.

When the Garland brothers first presented their case against sunscreens at the 1990 meeting, a few epidemiologists expressed guarded interest. Dr. Leonard Kurland of the Mayo Clinic called their analysis "intriguing and worth exploring further." But most supporters of the sunburn theory considered the brothers' argument ludicrous.

The Garlands openly admit that the case against sunscreens is not airtight. The controversial assertion that melanoma has a brief lag time needs corroboration. The study showing that UVA promotes squamous cell tumors in sun-exposed mice may not be applicable to human beings. And a recent study showed no correlation between vitamin D levels and melanoma risk.

But the best theory is the one that answers the most questions, and the sunburn/long-lag-time theory looks shaky. It ignores the studies showing a brief lag time. It doesn't address why sunburn rarely caused melanoma before the 1950s. It sheds no light on why melanoma risk is linked to income. And it fails to explain why increases in the melanoma rate have so closely paralleled the rise in sunscreen use.

Despite these shortcomings, the sunburn theory continues to be the dominant scientific theory, and it often takes decades to overturn a dominant theory. It took almost twenty years for researchers to accept a connection between sunburn and melanoma, and no one was out there saying, "Get burned. It's good for you." Today leading scientists *are* saying, "Use sunscreens. They're good for you." If sunscreens provide a false sense of security, or worse, promote melanoma, convincing the scientific establishment could take well into the next century.

Uninvited Guests

You could be sharing your next meal with a dangerous microbe

Winifred Conkling

Winifred Conkling is a health writer in Vienna, Va.

You can't see them, but they're everywhere: on the chicken you just brought home from the market, the leftover meat loaf in your refrigerator and the hamburger patty you're about to broil. Disease-causing microorganisms can invade your food, and you won't even know it because they can't be detected by sight, smell or taste. But if you ever eat a microbe that makes you sick, you'll never forget the consequences.

Microbial contamination is considered by health experts to be the greatest safety threat to today's food supply. The U.S. Department of Agriculture estimates that up to 40% of the poultry sold in this country is infected with dangerous *salmonella* bacteria. And outbreaks of illness from a deadly strain of *Escherichia Coli* (E. coli) bacteria in ground beef are creating a national health crisis. But while the risk is real—approximately 9,000 Americans die annually of food-borne illness and an estimated 80 million others fall ill—you don't have to stop eating.

"Your risk of choking to death on food is about 20 times greater than your risk of dying from food-borne illness," says Dr. Dean Cliver, a food microbiologist at the University of Wisconsin at Madison. Most food-borne illness can, in fact, be avoided by proper food handling and common sense.

There are many toxic microbes in the environment (see "Common Culprits"). Animals are common carriers, but so are kitchen knives, cutting boards and human hands. Most of these microbes grow in warm temperatures, which is why a bacterium such as *Staphylococcus aureus* thrives when potato salad sits out for hours. But others, such as E. coli and *Listeria monocytogenes,* can survive and grow even in the refrigerator. And while most bacteria are destroyed by freezing, E. coli and Listeria are among those that survive.

Microbes make you sick by attacking your digestive tract or producing toxins that damage your body. Small numbers of microbes may pass through the digestive tract unnoticed. Problems typically arise when the organisms multiply to levels high enough to cause illness. Generally, the more microbes you ingest, the more likely you are to become sick.

The effects of food-borne illness range from minor gastrointestinal distress to severe diarrhea causing dehydration, neurological damage, kidney failure and death. Symptoms may develop immediately, or they may not show up for days or even weeks. For most healthy adults, the problems are neither long-lasting nor life-threatening. But for infants, small children, the elderly, pregnant women and people with weakened immune systems, food-borne illness can be severe or even fatal.

Fortunately, practicing germ warfare at home is relatively easy. Most often, humans become sick when food is improperly cooked or stored or when it's contaminated by unwashed utensils, countertops or hands. Here's how to win the war against toxic microbes:

- Shop with care. Don't buy food in dented or bulging cans.
- Look for fresh seafood and keep up with local health department reports about infected waters.
- Don't buy fish piled high on a bed of ice; those at the top may not be cold enough to prevent microbial growth. Cooked fish lying on the same bed of

From *American Health,* October 1994, pp. 50, 52.

common culprits

		[Source]	[Symptoms]	[Onset]	[Prevention]
BACTERIAL	CAMPYLOBACTER JEJUNI	Bacteria on poultry, cattle and sheep that can contaminate the meat or milk of these animals.	Diarrhea, abdominal cramping, fever and/or bloody stools.	Two to five days.	Cook foods thoroughly; drink pasteurized milk.
	CLOSTRIDIUM BOTULINUM	(causes botulism) Improperly canned foods, luncheon meats, ham, sausage, lobster and smoked or salted fish.	Double vision, weakness, dry throat, inability to swallow and/or paralysis.	Four to 36 hours.	Cook foods thoroughly; avoid dented or bulging cans.
	CLOSTRIDIUM PERFRINGENS	Food left at room temperature.	Abdominal cramps, diarrhea, nausea and/or vomiting.	Eight to 12 hours.	Heat foods thoroughly; refrigerate leftovers at once.
	ESCHERICHIA COLI (E. coli)	Water, raw or undercooked meat and cross-contaminated foods.	Watery or bloody diarrhea, abdominal cramps or vomiting.	10 to 72 hours.	Cook foods thoroughly; wash hands well.
	LISTERIA MONOCYTOGENES	Soft cheese, raw milk, meat, ice cream, imported seafood, partially cooked frozen crab, shrimp and imitation shellfish.	Fever, headache, nausea and/or vomiting.	Two to three days.	Cook foods thoroughly; drink pasteurized milk.
	SALMONELLA	Raw or undercooked meat, poultry or eggs and unpasteurized milk.	Nausea, abdominal cramps, diarrhea, fever and/or headache.	Five hours to four days.	Cook foods thoroughly; drink pasteurized milk.
	SHIGELLA	Potato, chicken and tuna salads and raw foods such as lettuce and oysters.	Diarrhea, fever, nausea and/or cramps.	12 to 96 hours.	Cook foods thoroughly; wash hands well.
	STAPHYLOCOCCUS AUREUS	Food left too long at room temperature, including meat, poultry or egg products, tuna, potato or macaroni salad, and cream-filled pastries. Unlike other bacteria, staphylococci grow well in foods that are high in sugar or salt; any food can be contaminated by infected food handlers.	Vomiting, nausea, diarrhea, abdominal pain and/or cramps.	30 minutes to eight hours.	Cook foods thoroughly; refrigerate leftovers immediately; wash your hands before and after handling food.
	VIBRIO VULNIFICUS	Oysters, clams, mussels and other "filter-feeding" organisms, which absorb anything in seawater, including bacteria, viruses and chemicals.	Chills and/or fever; can be fatal.	Immediate.	Buy fresh fish and seafood, and cook thoroughly.
NONBACTERIAL	CIGUATERA TOXINS	Reef fish such as grouper, surgeonfish, barracuda or snapper.	Nausea, vomiting, diarrhea, numbness and tingling in the face.	One to six hours.	Pay attention to media reports about infected fishing areas.
	HEPATITIS A VIRUS	Oysters, clams, mussels or scallops that come from waters polluted with untreated sewage, and improper food handling with unwashed hands.	Weakness, appetite loss, nausea, vomiting and fever; jaundice may develop.	15 to 50 days.	Buy seafood from reputable markets; wash hands well.
	SCOMBROTOXIN	Tuna, mackerel, mahimahi or bluefish; the illness is caused by a histamine produced when bacteria multiply in fish left unrefrigerated.	Nausea, vomiting, diarrhea, asthma, cramps, flushing and/or burning in the mouth.	Within an hour.	Refrigerate fish immediately when purchased or caught; the toxin cannot be destroyed by cooking.
	TRICHINELLA SPIRALIS	(causes trichinosis) A parasite found in raw or undercooked pork or carnivorous animals.	Muscle pain, swollen eyelids and/or fever; can be fatal.	Eight to 15 days.	Cook meat thoroughly.

ice as raw fish could be contaminated.

- Add frozen foods, meat, poultry and seafood to your shopping cart right before you check out. Slip these products into separate plastic bags so that drippings won't contaminate other foods.
- When you get home, refrigerate or freeze perishables right away.
- Thaw food in the refrigerator or, if you need it right away, in the microwave oven, not at room temperature.
- Thoroughly wash cutting boards, kitchen counters and utensils that come in contact with raw meat, poultry and eggs with hot, soapy water before using them with any other food. Switch to a clean sponge or dishcloth after you work with raw meat or poultry. Wash your hands with soap and water for at least 20 seconds before preparing food, before working with a new food, after you finish food preparation, before you serve food, and, of course, after you use the bathroom.
- Wash fruits and vegetables before cutting, even if you plan to peel them.
- If a recipe for an uncooked dish calls for raw eggs, use pasteurized eggs, which are sold as a refrigerated or frozen liquid egg mixture. Use powdered egg-white products for meringue icings. Discard cracked eggs.
- Cook animal foods thoroughly. The internal temperature of a beef, pork or lamb roast should be at least 160°; poultry, 165°. Cook ground meat until it's no longer pink in the middle. Fish is done when the thickest part is opaque. Simmer shrimp three to five minutes, or until the shells turn red.
- Keep hot foods hot and cold foods cold until ready to serve. Store leftovers promptly. Discard any cooked foods that have been sitting at room temperature for two hours or longer.

Allergies

Nothing to sneeze at

A growing arsenal of sprays and tablets can help make your allergy season bearable

Larry Katzenstein

Larry Katzenstein is a Senior Editor at AMERICAN HEALTH.

Bill Clinton's fall campaign was rigorous, but spring and summer could prove even tougher. That's when some of the President's most formidable adversaries breeze into the nation's capital: weed pollen, grass pollen and mold spores. (President Clinton is moderately allergic to cat dander as well, but Socks, the first feline, seems in no danger of a Presidential veto.)

Allergies afflict not only presidents—former President Reagan has them too—but also more than 50 million of their constituents, who are tormented by the same garden-variety allergens that affect President Clinton, plus numerous others, including copper coins, nickel-coated earrings, mangoes, insect stings, heat, cold and even sperm. Reactions range from the merely annoying to the life-threatening.

The tendency to develop allergies is clearly inherited: If one of your parents has allergies, you have a one-in-three chance of developing them too (although not necessarily the same ones); with two allergic parents, it's almost a guarantee. Allergies usually show up by the time you're 30, although even people well into their 80s can become first-time sufferers. On the other hand, people tend to outgrow their allergic symptoms as they get older.

All allergies result from the same basic cause: an immune system unable to distinguish between the benign and the harmful. The immune system's crucial task is to produce antibodies that protect the body from disease-causing bacteria and viruses. But in allergic people the system also makes antibodies against seemingly innocuous substances, such as pollen grains.

The antibodies responsible for allergies belong to a class known as immunoglobulin E (IgE). Everyone makes some IgE, but allergic people make about 10 times as much as people unaffected by allergies.

The first encounter with an allergen—the name for a substance that trig-

Sniffler in Chief

HE HAD *a history of nasal congestion, swelling of his eyes and difficulty breathing through his nose. He gave a history of blowing his nose frequently, and the congestion was so severe during the spring he had difficulty running. ..."*

If proof were ever needed that commanders in chief are all too mortal (never mind fallible), this description of President Clinton's hay fever should suffice. It was written by his allergist, Dr. Kelsy Caplinger of Little Rock, Ark., and published earlier this year in *Physician's Weekly*.

At a consultation on August 27, 1991, with then-Governor Clinton Caplinger carried out skin tests and then started him on allergy shots using extracts of the inhalant allergens to which Clinton had reacted: mold spores, cat dander, weed pollen, grass pollen and house dust. To provide more immediate relief for his patient, Caplinger chose liberally from modern medicine's armamentarium and prescribed:

- ▶Hismanal, a nonsedating antihistamine tablet;
- ▶Deconsal II, a sustained-release decongestant tablet;
- ▶Vancenase AQ, a steroid nasal pump spray.

In addition, Caplinger told AMERICAN HEALTH, he gave his patient detailed written instructions for limiting his exposure to the allergens to which he's sensitive. "Avoidance is by far the best treatment for any allergy problem," he says—and his patient has complied: "I know for a fact that the President now uses dust- and allergy-proof mattress and pillow covers at the White House."

And as for Socks? Allergist Caplinger answered the question diplomatically: "Obviously, anyone allergic to cats shouldn't be around cats."

From *American Health,* May 1993, pp. 44-49.

Of Mites And Men

Do motes dance in the shaft of sunlight streaming through your bedroom window? If so, they could be causing your year-round hay fever or your child's asthma.

House dust is now recognized as a major cause of allergic disease. Inhaling it can cause symptoms ranging from mild irritation to incapacitating airway constriction. From 40% to 80% of all asthmatics, for example, react to one or more of its unsavory ingredients.

House dust components include human and animal dander, mold, lint and—most of important of all—dead dust mites: their powdery remains and especially their airborne feces, which are the main provokers of dust-mite allergy. The microscopic mites thrive in the summer, feasting primarily on human dander, and die in the winter.

"Dust mites are porbably the most important allergen in the world," says Dr. Michael Kaliner, head of the allergy disease section of the National Institute of Allergy and Infectious Diseases. "All temperate regions are afflicted with the pests, which live in carpeting, mattresses, pillows and upholstery." (Arid areas are spared, since mites can't survive when the relative humidity is below 50%).

"Most people can't control the dust conditions under which they work," says Kaliner, "but they can do something about the bedroom, where they spend six to eight hours a night and where dust mites most often reside." To this end, he offers the following suggestions for maintaining a dust-free bedroom:

►Keep carpets out of the bedroom. They trap dust—particularly shag rugs, the worst type for a dust-sensitive person.

►Buy products that kill dust mites, known as acaricides, which are now available in drugstores and can help control mites in carpets as well as in mattresses and sofas.

►Encase the bed's box springs, mattress and pillows in dust-proof zippered covers. (You can buy dust-proof fabric covers, which are more comfortable than the plastic variety.)

►Use window shades instead of Venetian blinds, which are dust traps. Other dust magnets include down-filled or fuzzy wool blankets or comforters, feather pillows (use Dacron), closets full of clothing, and dogs and cats. Keep all animals with fur or feathers out of the bedroom.

► Use only washable materials on the bed, and wash bedding weekly in hot water (above 130°). Warm or cold water won't kill mites. Also wash curtains weekly in hot water.

► Keep toys that gather dust—particularly stuffed ones—out of any bedroom that belongs to a dust-sensitive child.

► Clean the room daily, wiping down surfaces with a damp cloth or oil mop. Do a thorough cleaning once a week. Dust-sensitive people should avoid vacuuming, which may churn up more dust than it removes.

► Try to eradicate cockroaches, which are also important in causing allergies and asthma, particularly among urban children, who are often exposed to them.

► Consider purchasing a high-efficiency particulate arresting (HEPA) filtering unit, a device that can help reduce airborne allergens.

gers an allergic response—may prompt the body to begin churning out IgE against it. These antibodies attach to special cells known as mast cells, millions of which line the respiratory and digestive tract; millions more are found in the skin. The mast cells with their antibody coatings resemble mines bristling with detonators, ready to ambush the allergen if it reappears. And they can wait a long time.

Most antibodies last in the body only about three weeks, but IgE's can persist for months or years—and so can the mast cells they sit upon. "That's why someone who had an allergic reaction to penicillin as a child could still be allergic to the drug as an adult," explains Dr. Michael Kaliner, head of the allergic diseases section at the National Institute of Allergy and Infectious Diseases in Bethesda, Md. "The IgE antibody he made as a six-year-old could still be present at age 40, sitting on mast cells and conveying incredibly long-lived sensitivity to the allergen."

Generally, however, it takes several exposures to an allergen—two to five seasons in the case of tree or ragweed pollen, for example—before a person makes enough IgE to produce allergic symptoms. Then, when the allergen comes along, its encounter with IgE will trigger mast cells to release powerful chemicals such as histamine, which engage the "enemy" allergen but also inflame and damage surrounding tissue.

A person's symptoms depend on where in the body these chemicals are released. Allergies to foods or drugs can manifest themselves in hives (itchy skin welts) or intestinal upsets, including vomiting and diarrhea. Inflammation of tissue lining the air passages results in the wheezing, coughing and labored breathing of asthma.

And then there's the champion allergic malady, hay fever, which inflames the lining of the nose, sinuses and eyelids, producing watery, puffy or itchy eyes, sneezing fits and a runny, stopped-up or itchy nose. The culprits in hay fever are microscopic airborne allergens. They affect 35 million Americans, making hay fever the most common of all chronic diseases.

Hay fever is singularly misnamed, since it isn't caused by hay and doesn't involve fever. The more accurate term is allergic rhinitis, meaning nasal inflammation due to allergy. For most sufferers, hay fever signifies seasonal torment caused by pollen. But thanks largely to indoor contaminants, hay fever can affect people year-round as well.

Seasonal hay fever victims are usually afflicted in the fall or spring, or both, when the air is awash in pollen: grass and tree pollens in the spring and ragweed in late summer or early fall. Summer allergies can be caused by mold spores spawned by humidity, and winter allergies from dust in tightly shut houses.

In some people, dust and mold can also cause year-round hay fever, a problem that can be brought on by pets as well—particularly cats, whose skin and saliva are notorious for provoking misery. (President Clinton's puffy eyes, for example, probably are as much due to

Socks as to his propensity for burning the midnight oil.)

The best way to treat any allergy is to avoid the allergens that cause it. Seasonal hay fever sufferers know that avoiding pollen is easier said than done, but staying inside for part of the day and turning on the air conditioner can help: Pollen counts are highest in the early morning, and air conditioning filters out more than 99% of pollen in the air.

But for some allergic people—particularly those with year-round hay fever and asthma—staying inside just makes things worse. Microscopic menaces in household air play key roles in perpetuating symptoms, and eliminating them can markedly improve health.

If avoidance isn't feasible or doesn't work, the next choice should be medication to relieve symptoms. Recently introduced drugs have revolutionized hay fever treatment, but many people don't know about them. The following is a brief summary of available medications and what they can do for you.

▶**ANTIHISTAMINES** are the most frequently used drugs in hay fever treatment. As their name implies, antihistamines counteract histamines, the chemicals responsible for several hay fever symptoms, including runny nose, sneezing, and itching eyes and throat.

First-generation antihistamines include several types of nonprescription tablets such as brompheniramine (available in Dimetane and Nasahist B), chlorpheniramine (Chlor-Trimeton) and diphenhydramine (Benadryl and Benylin). Many of these products are also sold in generic form. All begin providing relief within 15 to 30 minutes, but they have a serious drawback: They often cause drowsiness. Several antihistamine ingredients, in fact, are also sold as sedatives.

Two newer, prescription-only antihistamines—terfenadine (Seldane) and astemizole (Hismanal)—don't cause that problem. These nonsedating antihistamines are as effective as their older brethren but are also much more expensive. They're not identical: Although Seldane starts working faster than Hismanal (within one or two hours vs. up to four hours), a dose of Seldane doesn't last as long (about 12 hours vs. 24 hours or longer). The recently introduced Seldane-D adds a dollop of decongestant. You can economize on antihistamines by taking a nonsedating antihistamine during the day and one of the sedating varieties before bed. A word of caution: Last year the Food and Drug Administration warned that Seldane, Seldane-D and Hismanal can cause abnormal heart rhythms when taken in excessive doses or when used with either ketoconazole (an antifungal drug) or the antibiotic erythromycin.

▶**DECONGESTANTS** relieve another symptom: nasal congestion, so common in hay fever and often not helped by antihistamines. They come in tablets, sprays and drops.

The decongestant sprays and drops typically contain either xylometazoline (Neo-Synephrine II long-acting nasal spray) or oxymetazoline (Afrin, Allerest 12-Hour, Dristan long-lasting nasal sprays and many others). They start acting immediately but must be used sparingly; if taken for more than three or four days in a row, the nasal decongestants often cause rebound congestion worse than the original problem.

Decongestant tablets don't work as rapidly as sprays but can be used for a longer time—although some people find their effectiveness diminishes after a couple of weeks. The tablets typically contain either pseudoephedrine (Sudafed and generic versions) or phenylpropanolamine (Propagest), which are equally potent. Oral decongestants can cause side effects including nervousness, restlessness and insomnia.

Drugstore shelves are swamped with cold and allergy tablets that combine a decongestant and an antihistamine: Chlor-Trimeton Decongestant, Contac 12-Hour, Dimetapp, Drixoral, Sudafed Plus, Tavist-D, Triaminic-12 and many others. If you really need both an antihistamine and a decongestant, these two-in-one products make sense. And the decongestant's "hyper" side effect may counteract the antihistamine's tendency to put you to sleep.

▶**STEROID NASAL SPRAYS,** introduced several years ago and available only by prescription, are the most effective of all hay fever drugs. Indeed, a recent article in *The New England Journal of Medicine* concluded that the drugs offer "excellent symptomatic relief" to "more than 90%" of hay fever patients. Steroid sprays work by reducing inflammation in the nasal passages. They complement antihistamines by relieving the nasal congestion that so often occurs in hay fever. Steroid sprays include preparations containing the steroids beclomethasone (Beclovent, Beconase, Vancenase AQ and Vanceril), flunisolide (AeroBid and Nasalide) and triamcinolone (Nasacort).

These steroids should not be confused with the hazardous anabolic steroids used by some athletes to gain strength: The chemicals are completely different. In addition, very little of the steroid in these sprays is absorbed into the body, making them much safer for regular use than oral steroid preparations, which can delay growth in children and cause bone thinning and other serious side effects when used for long periods.

The major drawback to steroid sprays is the long wait—about a week or more—before they become fully effective. (So it's best to start using them a few days before symptoms are expected—before the fall ragweed season, for example.) They're also expensive, and they cause sneezing, nasal irritation or burning in about 10% of users.

▶**CROMOLYN SODIUM** is another type of anti-inflammatory drug used in treating respiratory problems. It comes in several forms including an inhaler (Intal) and a nasal solution (Nasalcrom). Cromolyn sodium is somewhat less potent than steroid sprays, but its lack of side effects makes it particularly appropriate for children.

Most hay fever sufferers should obtain considerable relief from the drugs now available. Unlike allergy shots, they work against symptoms caused by a wide variety of allergens. In some cases a combination may be needed: an antihistamine for a runny nose and a steroid spray for congestion, for example.

Although today's drugs excel at handling symptoms, allergy shots are the only known "cure" for allergies. Patients receive regular injections of extracts of the allergens that irk them. "The shots desensitize a person to these allergens by reducing his production of IgE antibodies and increasing levels of another class of antibodies, the IgG's, which actually protect people from allergic disease," Kaliner says.

Shots are especially useful for people strongly allergic to stings from bees and other insects. They're also suited for people who, like President Clinton, have year-round allergy symptoms: "We generally use shots when people have problems for two seasons of the year or longer," Kaliner says. "Those with single-season allergies are usually treated with medication, but if they're really bothered in a major way, we'll

Asthma and The Allergy Connection

ASTHMA, A DISEASE marked by shortness of breath and wheezing, is affecting more Americans, especially younger ones. Some 3.7 million children and adolescents now have asthma, up sharply from 2.4 million in 1980. Possible reasons for the increase include tighter, better insulated homes (which trap allergens and other pollutants) and respiratory infections linked to day care. About 15 million Americans have asthma, and more than 4,000 die from it each year.

Asthma affects the tubes that bring air to the lungs, known as bronchi, which become narrowed in several ways: The muscles surrounding them constrict; their lining becomes inflamed and swollen; and excess mucus threatens to clog whatever space is left.

While asthma and allergy are distinct conditions, they do overlap, especially among asthmatics 15 and younger. Ninety percent of asthmatic children have allergies, and evidence suggests that their allergies are often the cause of their asthma. A recent study, for example, found that children exposed to high levels of airborne dust mites as infants were at increased risk of developing asthma; another study found that childhood exposure to cat dander had the same effect.

But while allergies seem responsible for many cases of asthma, not all asthmatics have them. Other causes include respiratory infections, chemicals in the workplace and childhood exposure to cigarette smoke.

The big news in asthma is the change in the way it's treated—or should be treated. Until recently, treatment emphasized bronchodilators—drugs that widen the airways by relaxing their surrounding muscles. But researchers have discovered that asthma is primarily a disease of airway *inflammation*, which persists even when the asthmatic person seems fine. Inflamed bronchial tissue is hyperreactive to things that can trigger asthma attacks, including pollen and other airborne allergens, exercise, aspirin, sulfites and pollutants such as cigarette smoke.

In 1991 recognition of asthma as an inflammatory disease led the National Institutes of Health to call for greater use of anti-inflammatory drugs to treat it. For most asthmatics, that means regular use of inhaled steroids or inhaled cromolyn sodium to control airway inflammation (see main story).

use shots to lower their need for drugs."

Shots reduce symptoms in about 85% of people who receive them for hay fever caused by grass, ragweed, trees and dust mites. And people whose asthma is provoked by such allergies can also benefit from shots. On the negative side, shots are expensive, occasionally cause allergic reactions themselves, and require frequent office visits. What's more, it usually takes a year or more before a patient experiences maximum symptom relief.

Contact the following organizations for further information on allergies:

▸**The National Jewish Center for Immunology and Respiratory Medicine, 800-222-LUNG.** Nurses will answer questions Monday through Friday, 8 a.m. to 5 p.m. Mountain Time.

▸**The Allergy and Asthma Network/Mothers of Asthmatics, 800-878-4403.** Staff members will answer general questions Monday through Friday, 9 a.m. to 5 p.m. Eastern Time. Or send a business-sized SASE with 52¢ postage **(3554 Chain Bridge Rd., Suite 200, Fairfax, VA 22030; Attention: AMERICAN HEALTH)** to receive a description of membership benefits ($25 a year), a sample newsletter and a flyer on allergies.

▸**American Academy of Allergy and Immunology, 800-822-ASMA.** Call at any time for a list of allergists in your area and basic information.

▸**University of California at Davis's Pet Loss Support Hotline; 916-752-4200.** If allergies force you to give up your pet, you can call this center Monday through Friday, 6:30 p.m. to 9:30 p.m. Pacific Time.

▸**Allergy Control Products, 800-422-DUST.** Call Monday through Friday, 8:30 a.m. to 8 p.m. Eastern Time, and Saturday, 9:30 a.m. to 5 p.m. for information and a free catalog of dust-proof covers, acaricides and other allergy products.

Return of THE GERM

Antibiotics were supposed to wipe out infectious bacteria. What went wrong?

Richard Saltus

Richard Saltus is a science writer at The Boston Globe.

FLESH-EATING BUG KILLED MY MOTHER IN 20 MINUTES . . . KILLER BUG ATE MY FACE . . . I WATCHED KILLER BUG EAT MY BODY. . . .

Last June a cluster of 11 deaths in England triggered sensational tabloid headlines there that terrified large segments of the public. The publicity soon spawned news of similar cases—and similar headlines—in many other countries. (FLESH-EATING VIRUS INVADES THE U.S., proclaimed the *Weekly World News.*)

What prompted all this fuss was actually not a virus at all but a type of bacteria, *Streptococcus pyogenes* (see "Fleshing Out the Flesh-Eating Bug"). It's just the latest example of an alarming phenomenon: lethal infections emerging seemingly from out of nowhere.

Experts date this microbial resurgence to the late 1970s and early '80s, with the appearance of Lyme disease, Legionnaires' disease, toxic shock syndrome and—most notorious of all, of course—AIDS. Now the pace seems to be quickening, judging by developments over just the past two years:

•**1992.** Tuberculosis, a disease all but eliminated in the U.S., becomes a public health crisis when bacterial strains that can resist drugs used to treat it emerge. In New York City that year, the new strains cause an estimated one of every three newly diagnosed cases of TB.

•**December, 1992.** Some 500 people become ill—41 of them with acute kidney failure—and four children die from contaminated hamburgers served at Jack in the Box restaurants in the Northwest. The villain—also linked to outbreaks involving home-cooked hamburgers—was a recently discovered, virulent strain of common E. coli bacteria, which live in the intestines of humans and animals but sometimes get into hamburger meat.

•**March, 1993.** In Milwaukee 403,000 people—nearly half the city's population—become ill, 4,400 are hospitalized and 104 die in the largest recorded outbreak of water-borne disease in U.S. history. The illness is traced to *Cryptosporidium,* a one-celled intestinal parasite that somehow turned up in Milwaukee's drinking water system. The parasite survives chlorination and can be removed only by filtration.

•**May, 1993.** The nation learns of a mysterious respiratory illness that is killing Native Americans and others in the Southwest. The cause is soon found: a previously unknown member of the hantavirus family of viruses. The virus, carried by deer mice, has so far been linked to 80 illnesses, including 44 deaths, in 19 states.

•**June, 1994.** *The Journal of the American Medical Association (JAMA)* reports that strains of drug-resistant pneumococcus bacteria—once considered medical curiosities—have become widespread in the U.S. The finding is alarming, since this species causes several million cases of middle-ear infections each year in children, it's the most common cause of pneumonia (half a million cases yearly in the U.S.) and it causes 50,000 bloodstream infections and 5,000 to 6,000 cases of meningitis a year.

•**July, 1994.** Researchers report in *JAMA* that they've detected a new and sometimes fatal tick-borne bacterial disease in the upper Midwest. Also that month, a cruise ship to Bermuda is evacuated and disinfected after passengers develop Legionnaires' disease, a bacteria-caused respiratory illness fatal in up to 15% of cases.

A usually mild infection had boiled into meningitis.

The dangers of resurgent infections were strikingly illustrated last spring in the case of Meghan Sullivan, an 11-year-old from Duxbury, Mass. Until she awoke on April 4th with a soaring fever and delirium, Meghan had been a bright, active sixth grader with no unusual health problems. But by the time her parents got her to a hospital in nearby Plymouth, she was already slipping into a coma. A usually mild infection had boiled into a raging case of meningitis. Two days later, Meghan was dead.

"She was perfect, she was sweet, she was caring, she was considerate," said Michael Sullivan, anguished father of the honor student, athlete and musician. "She was my baby girl."

A half-century ago, the grief of Meghan's parents would have been just as sharp, but her death would not have been so shocking. Until World War II, infectious diseases were all too prevalent; they were, in fact, the major cause of death in the U.S. Then, beginning with the introduction of penicillin in the 1940s, came the era of antibiotics, the most important development ever in the battle against infectious disease.

Penicillin was soon joined by other compounds such as streptomycin, erythromycin and tetracycline. More potent second- and third-generation antibiotics were added later, and together they defeated pneumonia, tuberculosis and other notorious killers.

By 1969 it was possible for Surgeon General William Stewart to survey the landscape and declare, "It is time to close the book on infectious disease." He and many others believed that medical research should be retargeted to the stubborn and chronic diseases of a postindustrial society: cancer, heart disease and the degenerative diseases afflicting an aging population.

That optimism has now been shattered. Last April scientists from the Centers for Disease Control and Prevention (CDC) warned that we've entered an era when "the spectrum of infectious diseases is expanding, and many infectious diseases once thought to be controlled are increasing."

Just why are they making a comeback? Medical historians, pointing to the rise and ebb of diseases throughout history, say such resurgences are probably inevitable. Nevertheless, the social and environmental turbulence that marks the end of the 20th century is clearly playing a role.

"Human populations—immigrants and refugees—are moving in unprecedented numbers across borders and into areas where they may be exposed to new infectious agents," says Dr. Mary Wilson, a member of the working group on new and resurgent diseases at the Harvard School of Public Health. In addition, jet travel and the surge in global commerce have brought us closer to dangerous microbes as well as to each other. "Viruses don't need visas," one scientist notes.

Changes in land use also fuel the rise or return of diseases. Consider Lyme disease, first identified among residents of Lyme, Conn., in 1976. It's caused by a spirochete (a kind of bacterium) carried by deer ticks whose bites transmit the infection to humans. The chronic symptoms include fatigue, painful joints and impaired memory. Experts trace the rise and spread of this new disease to the changing New England landscape.

Deer ticks latch onto and are carried by white-tailed deer. Thanks largely to reforestation of abandoned farmland over the past 100 years, the deer population has exploded, vastly increasing opportunities for ticks to infect people, who at the same time were moving to suburbs bordering woodland areas. More than 50,000 cases of Lyme disease have been diagnosed since its discovery less than 20 years ago.

AIDS, the most devastating new epidemic, may also have been spawned by environmental changes encountering social ones. Viruses closely related to HIV, which causes AIDS, are believed to have been present for centuries in African primates. Humans turning jungle into farmland encroached on these animals' territory. A monkey bite, some experts believe, may have first introduced HIV into the human population.

According to this theory, infected people moving from rural areas to cities brought the virus with them. Changing sexual mores in Africa—a rise in prostitution, associated with an increase in sexually transmitted diseases and the open lesions they cause—allowed the infection to spread. And finally, rapid global travel introduced the virus to Western countries, where in the early 1980s AIDS first exploded among gays through promiscuous sexual activity and among IV drug users sharing needles.

The emergence of AIDS and other new infections and the resurgence of old ones like TB have underlined the need for an early warning system to spot such threats when they first arise. Last April the CDC announced plans for a global network (see "Early Warning System,") that should help detect such outbreaks early, when they can still be contained.

Just as frightening as the emergence of new infections is the fact that antibiotics, our shield against infection for 50 years, are losing their power. Microbes that readily succumbed to antibiotics a few years ago have evolved strains that resist them.

A decade go, for example, drug-resistant TB was practically unheard of but now accounts for 14% of cases nationwide. And in an outbreak in a Westminster, Calif., high school, 12 of 17 cases of active TB are drug-resistant.

Ironically, the rise of antibiotic-resistant strains is partly due to medical progress: Hospitals housing patients with weakened immune systems have become major breeding grounds for resistant strains.

An antibiotic won't kill all of the millions of microbes against which it's targeted; a healthy immune system is needed to mop up hardier ones that are

Fleshing Out the Flesh-Eating Bug

The tiny bug that made giant headlines last spring isn't as fearsome as it sounds. It can maim and kill—but so can being struck by lightning, and your chances of being felled by either are about the same.

The bug, *Streptococcus pyogenes,* is part of the streptococcus family known as strep A; another family member caused the overwhelming pneumonia that killed Muppeteer Jim Henson in 1990.

These strep A bacteria are by no means new or even exotic. Their "flesh-eating" ability was first described in 1924, and at any one time, 5% to 10% of Americans carry strep A around in their throats. But most people have no symptoms or just a sore throat. We often have strep A bacteria on our skin as well, and they can enter the body when the skin is cut, scraped or burned, causing the sorts of infections that have created the recent headlines. But for reasons not understood, a strep A infection harmless to most people can cause severe problems in others.

The Centers for Disease Control and Prevention estimates that 10,000 to 15,000 severe strep A infections occur each year in the U.S. Just 500 to 1,500 of those infections are the so-called flesh-eating kind (known technically as necrotizing fasciitis), and about 30% are fatal. The microbes don't actually eat flesh. Rather, once they encounter muscle or fat, the bacteria secrete a toxin that kills the tissue, which must then be surgically removed; in some cases the toxin and bacteria enter the bloodstream, traveling to other parts of the body and causing the lungs, kidneys or other vital organs to fail.

To defend against infection, wash broken skin promptly with soap or an antiseptic skin cleanser such as Betadine and apply a bandage. Infections will respond to antibiotics, but the earlier the treatment starts, the better.

Early Warning System

A new strain of cholera in southern Asia...yellow fever in Kenya...Rift Valley fever in Egypt...multidrug-resistant dysentery in Burundi...dengue fever in Costa Rica...diphtheria in Russia....

The Centers for Disease Control and Prevention (CDC) reports that all these infections emerged overseas in 1993 alone.

"AIDS was a wake-up call that showed us we really won't conquer infectious diseases this century or in our lifetime," says Dr. Ruth Berkelman, deputy director of the CDC's National Center for Infectious Diseases. "But these more recent outbreaks have revealed our complacency in detecting infectious disease threats, and detection is really the key step in controlling them."

A plan proposed last April by the CDC should help bolster surveillance for infections. Its cornerstone is the creation of national and global networks to provide early warning about new threats: emerging, resurgent and drug-resistant infections. Detected early, such infections could then be stopped before they have a chance to spread.

Four U.S. emerging infection centers will be created to investigate disease outbreaks, test microbes for resistance to antibiotics and create projects to prevent diseases from spreading. The CDC will also link up research centers around the world to create a global consortium for detecting and investigating infections that could affect the health of Americans.

The CDC's beefed-up effort against infectious disease will cost up to $125 million. Among its goals:

- Improve public health laboratories and train infectious disease specialists.
- Strengthen disease surveillance at the state and local levels.
- Work with the U.S. Department of Agriculture and the Food and Drug Administration to combat food poisoning.

not susceptible. But many hospitalized patients can't shake those surviving microbes because their immunity is impaired. People with AIDS, trauma and burn patients, organ transplant recipients, chemotherapy patients, the elderly and premature babies can all foster antibiotic-resistant strains.

Unfortunately, the massive amounts of antibiotics used in hospitals (about one-third of patients get them) creates a "survival of the fittest" situation that encourages drug-resistant bacterial strains to evolve, flourish and spread from patient to patient. Each year about 2 million patients—5% of all people hospitalized—suffer hospital-caused infections, which result in about 60,000 to 70,000 deaths. An estimated 50% to 60% of hospital infections involve bacteria resistant to one or more antibiotics. Seriously ill patients with weakened immune systems are most susceptible, but even patients checking in for elective surgery are at risk.

The drug resistance problem is actually not new, having first turned up shortly after penicillin was introduced. "If you use an antibiotic, you will see resistance," says Dr. Robert Gaynes, an epidemiologist with the CDC's hospital infections program. "What other class of drugs starts losing their effectiveness as soon as they're approved by the Food and Drug Administration?"

Until recently, researchers stayed one step ahead of resistant strains by coming up with new antibiotics to handle them. But in the 1980s, drug companies started giving antibiotic research a low priority and instead emphasized new treatments for chronic diseases. The most recent class of antibiotic, the quinolones, was introduced in the 1980s, and no significant ones are now in the pipeline.

"What we need is an entirely new class of drugs," says Dr. Mitchell Cohen, director of the CDC's division of bacterial and fungal diseases. "But it will probably take four or five years to get such drugs on the market, which means we'll be vulnerable for a while longer." Unfortunately, recent insights into bacterial behavior suggest that the task of keeping up with the microbes could prove daunting.

The one microbe in a million that survives an antibiotic attack may have a mutation making it more resistant than its fallen comrades. Or it may possess a resistance plasmid (a circular ring of DNA outside its nucleus). A gene in that plasmid produces a protein that can neutralize the antibiotic.

It's bad enough that the lucky survivor can go on to produce millions of antibiotic-resistant offspring. But even more ominous is the ability of bacteria to swap resistance plasmids with other bacteria, including those of other species. This microbial cooperation has hair-raising implications, as the bacterium *Enterococcus faecium* shows.

Enterococcus readily spreads among patients in hospitals, where it's responsible for many gastrointestinal infections. And it recently achieved a unique notoriety: Some of its strains have acquired resistance to all antibiotics, including vancomycin, the drug of last resort. In a particularly scary finding last July, researchers in Philadelphia reported on patients with enterococcal infections that not only resisted vancomycin but actually turned out to *require* it to grow and thrive.

More alarming, however, is the recent lab finding by British researchers that enterococci can donate their resistance plasmids to a far more fearsome bug: *Staphylococcus aureus,* the main cause of deadly wound and bloodstream infections in hospitalized patients.

Many staph strains are already resistant to nearly all antibiotics. In a patient infected with both enterococcus and staph aureus, the vancomycin resistance plasmid could jump over to the staph. Once that happens—most specialists believe it's only a matter of time—doctors will have nothing left to combat these dreaded staph infections.

"Everyone is really holding their breath, hoping this won't happen."

"This is really frightening," says Dr. David Hooper, a member of the infection control department at Massachusetts General Hospital in Boston. "Everyone is really holding their breath, hoping that this won't happen in hospitals. If it does, these staph infections will be extremely difficult to treat—in fact, almost impossible."

Hospital-bred "superbugs" readily travel into communities. But they're not solely to blame for today's worrisome increase in antibiotic-resistant bacteria. Experts also point to day care centers as prime "clearinghouses" for spreading antibiotic-resistant infections.

Samples taken in day care centers often turn up antibiotic-resistant strains of pneumococcus and of the intestinal microbe E. coli. Two factors are to blame, says the CDC's Cohen: Pediatricians set the stage for drug-resistant infections by indiscriminantly prescribing antibiotics for children (particularly for middle-ear infections), and children congregating in day care centers pass on resistant bugs to each other and later to their families and society at large.

Cohen acknowledges that doctors feel pressure to prescribe *something* when children have ear infections, even when they suspect a virus is to blame (antibiotics have no effect on viruses). But antibiotic overuse helps create the superbugs that now shrug off treatment.

"Twenty years ago, if a child developed bacterial meningitis, you'd put her on ampicillin and that would take care of it," notes Dr. Edward O'Rourke, a pediatric infectious disease specialist at Children's Hospital in Boston. "But pneumococcus bacteria have acquired resistance to ampicillin, and more recently to more potent drugs. We can use vancomycin, but it's difficult to use for meningitis since it doesn't penetrate well into the spinal fluid. So we may use rifampin, because it penetrates well, but you get resistance very quickly with that drug."

As the resistance problem worsens, vaccines—administered to bolster immunity to particular diseases—could prove to be saviors. Until a few years ago, for example, the bacterium *Haemophilus influenzae* type b was the leading cause of bacterial meningitis in American children under five. The infection had proven resistant to the usual treatments, penicillin and amoxicillin. But after a vaccine was introduced in 1988, H. influenzae infections dropped dramatically. Diseases caused by the bacteria are now targeted for elimination by 1996, according to the CDC.

Until more vaccines arrive, two of the best ways to slow antibiotic resistance are for doctors to prescribe the drugs more sparingly, and for patients to stop demanding them.

In European countries, O'Rourke points out, antibiotics are much less routinely prescribed for a child's ear infection. Instead doctors treat the pain and give the infection a few days to clear up by itself, which happens more than half the time. Since middle-ear infections are now the most common reason U.S. children visit doctors, such a practice could substantially reduce antibiotic use, and with it the opportunity for resistant strains to arise. Last July a federal agency recommended that doctors be less aggressive in prescribing antibiotics for children with fluid in their middle ears.

The threats we now confront—new infections emerging and old ones becoming resistant to antibiotics—are serious indeed. But while scientists try to come up with answers, there are steps you can take to minimize your risk, as well as the risks to society:

- **Make sure you and your family get all your immunizations.** This is critical—and something many people don't do. For example, a vaccine is available against pneumococcal pneumonia, and it can even protect against antibiotic-resistant strains that are now widespread. Those most susceptible are people over 65, and people with serious chronic health conditions, compromised immune systems or respiratory problems. The CDC recommends that such individuals get vaccinated, but compliance reportedly is dismal.
- **Recognize that antibiotics won't work against viruses.** Asking the doctor to prescribe them for colds and other viral infections wastes money and contributes to the resistance problem.
- **If a physician does prescribe** an antibiotic, take the pills for the length of time prescribed, even if you feel better sooner. Incomplete antibiotic therapy results in a greater number of surviving microbes, which may lead to the creation of resistant strain in your body. (Poor compliance with tuberculosis treatment has helped create today's multidrug-resistant strains of TB.)
- **Be vigilant about microbes on produce.** "We should take precautions like washing fruits and vegetables" to reduce the risk of ingesting dangerous microbes, says Dr. Ruth Berkelman, deputy director of the CDC's National Center for Infectious Diseases.
- **Be sure to cook all meat thoroughly,** to prevent serious illnesses such as those caused by undercooked fast-food and home-cooked hamburgers. Last July a panel of federal, industry and health officials recommended that hamburger meat be irradiated to kill off the strain of E. coli that poses a threat. Studies have shown that this strain is extremely sensitive to irradiation, a process that does not make food radioactive and that is widely used in other countries to safeguard food.
- **When traveling to other countries,** find out which disease organisms are currently causing problems, and get immunized against them.
- **Make sure your dogs and cats** are properly immunized, since they can carry serious diseases such as rabies.
- **Avoid contact with mice** and other rodents (other than pets). The deadly hantavirus, for example, is carried by mice, and people become infected mainly by inhaling viruses the rodents have shed.

Sleeping With the Enemy

Be careful out there; there's much more to watch out for than AIDS

Five years ago, stunned by the fact that 25,000 Americans had developed AIDS, health experts warned that the disease could eventually claim more lives than the Korean or Vietnam War. Today the death toll from AIDS stands at about 120,000—more than the two wars combined—and it's still accelerating: more Americans will die of AIDS in the next two years than have died in the past 10. But AIDS isn't the only argument for safer sex. The genital tract can harbor a menagerie of disease-causing organisms, and though none of them is as deadly as HIV, their consequences are often devastating. Gonorrhea and chlamydia are leading causes of infertility. Untreated syphilis can ravage the heart and brain. The sexually transmitted viruses that cause hepatitis and genital warts also foster certain cancers. And many venereal infections can pass from mother to child at birth, leaving the baby blind, brain damaged or dead. All these diseases are preventable, and some are easily cured. Yet many are on the rise. They strike 12 million Americans, including 3 million teenagers, every year.

1 Syphilis

Annual incidence: 130,000 cases

Unleashed on the world five centuries ago, apparently after Spanish explorers took it home from the Americas, venereal syphilis spread largely unabated until the 1940s. Penicillin tamed the disease during the '50s, and it was largely forgotten until the mid-1980s, when drug abuse, poverty and declining health care fueled new inner-city outbreaks. Syphilis is still rare compared with other sexually transmitted diseases, but reported cases have doubled since 1984. The rate among black males (157 cases per 100,000) is now more than 54 times the corresponding rate for whites.

The syphilis bacterium *(Treponema pallidum)* often causes genital lesions known as chancres within six weeks of infection. The sores heal readily by themselves, but without treatment the disease advances. Within 12 weeks, most sufferers experience fevers, aches, rashes, hair loss and mouth sores. Only at later stages does syphilis invade the heart, eyes, brain and other organs. The greater risk is that an infected woman will unknowingly pass the disease to her unborn baby. The germ can cross the placenta any time after the fourth month of pregnancy, causing meningitis, deformities or stillbirth. Antibiotics can stop the disease at any stage, but they can't undo its damage. Syphilis testing is a good idea for any sexually active person who develops genital sores or who learns that a partner was infected. Blood tests can detect antibodies to the bacterium, but antibodies may not show up in the blood for six weeks or more. Specialized microscopes can spot the bacterium in tissue taken from a chancre.

2 Gonorrhea

Annual incidence: 1.4 million cases

Gonorrhea declined markedly during the 1980s, suggesting that large segments of the population have gotten the message about safer sex. But the disease is still 10 times as common as syphilis, and the racial disparities are more striking than ever. The rate of new infections, 12 times higher among blacks than whites a decade ago, is now 39 times higher. Like syphilis, the condition is easily treated with antibiotics.

The gonococcus bacterium thrives in moist, warm cavities, including the mouth and throat as well as the rectum, cervix and urinary tract. Genital symptoms such as burning, itching or unusual discharge normally show up two to 10 days after infection. If those symptoms go unnoticed, as often happens in women, the infection can spread into the fallopian tubes, causing such complications as infertility and tubal pregnancy. Doctors can readily detect gonococcal infection by analyzing penile or cervical discharge under a microscope. Testing is recommended for anyone who experiences symptoms or who has unprotected sex with more than one partner. Since the germ can infect a child's eyes at birth, many experts also favor testing for all pregnant women and antibiotic eyedrops for all newborns.

3 Chlamydia

Annual incidence: 4 million cases

The government has never tracked chlamydia as closely as syphilis, gonorrhea or AIDS, but health officials rank it the nation's most common sexually transmitted disease. An estimated 4 million Americans contract this bacterial infection each year. The most common symptom is an inflammation of the urethra that causes painful urination or a discharge of pus or mucus. In addition to painful urination and vaginal discharge, women sometimes experience general pain in the lower abdomen. Like gonorrhea, chlamydia can lead to sterility in women who don't receive treatment.

Unfortunately, the disease is easy to miss until complications set in. One in four infected men, and at least half of all infected women, experience no initial symptoms at all. So experts recommend that anyone with more than one sex partner—especially women still in their childbearing years—be tested annually. Until recently, testing for chlamydia involved culturing genital secretions. The process took several days, and because gonococcal bacteria don't grow readily in culture, the results were unreliable. Using new diagnostic techniques, doctors can reliably analyze the secretions in the course of a 30-minute office visit. Tetracycline is the usual treatment for chlamydia. The drug can't be taken during pregnancy, but substitutes are available.

4 PID

Cases treated annually: 420,000

Gonorrhea and chlamydia can both lead to pelvic inflammatory disease, or PID, the most frequent complication of sexually transmitted disease in women. The trouble begins when an infection spreads from the cervix into the fallopian tubes (a process that vaginal douching and the use of intrauterine devices may hasten). The tubes become scarred, and the scar tissue impedes passage of fertilized eggs to the uterus. Besides obstructing pregnancy, PID can cause fertilized eggs to lodge in the wall of the fallopian tube, destroying the embryo and endangering the mother's life.

PID seems to be waning along with gonorrhea; a recent study by the Centers for Disease Control showed a sharp drop in incidence between 1982 and 1988. But the disease still afflicts nearly 11 percent of the nation's childbearing-aged women—one in 10 whites and one in six blacks. Some 420,000 sufferers seek treatment every year, at a cost of $2 billion. The warning signs of PID, easily spotted during a routine pelvic exam, include swelling or tenderness in the cervix, uterus or surrounding tissue. A cervical smear can confirm that the lower reproductive tract is infected or inflamed. But diagnosing more widespread PID often requires laparoscopy, an outpatient surgical procedure that involves inserting a scope into the abdomen through a small incision below the navel. Antibiotics can stop the disease. To avoid reinfection, women who develop PID should get their partners tested for the responsible bacteria.

5 Genital Herpes

Annual incidence: 500,000 cases

Unlike a bacterial infection, genital herpes can't be cured with antibiotics. Once infected with a herpes simplex virus, you're infected for life. Some 30 million Americans carry these common pathogens (there are two types), and most never suffer any consequences. But an estimated half-million people develop new cases of active genital herpes each year. The number of patients seeking treatment has grown sevenfold since the late 1960s.

In adults, the condition is more an annoyance than a health threat. The virus causes cold-sore-like lesions on the genital area. They normally appear within 10 days of infection and heal within three weeks. But many carriers experience occasional flare-ups, and anyone with an active lesion can pass the virus to a sex partner—even if the lesion is unnoticeable. Women with active herpes can also infect their babies during delivery, causing brain damage or death. Though no drug can root out the infection, daily doses of acyclovir, an antiviral drug, can help control it. And Caesarean delivery can reduce the risk to a newborn.

6 Genital Warts

Annual incidence: 1 million cases

Like herpes sores, genital warts are caused by viruses that medical science has yet to tame. No one knows just how many people carry the culpable strains of human papilloma virus (HPV). Nor is it clear whether symptom-free carriers can spread the infection. But health officials estimate that 1 million Americans develop active warts every year and that two thirds of their sex partners contract the infection. The hard, fleshy bumps typically appear within three months of exposure to the virus, and they can show up well inside the vagina or the cervix, making self-diagnosis difficult for women.

The warts themselves are more unpleasant than dangerous; doctors can usually remove them by freezing, burning, chemical solutions or, when necessary, surgery. But experts worry about possible links between HPV and cancers of the penis, vulva and cervix. Cervical cancer strikes 14,000 American women a year, and kills 6,000. The malignancy is treatable if detected early, so women with a history of genital warts should have annual Pap smears as a precaution.

7 Hepatitis B

Annual incidence: 300,000 cases

Hepatitis B isn't generally thought of as a sexually transmitted disease, but it should be. The virus infects an estimated 300,000 Americans every year, causing 5,000 deaths, and sex is the leading mode of transmission. Overall incidence hasn't changed much in recent years. But while the rate among gay men plummeted during the '80s—apparently in response to AIDS-inspired precautions—heterosexual transmission surged by 38 percent. Anyone with more than one partner is at risk.

The hepatitis B virus (HBV) attacks the liver, causing a tenacious flulike illness marked by jaundice. There is no cure; most people recover naturally and develop immunity to future infection. But HBV can take root in the body, remaining contagious and leading slowly to cirrhosis or liver cancer. There is a proven hepatitis B vaccine; the government recommends it for all sexually active gay men and for heterosexuals with more than one partner. But while 28 million heterosexuals are at risk, less than 1 percent have taken advantage of it.

8 AIDS

Total U.S. cases: 199,406*

An estimated 1 million Americans are infected with the AIDS virus—many of them unknowingly—and any infected person can pass the virus to sexual partners. Gay men still constitute the largest risk group for AIDS, followed by intravenous drug users. Only 6 percent of all U.S. cases have been traced to heterosexual contact. But heterosexual transmission is the norm throughout much of the world, and experts agree it will become more common here as the epidemic matures.

HIV often causes a brief, flulike illness at the time of infection, but it can remain silent for a decade or more before causing the fatigue, fevers, diarrhea, weight loss and susceptibility to infections that mark the onset of full-blown AIDS. Within a month or two of infection, the body produces antibodies that a blood test can detect. Testing is recommended for anyone with multiple partners or a history of sexually transmitted disease. The antiviral drugs AZT and ddI can slow the progress of HIV disease, and new treatments have made some AIDS-related infections more manageable. But safer sex is still the best medicine. The disease is incurable, and unlike the others, it always kills.

Geoffrey Cowley *with* Mary Hager

*Through October 1991.

what every woman needs to know about personal Safety

Are you scared silly? It's time to get scared *smart.* Trade fear for caution by understanding when and where you're most at risk and how to protect yourself against crime.

Lauren David Peden

Are you afraid to walk down the street alone at night? Let a repairman into your house when your husband isn't home? Accept help from a stranger if your car breaks down on the road? More women than ever answer yes. They're scared, and for good reason. One violent crime is committed every 17 seconds in the United States, with the number of murders and rapes each increasing 9 percent from 1989 to 1990.

And everywhere a woman turns, it seems, she is reminded of the danger. Switch on the television or go to your local movie theater and you're confronted with a slew of "jep" movies—the name that the entertainment industry gives to films in which a woman is in jeopardy of being raped, mugged, beaten, duped or worse. Movies such as *Cape Fear, Sleeping With the Enemy* and *The Hand that Rocks the Cradle* send shivers through female viewers by implying that they could be next. Even everyday life seems more dangerous. Newscasts, top-heavy with stories of crime and tragedy, compound the scare factor with "special reports" on the perils of everything from eating fresh fruit to shaving your legs.

The result of such menacing messages? Mean World Syndrome, a perception that danger lurks around every corner and that one is perpetually on the verge of being victimized. "Basically we're terrorized by the media," says George Gerbner, professor emeritus of communications at the Annenberg School for Communication in Philadelphia, who coined the term and has studied the phenomenon extensively. "Television shows are full of violence, and news programs dole out risk information without comparison, context, perspective or other relative values. It makes people panicky, particularly women." According to Gerbner, women are afflicted with the syndrome more than men and children primarily because of Hollywood's unnerving depiction of females. "On a typical TV drama, male characters outnumber females by three or four to one, but when there's violence, women are more often portrayed as victims," he explains. "In turn, women perceive the world as fraught with more danger than really exists." And Gerbner's studies have shown that the more hours women log watching TV, the more they suffer from Mean World Syndrome.

But experts are quick to point out that while these fears are exaggerated, they are still very real. It's how women put them in perspective that makes the difference between being reasonably cautious and hyper-afraid. The fact is, a woman *does* have a one in three chance of being raped in her lifetime and a one in 348 chance of being murdered. But when these statistics are stacked up against other odds, they're easier to live with. Overemphasized risks may be inconsequential, and underemphasized ones may deserve more attention. For instance, while you have only an 82 in 100,000 chance of being struck by lightning (an oft-depicted tragedy on reality-based TV shows like *Rescue 911*), your chances of drowning are significantly higher at 4,199 in 100,000.

The key, then, is knowing where your real risks lie and keeping your guard up in those situations but relaxing in others. Statistics show that terrible things happen to good people, but they're not inevitable. In fact, sometimes they're *very* unlikely. We'll discuss the most common dangers you should be concerned about and what you can do to minimize them. So you can learn to look over your shoulder prudently, not constantly, and concentrate on the good things in life.

Reprinted with permission from *McCall's* magazine, May 1992, pp. 72, 74, 76, 78. © 1992 by the New York Times Company.

How to Feel Safe in Your Home

Crime hits hard on the home front, and Americans know it. We spent $3.4 billion on home burglar-alarm systems in 1991. Are such security systems worth the money? Maybe, but before you get out the checkbook, consider this: When criminals were asked what *they* would use to protect their homes, they said dogs, not alarms. Here are the biggest risk factors and some smart measures to keep you safe and sound at home.

• **Fifty-five percent of all burglars enter homes through an unlocked door or window,** says the National Crime Prevention Council. Keep all points of entry locked at all times. And be vigilant about it. Instill the habit in your kids too.

• **In almost all other cases, burglars enter homes through forced entry—**bashing in a window, prying a door away from its frame. Make sure the locks on doors are heavy-duty dead bolts and that the doors themselves are made of metal or solid-core wood that is at least 1 3/4 inches thick. Bolster window safety by installing specially designed pins through the casings to prevent windows from being opened from the outside (contact your local fire department for instructions). In suburban areas, thieves often enter houses by kicking in a basement window. Install bars over cellar windows that thwart break-ins.

• **A criminal may disguise himself to get into your home.** Criminals have been known to masquerade as salespeople, police officers and even victims of car accidents. *Never open your door to strangers.* First look through a peephole or window to see who it is. If you don't know the person, either ignore him until he goes away or ask what he wants through the locked door.

A New Kind of Street Smarts

Even if you don't live in a big city where street smarts are the way of the land, chances are you don't feel completely comfortable walking down the street alone at night (or even during the day in some areas). In fact, according to the National Victim Center, women are so concerned for their safety that 75 percent of them say they limit the places they go by themselves. Over half of all robberies and muggings occur on a street or highway, and driving doesn't afford any additional protection. Carjacking (stealing cars from drivers at gunpoint) is a growing phenomenon, so new that statistics on it aren't yet available. Here are three common crimes that women need to be on guard against.

• **Purse snatching.** The safest way to carry your purse is tucked snugly under your arm like a football with the strap wrapped around it. If the bag has a clasp closure, carry it clutched in your dominant hand, clasp side down. Should someone try to grab it, release the clasp and let the contents spill on the ground. A thief usually won't stop to sift through the mess.

• **Robbery by force or weapon.** Criminals scope out *easy* targets. Appear confident by walking with a strong gait, your hands out of your pockets. If you suspect you're being followed, don't go home. Even if the criminal passes you up, he'll learn where you live. Instead, cross the street, abruptly change direction or head toward an open store, restaurant or well-lit residence and call the police.

• **Carjacking.** According to the FBI, more than 1.6 million cars were stolen in 1990, a jump of over 50 percent since 1981. Increasingly, thieves are stealing cars from their owners right on the road. When you're driving, always keep doors locked and pay attention to other cars and pedestrians around you, particularly at traffic lights and stop signs. If a suspicious person approaches your car, lean on the horn and drive away, even through a red light if necessary. If the person threatens you, relinquish your car to minimize your chances of being hurt.

How to Feel Safe at Work

According to the U.S. Department of Justice, a surprising 13 percent of all violent crimes and 20 percent of all thefts occur on the job. Why the office? It's a contained environment where people spend at least eight hours a day—and it's easy for a criminal to blend in with the crowd or hide in isolated areas, such as rest rooms and stairwells. Here are two concerns to be especially aware of in the workplace.

• **Theft.** The simplest deterrent: Hide all valuables. Keep your purse and other important items in a locked desk or file-cabinet drawer, *not* on the floor under your desk.

• **Physical assault.** In this case, you're most at risk before and after regular hours. Stay alert when coming in early or staying late. Lock your office door while you're working if you're alone or in the company of other employees you don't know well. Keep the phone number for building security taped to your telephone. If your building doesn't have guards at the main entrance, make sure that door is locked too, if possible. And wait to use the bathroom until co-workers arrive or, if you'll be working late, use it before everyone has left for the day.

Stress and Mental Health

Years of medical research have significantly advanced our knowledge and understanding of the human body to a point where not only can organs be transplanted, but machines can be built to replicate their functions. The one organ that still mystifies and baffles the scientific community, however, is the brain. While more has been learned about this organ in the last five years than in all the rest of recorded history, our understanding of this complex organ is still in its infancy. What has been learned, however, has spawned exciting new research and has contributed to the establishment of new disciplines such as psychophysiology and psychoneuroimmunology (PNI).

Traditionally, the medical community has viewed health problems as either physical or mental, treating each type separately. This dichotomy between the psyche (mind) and soma (body) is fading in light of scientific data revealing profound physiological changes associated with mood shifts. The discovery of this complex interaction between mind and body has stimulated intense research regarding the role of stress in health. The articles "Does Tension Cause Hypertension?" and "Stress" explore the psychophysiology of emotions and their impact on one's health.

Hans Selye, the father of stress research, described stress as a nonspecific physiological response to anything that challenges the body. Dr. Selye demonstrated that this response could be elicited by both mental and physical stimuli. Some general characteristics of this response include increases in heart rate, muscle tension, blood pressure, blood sugar, blood fats, and blood coagulability. While these responses are adaptive during times of crisis, Dr. Selye found that these same mechanisms could provoke physiological dysfunction if they persisted for prolonged periods of time. These findings clearly suggested that stress could play a crucial role in the etiology of various diseases.

Today researchers are examining the role stress may play in a variety of illnesses. Physical ailments currently believed to be associated with emotional stress include coronary heart disease, hypertension, obesity, diabetes, asthma, tension headaches, migraine headaches, ulcers, cancer, and a general increased susceptibility to infectious illnesses. If stress is a generalized physiological response, why then are there so many different illnesses associated with it? While this question has not been conclusively answered, most experts think the explanation may be "the weak organ theory." According to this theory, every individual has one organ system that is most susceptible to the damaging effects of prolonged stress. Should the individual be subjected to such stress, this organ system will be the first to manifest some dysfunction. If this theory is correct, it may explain why different individuals exposed to the same stressor develop different illnesses. Elizabeth Stark's article "Stress" discusses how genetics may play a role in determining both an individual's tolerance for stress and the organ system most susceptible to the damaging effects of prolonged stress. "Energy!" by Gini Kopecky discusses how genetics, diet, sleep, exercise, environmental stimuli, mental set, and perceived stress can affect your energy level.

Mental illness, which is generally regarded as a major dysfunction of normal thought processes, has no identifiable etiology. One may speculate that this is due to the complex nature of the organ system involved. It may also be that many conditions labeled as mental illnesses are not really illnesses at all, but rather behaviors that society has deemed unacceptable. While the latter seems to be true for conditions and behaviors such as homosexuality, drug abuse, child abuse, and sexual dysfunction, there is mounting evidence to suggest an organic component to the more traditional forms of mental illness such as schizophrenia, chronic depression, and manic-depression. Even as researchers are identifying specific neurochemical disturbances associated with these conditions, experts are locked into a debate as to whether these findings represent the cause or the effect of the mental illness.

The fact that certain mental illnesses tend to occur within families has divided the mental health community into two camps: those that believe there is a genetic factor operating in mental illness, and those that see the family tendency as more of a learned behavior. Regardless of which side is correct, the evidence strongly supports mental illness as yet another example of the weak organ theory.

While the media has alerted the public to the dangers of stress, it has also created the belief that all stress is bad and should be avoided. Avoiding all stress is not only an impossible task, but an undesirable goal as well. Current thinking on this issue has changed the focus from the elimination of stress, to an approach that views stress as an essential component of life and a potential source of health. The notion that stress could serve as a positive force in one's life was presented by Dr. Selye in 1974 in his book *Stress Without Distress*. Dr. Selye felt that there were three types of stress: negative stress (distress), normal stress, and positive stress (eustress). He maintained that positive stress not only increases a person's self-esteem, but inoculates him or her against the negative effects of distress. The distinction between these two types of stress is a subjective assessment based solely on the perception of the individual. If these assumptions are correct, then

Unit 3

the most effective way to change distress into eustress is to work on changing the context or mind-set.

Recent studies in the area of occupational stress strengthen the assertion that perception plays a vital role in the stress equation. These studies also challenge the commonly held notion that executive jobs are the most stressful due to the decision-making requirements of these jobs. Current findings suggest that while executive positions do entail a relatively high level of stress, this stress is generally of the eustress variety. This is in sharp contrast to the distress experienced by workers at the bottom of the job ladder. These jobs emphasize performance and provide little latitude for decision making or control. Interestingly, it is this perceived lack of control that makes these jobs particularly stressful.

According to a recent government document, the incidence of mental illness among adult Americans is approximately 19 percent and growing. This statistic is based on a broad definition of mental illness that includes some 230 separate categories, such as tobacco dependence, sexual dysfunction, and developmental defects. Reports such as this, coupled with increasing evidence that mental stress is a contributing factor to many health problems, is prompting researchers to develop therapeutic interventions that will protect individuals from the damaging effects of stress, as well as treat those already experiencing some degree of dysfunction. While tranquilizers have been the traditional treatment of choice, a new branch of medicine termed "behavioral medicine" is utilizing techniques such as biofeedback, meditation, self-hypnosis, mental imagery, progressive relaxation, exercise, and nutrition counseling to control stress. In addition to these techniques, many stress management programs include time management training, assertiveness training, and goal setting as stress control strategies. While all of the aforementioned techniques may serve a valuable function in a stress management program, none of them is universally effective. "Out of the Blues" by Kathleen McAuliffe discusses how exercise such as walking can provide therapeutic benefits to those suffering from depression. According to McAuliffe, walking ranks with the best talk therapies as a mode of treatment for those suffering from depression. This finding provides additional support for a unified mind-body concept by demonstrating that mental disorders can be treated by actions that alter one's physiological state. In "Depression: Way Beyond the Blues," Sandra Arbetter examines various aspects of depression and suggests things that you can do to help a friend who is depressed.

While significant gains have been made in our understanding of the relationship between body and mind, much remains to be learned. What is known suggests that the mind-set of an individual is the key factor in shaping one's response to stress. In order to be successful in converting distress into eustress, some people may need to reevaluate their approach to life so that they can experience a sense of direction and purpose.

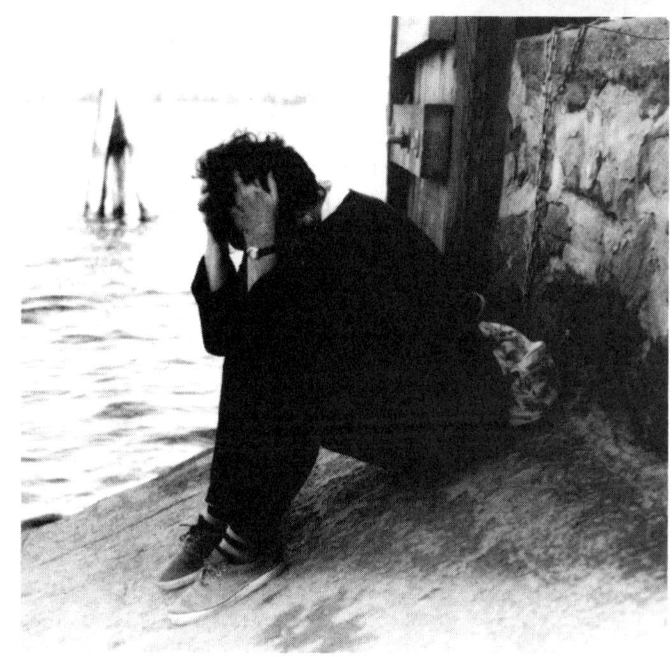

Looking Ahead: Challenge Questions

How have humankind's stressors changed over the last 5,000 years?

How do you manage the stress in your life?

Discuss how positive affirmations and feeling a sense of purpose in your life can help to reduce stress.

How can one gain a sense of purpose and direction by which to live one's life?

Why do different people respond to stress differently? How do genetics and perception influence one's response to stress?

What can you do to help someone who is suffering from depression?

How is emotional stress linked to both hypertension and coronary heart disease?

Why are activities such as walking effective in treating mood disorders such as depression? What is the mechanism by which they work?

If perception is a major component in the stress equation, is there anything one can do to alter one's perception?

STRESS
It's All Relative . . . and Relatively Easy to Manage

Elizabeth Stark

Elizabeth Stark is a freelance writer specializing in health and behavior.

It's that time of year again: time to send out your holiday cards, buy presents for everyone from your mother to your mail carrier, wrap those gifts, rush from one holiday party to another, travel to see friends and family, and, most likely, eat and drink too much. Is it any wonder that many people consider this the most stressful time of year?

Lest holiday demands turn you into another Ebenezer Scrooge, you should know that you have more control over stress than you may think. And contrary to popular belief, stress often isn't caused so much by external events—such as standing in line for an hour at the post office—as by the way we perceive and cope with them.

Many of us view stress as the unavoidable price of modern life. Nearly nine out of 10 Americans say they experience high levels of it at least once or twice a week, and one in four complains of high levels every day. In the late 1960s, psychiatrists Thomas Holmes and Richard Rahe created a "life stress scale" that listed dozens of events, ranging from things like getting a promotion to the death of a spouse; they assigned each a certain number of points. By checking off those you had experienced in the preceding year and adding up your score, the test implied, you could assign a number to your stress level.

The problem with tidy stress charts is that our reactions to events vary from person to person. What frazzles one may excite or challenge another. Research increasingly shows that it's not the amount of stress that matters, but one's ability to control the situations that engender it.

Understanding stress is further complicated by the fact that the term itself is "one of those words that everyone knows the meaning of but no one can define," says psychiatrist Sanford Cohen, director of the Stress and Clinical Biobehavioral Medicine Center at the University of Miami. For example, many of us refer to upsetting external events as stress, when those are in fact *stressors*. To a psychologist, stress describes the body's reaction to such events. Dr. David Jenkins, a professor of psychiatry at the University of Texas Medical Branch at Galveston, likens stress and an individual to water in a bathtub: "Just as whether the water spills over the top depends in part on the tub's size, people who have a large capacity to deal with challenge may not 'overflow' under stress."

But what happens when your body *does* overflow with stress? First the voluntary nervous system, which responds to sensory input and controls intentional movements, sends messages to your muscles, preparing you—as in prehistoric days—to fight or flee. Then the autonomic nervous system, which regulates involuntary body functions, sends extra blood to your muscles to get you going and slows down other bodily functions such as digestion. In addition, the neuroendocrine system releases adrenaline, the hormone that primes the body for action, and cortisol, another hormone that magnifies and prolongs adrenaline's effect.

> Often, external events don't cause stress. How we perceive and cope with them does.

This surge of chemicals may have ensured our early ancestors' survival in dangerous situations, but it can wear us down when it results from the unremitting saber-toothed tigers of today: anything from financial woes to that most modern lament, "too much to do, too little time." Bodies exposed to constant, unresolved stress never have a chance to recover. The symptoms that result include headaches, backaches, insomnia, anxiety, depression, arthritis, asthma, gastrointestinal upsets, skin disorders, weight problems and drug and alcohol abuse. In fact, according to the American Institute of Stress (AIS) in Yonkers, N.Y., 75% to 90% of all visits to physicians involve stress-related complaints.

Researchers in the field of psychoneuroimmunology, the study of the relationship between our health and emotions, have even linked stress to specific illnesses. "We now know the mechanisms of many stress-related disorders," says Dr. Paul Rosch, president of the AIS and a professor of medicine and psychiatry at New York Medical College in Valhalla. He believes that chronic, insidious types of stress such as lone-

From *American Health,* December 1992, pp. 41-42, 44-47.

liness and poverty can affect the immune system; some studies indeed suggest that stress can increase the risk of catching a cold, perhaps even of being struck by cancer or AIDS. Anger, on the other hand, may increase production of hormones such as adrenaline and noradrenalin, which also reduce the body's ability to fight disease and can lead to higher blood pressure and heart attacks as well. Anxiety, another common stress symptom, often affects the gastrointestinal system, contributing to the development of ulcers, colitis and irritable bowel syndrome.

A growing body of evidence indicates that some people are biologically more stress-resistant than others. Genes may play a role. "There seem to be heritable differences in the degree of activity of different body parts," Cohen says. "One family may be susceptible to gastrointestinal reactions, while another gets high blood pressure or headaches."

Research is also focusing on temperament's role in stress reactions. People who seek out challenges that many others would find upsetting fall into a category that Dr. Frank Farley, incoming president of the American Psychological Association and a professor of psychology at the University of Wisconsin in Madison, calls "Type T," for thrill-seeking and risk-taking personality. Partly for physiological reasons, he argues, such people tend to be more creative and extroverted and to take more risks than others, whether positive or negative. A new University of Washington study of high school athletes highlighted a particular dimension of Type T stress resilience: Players who fit Farley's criteria lost less time because of injuries than those with a lower threshold for thrills, probably because they're more tolerant of negative events.

Contradicting a popular prejudice, recent studies by Dr. Redford Williams, a behavioral medicine researcher at Duke University, suggest that having a hurried, impatient Type A personality doesn't necessarily put one at risk for coronary disease. Says Williams: "If you're racing around because you're a go-getter—you're enthusiastic, you're positive—the evidence is that it doesn't hurt you." So-called hostile Type A's, on the other hand, react to anger with an excessive surge of adrenaline; moreover, the neurological responses that normally counter this reaction are weaker in these people. Compared with others, hostile Type A subjects in Williams' studies were also more overweight, consumed more alcohol, smoked more cigarettes, had worse lipid profiles and consumed more caffeine. "Our findings suggest that the hostile Type A's autonomic nervous system is balanced differently," Williams says. "Since that's a biological characteristic, it does make you think that genetic factors play a more important role in stress than previously thought."

Although biology may lay the foundation for how well we deal with life's stressors, the ways we've learned to defuse them dramatically affect our resilience too. After looking at 1,200 men and women who deal well with stressful situations, Dr. Raymond Flannery, an assistant clinical professor of psychology at Harvard University Medical School, found that they tend to control their lives and look for active solutions to problems; they're committed to meaningful goals; they use little nicotine and caffeine, relax at least 15 minutes a day and get regular aerobic exercise; and they're actively involved with others. "People who live by these principles have better physical and mental health and a greater sense of well-being," Flannery says. When others learn the precepts in his 10-week program, called Project SMART (Stress Management and Relaxation Training), they too report better functioning at home and work and improved health.

While most of us have developed some skills for dealing with stress, says Flannery, we tend to underestimate the importance of social interaction. "Studies show that social contact may lower pulse rate and blood pressure, enhance the immune system and boost the production of endorphins—neurochemicals that make us feel good. When you're in a caring relationship with another person, all these health benefits can accrue."

When your stress load weighs especially heavily, the first step is "to distinguish between things you can do something about and things you can't," the AIS's Rosch says. "Otherwise, you'll be constantly frustrated." He recommends making a list of your stressors, then separating them into those two categories. As simple as this process sounds, he says, many people don't take the time to think in these concrete terms. Yet, as Flannery says, "none of us can have it all. Life requires each of us to make choices."

Those who learn certain precepts report better health.

One of the major sources of stress is the workplace, where picking and choosing aren't always possible. More than a quarter of the respondents to a 1990 survey from Northwestern National Life, a Minneapolis-based insurance company, said job stress was the single greatest strain in their lives; seven out of 10 said it lowered their productivity and caused frequent ailments. "There are many unhappy, ineffective workers," says Wisconsin's Farley. "I think much of that problem can be laid at the doorstep of an ill-fitting interaction between a person and his environment. People often choose jobs unwisely because they don't know enough about themselves." He cites those ubiquitous lists of the "10 Most Stressful Jobs," which usually include air-traffic controller and police officer. The problem, says Farley, is that some people crave the excitement and danger of being a cop, while others need the familiarity and predictability of, say, an assembly line job. He proposes that "there aren't that many absolute stressors. Stress is an outcome of who you are and what you are doing." That's why, says Rosch, "Type A's thrive in highly demanding jobs as long as they're in control."

Of course, some sense of control is important to *all* workers. Studies have shown that those who feel they have a lot of responsibility and yet have little or no say over decisions that affect them suffer the most stress. Even race-car drivers often say that they feel far more stress sit-

Holiday Stress

Supposedly all-joyous celebration, the holidays are often a time of tremendous tension. Who hasn't experienced that feeling in the pit of the stomach upon realizing it's December 15th and there's still a mountain of gift buying, card sending and cooking ahead?

At this time of year, a big part of the stress load is physical—eating and drinking too much at parties, battling crowds and squeezing just one more event into the day. More insidious is the psychological strain. Merchants and media dictate an impossible holiday ideal. Personal heartaches—about everything from people no longer with us to our unrealized dreams—tend to be magnified at this time. Add in our childhood memories of "perfect" holidays, and how can reality measure up?

Changing demographics have made many traditional holiday expectations unrealistic, says Jo Robinson and Jean Coppock Staeheli, authors of *Unplug the Christmas Machine* (William Morrow, 1991, $8.95). When they examined the causes of holiday stress among thousands of people, they found that in this age of divorce and widely dispersed relatives, the warm, fuzzy image of whole families gathered around groaning boards is long outdated. Considering that both parents in most families work outside the home, lavish feasts and elaborate decorations are also anachronistic.

To bring holiday expectations back down to earth, researchers offer these suggestions:

► **BE REALISTIC:** Set achievable goals. Don't expect to be happy every minute or for everything to be perfect.

► **SET PRIORITIES:** Take a hard look at how you've been spending holiday time in the past, and eliminate elements that aren't important to you.

► **SIMPLIFY:** Do you really need to serve three desserts? Can you scale back on gift giving? Some families draw names from a hat, and have each member buy one terrific gift for the person whose name they pull.

► **ENLIST THE HELP OF OTHERS:** Mothers often carry an unfair burden of holiday responsibilities. Ask other family members and friends to help.

► **TAKE CARE OF YOURSELF:** Try not to eat or drink too much. Keep your sleep schedule as regular as possible. Take time out for long walks or hot baths.

► **GET SOCIAL SUPPORT:** Spend time with those you care about. If you're lonely, seek out people and groups who can make the holidays warmer.

—E.S.

ting in the pit while the crew works on the car than when they're barreling around the track.

Still, there will aways be people doing jobs for which they're ill-suited and encountering stressful situations that can't be avoided. When you can't change the situation, stress experts recommend that you try to change your outlook. "Most people's problems have to do with faulty perception—perhaps unnecessarily seeing a situation as hopeless—and they have the power to change that," Rosch says. "You can develop certain cognitive skills, such as assertiveness or the ability to manage time better."

If psychological approaches don't appeal to you, you may want to try exercise. Along with providing physical release and mental distraction, it produces natural opiates that elicit calm and euphoria. Experts particularly recommend aerobic activities such as running and swimming. Techniques such as relaxation, biofeedback, visualization, yoga, massage or meditation can also be effective, but you may have to try various approaches to find the one that suits you best. The Type A person, for example, might have a difficult time meditating, even becoming more stressed in the process.

Before prescribing treatment for her clients, Dr. Suzanne Miller, an associate professor of psychology and medicine at Temple University, determines whether they are "monitors," who want as much information about a stressful situation as possible, or "blunters," who like to distract themselves from it. Because monitors do better with more intellectual, problem-solving approaches, one effective method for them is setting aside a certain period each day as "worry time." When fretful thoughts intrude at other moments, they write them down and go back to the business at hand. The blunter's coping style lends itself much more readily to relaxation and meditation techniques. Although blunters handle stress better in the short term, they often ignore its warning signs, only to find themselves faced with major stress-related ailments later on.

A high-tech way to handle stress, biofeedback allows us to monitor seemingly involuntary body functions. In a biofeedback session, the patient is hooked up to a machine with painless sensors attached to various parts of the body, such as the hands, arms and face. These sensors measure physiological reactions such as heart rate and muscle

Race-car drivers report more stress waiting in the pit than on the track.

tension, and produce a flashing light or a beep in response to changes. Using these signals as a guide, the patient learns to control his response, usually by controlling his thoughts. A trainer typically stands by to offer suggestions for improving performance.

If none of these strategies work, a stress-management program may help, particularly one offered by a major medical center or university hospital. Unfortunately, Rosch has found that many "stress-reduction experts"—who aren't licensed—are merely opportunists with little training.

Flannery suggests that if you're considering enrolling in a program, you should ask some questions first: Does the practitioner have a background in counseling or health psychology? Has he demonstrated some mastery in the field? Where was he trained? What does he consider to be reasonable expectations for the program? "A lot of these things are offered as four-hour, quick-fix workshops on a Saturday morning," Flannery says. "But it's going to take a lot longer to enhance your capacity to cope with stress. Look at how long it takes a person to get into physical shape. You'll feel better once you start, but expect to spend anywhere between six months and two years before you enjoy the full benefits." Still, Flannery believes that no one who goes the distance will regret it. "Once people start, they say, 'Why didn't I do this years ago?' And they don't go back to their old ways."

How the Body Responds

Much more than just a feeling of unease, emotional stress triggers a series of bodily responses: The heart races, blood pressure surges, breathing revs up and a rush of adrenaline primes the muscles for action. Embedded in our genes, this so-called fight-or-flight response was intended to protect us from predators. But in a world in which predators often wear pinstriped suits, it's more likely to trigger several physical illnesses.

► **HEADACHES.** "There's no question that emotional stress has an impact on headaches," says Dr. Ed Blanchard, a professor of psychology at the State University of New York at Albany. Stress, he says, is a major cause of tension headaches—the most common type of headache—and of migraines as well. Stress reduction techniques have been found useful in treating both kinds.

► **IRRITABLE BOWEL SYNDROME.** Almost everyone experiences gastrointestinal distress occasionally. But frequent problems, including abdominal pain, cramping, bloating, diarrhea and constipation, may be signs of irritable bowel syndrome (IBS), which afflicts 15% to 20% of Americans.

IBS has no known cause or cure, and physical exams usually don't detect it. The majority of those with the problem aren't under exceptional stress and don't even seek medical help. Yet studies have found that IBS patients are more prone than others to the effects of stress, particularly intestinal upheavals. In many cases the symptoms can be soothed by doing relaxation exercises, adding fiber to the diet and avoiding high-fat foods and caffeine. If the problem persists, a doctor may prescribe antidiarrheal or antispasmodic drugs.

► **ULCERS.** The excess stomach acid triggered by stress has long been considered a major cause of ulcers. But recent research has found stress to be more contributor than cause. The new prime suspect: a type of bacteria present in 70% to 80% of all stomach-ulcer patients and nearly everyone with duodenal (small intestine) ulcers.

"Stress itself won't cause ulcers," says Dr. David Graham, the gastroenterologist at the Veterans Affairs Medical Center in Houston who has been researching the bacterial species, known as *Helicobacter pylori.* "But if you have the bacterium in your system, the increase in gastric acid caused by stress can worsen the ulcer." A two-week antibiotic regimen can eliminate the bacteria.

► **HEART DISEASE.** Two key risk factors for heart disease—high blood pressure and elevated blood cholesterol levels—can both be exacerbated by stress.

Although elevated blood cholesterol stems mainly from a high-fat diet, a recent study found that people performing mentally stressful tasks experience a temporary rise in cholesterol levels. And earlier research detected a dramatic rise in blood cholesterol levels in income tax accountants every year just before the April 15th deadline.

Men in high-stress jobs are known to be three times more likely than their low-stress counterparts to have high blood pressure. Stress-management techniques such as biofeedback, meditation and yoga can sometimes help lower blood pressure, especially if used over the long term.

Growing evidence is confirming what researchers have long believed: Once people have heart disease, stress increases their chances of dying from it. In studies of heart disease patients, those who were socially isolated or financially strapped died much sooner than more fortunate patients.

Another kind of emotional stress—anger—may also be dangerous to the heart. In a recent study, men with mild heart disease were asked to describe an incident that made them angry. In response to the stress, the pumping efficiency of the men's hearts dropped significantly. The drop meant that the coronary arteries weren't providing the heart muscle with enough blood, perhaps because anger was sending the diseased arteries into spasm.

But many deaths from stress can probably be prevented. A recent study suggests that blood pressure drugs known as beta-blockers can prevent heart malfunctions that occur when cardiac patients are under emotional stress. And minimizing stress can also help: In another recent study, teaching heart attack survivors simple stress reduction techniques lowered their risk of cardiac death by half compared with a control group.

—Winifred Conkling

DOES TENSION CAUSE HYPERTENSION?

Stress can make blood pressure rise. In some people, it can cause a lasting rise.

At the climax of the movie "The Little Foxes," Bette Davis taunts her on-screen husband so viciously that he suffers a fatal heart attack. That chilling scene is not just the product of a melodramatic imagination—stress can indeed trigger a heart attack in someone who has coronary disease.

But stress can have a far more insidious impact on the heart. It now seems that prolonged tension—due to a demanding job, a rocky relationship, a chronically ill family member—can lead to persistently elevated blood pressure, or hypertension. And hypertension is a major cause of coronary disease and of heart attacks in those who have the disease.

The distressing evidence

When you're under stress, the body prepares for emergency action by flooding the blood with cortisol and adrenaline, hormones that boost blood pressure as well as blood-sugar levels, muscle tension, and heart rate. Those increases can last for hours, even after any obvious psychological pressure has eased. For some people, the psychological pressure seldom eases, so blood pressure seldom returns to normal. Eventually, the body may adjust to chronic stress by ratcheting its baseline blood pressure, or resting level, up into the hypertensive range.

In theory, even intermittent bouts of stress may lead to chronic hypertension, by changing the physical properties of the arteries. Studies have suggested that stress—or the surges in blood pressure triggered by stress—can eventually stimulate the growth of extra muscle in the artery walls. That additional bulk narrows and stiffens the vessels, increasing the resting blood pressure.

In the past year, three studies have provided the strongest evidence so far that chronic stress may indeed lead to chronic hypertension. In the most impressive of those studies, researchers from the ongoing Framingham Heart Study measured stress levels in some 1100 people and then checked their blood pressure annually for some 20 years. Middle-aged men (up to age 60) who scored highest on that stress scale were more than twice as likely to develop high blood pressure as the calmer middle-aged men.

While that study did not link chronic stress with hypertension in women, an earlier, three-year study of more than 450 middle-aged women by the same author, using the same psychological test, did find such a link. The author speculates that a stress-hypertension connection in women showed up only in the briefer study because that investigation started in the 1980s, when far more women worked outside the home than they did in the 1960s, when the longer study began.

ARE YOU STRESSED OUT?

The following test, used in the Framingham Heart Study, can provide a rough gauge of how much stress you experience. Answer yes or no:

___ Are you often troubled by feelings of tenseness, tightness, restlessness, or inability to relax?
___ Are you often bothered by nervousness or shaking?
___ Do you have trouble sleeping or falling asleep?
___ Do you feel that you are under a great deal of tension?
___ Do you often have trouble relaxing?
___ Do you often have periods of restlessness so that you cannot sit for long?
___ Do you often feel that difficulties are piling up too much for you to handle?

The more questions you answer "yes," the greater your probable level of stress, and the more you stand to benefit from stress-reduction techniques. The exact relationship between these test scores and the risk of hypertension is not clear for all age groups. But for middle-aged men and middle-aged working women, studies have shown that answering yes to at least five questions more than doubles the chance of developing high blood pressure.

Job stress may indeed play a major role in the development of hypertension, according to an ongoing series of studies from Cornell University Medical College. The researchers evaluated some 260 men who worked at various jobs in New York City. Those who had high-stress jobs—lots of pressure and little power to make decisions—were more than three times as likely to have hypertension as those in less stressful jobs. Three years later, the researchers retested nearly 200 of the men. The results, reported at an international conference in March, showed that resting blood pressure had increased in those who either stuck with a stressful job or switched to a more stressful one; those who shifted to a less demanding job now had lower blood pressure than before.

Of course, stress is partly subjective: What's stressful to one person—speaking in public, for example—may be routine or even enjoyable to another. Several small, prospective studies have found that people who react strongly to everyday frustrations like being stuck in traffic are at increased risk for developing hypertension. Late last year, the largest, longest study so far bolstered those findings. Researchers at the University of Pittsburgh School of Medicine measured the blood pressure of some 200 middle-aged people who were grappling with frustrating mental tasks while a computer punctuated every mistake by beeping. Those whose blood pressure jumped the most during that test experienced the greatest increases in resting blood pressure over the course of the next six years.

Taming stress

Those studies clearly support the notion that stress increases the risk of developing hypertension. Whether reducing stress actually reduces that risk is less clear. Here's a look at the evidence to date on the two major approaches to controlling stress.

■ **Learning to relax.** A grab bag of techniques known collectively as the cognitive-behavioral approach can help keep you calm: The cognitive part involves learning to think realistically, so you don't overreact when you're under pressure. The behavioral part mainly involves relaxation techniques, such as meditation, yoga, biofeedback, or muscle relaxation. Cognitive-behavioral methods can lower elevated blood pressure, at least temporarily; they can also help prevent stress from making blood pressure jump.

Consider, for example, the phenomenon of "white-coat hypertension." Roughly 20 percent of people who are diagnosed as hypertensive do not actually have sustained hypertension. They apparently get so nervous in potentially stressful situations—such as having a doctor or nurse strap a measuring cuff on their arm—that their blood pressure soars; if they take their own blood pressure at home, the readings are normal (see CRH, 2/94). Several studies have shown that those people can learn to keep their blood pressure normal in a stressful situation like being in a doctor's office by curbing fearful thoughts or by practicing relaxation.

The evidence is mixed on whether cognitive-behavioral methods can actually help prevent or treat hypertension. But studies may have failed to detect any sustained benefit from reducing stress simply because many of the people studied were not leading stressful lives in the first place. The few studies that have separately analyzed the results for tense individuals—those who have high levels of stress hormones or who easily get upset—do suggest that easing stress may lower resting blood pressure in people who are under a lot of stress.

■ **Working out.** Some physiological evidence suggests that aerobic exercise may blunt the transmission of the nerve signals that help spark physical and psychological tension. Whatever the mechanism, people do feel calmer, have lower blood pressure, and react less strongly to stress for several hours after they work out.

Some studies indicate that when people work out regularly, those benefits may persist. For example, at least four clinical trials have found that regular aerobic exercise helps keep blood pressure from jumping during a grueling, frustrating, or competitive test. That ability of exercise to blunt the effects of stress—combined with its apparent tendency to lower blood pressure regardless of stress—may help reduce the risk of hypertension. Three large observational studies, involving a total of some 25,000 people followed for as long as 15 years, have indeed found that physically fit individuals are less likely to develop hypertension than inactive individuals. However, intervention trials—the only way to confirm that connection—have not been performed.

A sensible step

Taking steps to control stress, either through cognitive-behavioral methods or exercise, seems like a sensible precaution. Stress may increase the risk of developing not only hypertension and coronary disease but also colon cancer (see last month's CRH). Stress may also impair immunity and increase susceptibility to infection. And stress can contribute to many lesser ailments, including asthma attacks, back pain, chronic fatigue, gastrointestinal symptoms, headaches, and insomnia. It stands to reason that reducing stress would reduce at least some of those risks. If nothing else, learning to stay calm will simply make you feel better.

ENERGY!

How to get more of it, use it better, keep it longer

GINI KOPECKY

Gini Kopecky is a New York City–based journalist who writes about health and human relationships.

How come some people have so much energy? Take Dr. Dean Ornish, president of the Preventive Medicine Research Institute in Sausalito, Calif. In a typical weekend he may travel from California to New York to Chicago and back to California. He directs six weeklong training programs a year for heart patients and others interested in improving their health, and he conducts seminars in hospitals in New York, Florida, Nebraska and Iowa teaching other practitioners to teach his training program, which has proven effective in reducing heart disease. He's developing a line of lowfat, vegetarian frozen dinners. He lectures, appears on television and serves as a dietary consultant to President and Mrs. Clinton and their chefs. And all of this is on top of his duties as an assistant clinical professor of medicine at the University of California at San Francisco School of Medicine and as an attending physician at California Pacific Medical Center in San Francisco. People sometimes say to him, "How do you keep up this pace?" His answer: "I don't feel stressed by it most of the time. When you can manage stress more effectively, you can accomplish even more without getting sick in the process."

Energy Types

Psychiatrist Ronald Fieve of Columbia University would probably classify Ornish as a hyperthymic personality—a type much admired in our culture. "These are the people who are slightly turned on or revved up," Dr. Fieve says. "They're highly motivated, active, successful, driven, interested in new things and involved in many things at once." Hyperthymics fall at the upper end of the normal range of human energy levels. (Some people whose energy is unnaturally suppressed by depression seem to be "transformed" into hyperthymics under the influence of antidepressant medications, but Fieve believes that such transformations only occur when a patient is genetically hyperthymic to begin with.) At the low end of the normal energy range are the hypothymics. "They're content to go to work, go home, go to bed," says Fieve. "Above the hyperthymics in energy are the hypomanics, who have even more energy but who start making judgment errors—getting speeding tickets, mismanaging money." Somewhere at this upper end of the human energy spectrum also come mild manic-depressives, who swing back and forth between energy highs and lows. "And then," Fieve says, "there's the full manic. That person goes to the hospital."

Nature and Nurture

Most of us occasionally visit the enviable hyperthymic energy state—when we're rushing to finish a pile of work before leaving on vacation, for example. But we can't live there full-time unless we've inherited the right energy genes, which developmental behavioral researcher Robert Plomin is now trying to locate in mice as a step toward locating them in humans. "Energy or activity level is probably more heritable than most personality traits," says Dr. Plomin, a professor in the College of Health and Human Development at Pennsylvania State University. "But that's not to say that environment has no influence."

Early environmental factors can foster or interfere with a high-energy life. But even negative factors can be overcome. Psychologist Mihaly Csikszentmihalyi of the University of Chicago, who has been studying people in their 70s, 80s and 90s who have achieved something important in life (such as earning a Nobel Prize), is surprised at how many were sickly children. "Some had life-threatening illnesses," he says. "And now they're so full of energy, you'd think they had that extra dose of health."

How did they become so energetic? How can we?

The Oomph of Optimism

Dr. Csikszentmihalyi believes that being raised with or cultivating a positive outlook, even in the face of adversity, fosters "un-self-conscious self-assurance," the opposite of a victim mentality, and he says it allows people to use their physical and mental energy to achieve their goals. Psychologist Michael Scheier of Carnegie Mellon University calls the same characteristic "dispositional optimism." When people who have it encounter setbacks, he says, "they renew their efforts and try to attain the goal," whereas those with negative expectations give up. "They'll put the problem out of mind and deny it exists, which, if the problem has a solution, is not an effective approach," says Dr. Scheier. An optimistic student who gets a poor grade, for example, might talk to the instructor about how to improve it or try studying differently, while a pessimistic student will ignore the problem or feel powerless to correct it.

"Optimism strongly affects achievement by increasing persistence," says Martin Seligman, a psychologist at the University of Pennsylvania. And optimism, he believes, can be learned. In his practice, Dr. Seligman encourages people to become more optimistic by having them challenge their negative beliefs—by asking themselves what evidence there is to support those beliefs, marshaling evidence to contradict them, devising less self-blaming or catastrophic explanations, and putting aside the negative thoughts when they hamper ability to perform.

Diet, Sleep and Exercise

Diet affects energy levels, and fat plays a particular role. "Fat makes you fat," says cardiologist James Rippe, director of the Center for Clinical and Lifestyle Research in Shrewsbury, Mass. "Ounce for ounce, it has more than twice the calories of carbohydrates or protein." Ever notice how quickly you tire when carrying a 10-pound bag of groceries? Carrying around an extra 10 pounds of fat has the same effect. The American Heart Association recommends that people reduce fat consumption to no more than 30% of their calorie intake. Rippe suggests 23%, and Ornish goes even lower, recommending a vegetarian diet high in fiber and complex carbohydrates and with no more than 10% fat. "If you go on a 30%-fat diet, in a way you get the worst of both worlds," says Ornish. "You're making big enough changes in your eating habits to feel a sense of deprivation but not enough to experience much benefit."

You can, of course, get a surge of energy from sugar or caffeine. But when the immediate effect wears off, you

Relax for Energy?

Strange as it may sound, learning to relax can boost your energy by enhancing your ability to focus and get things done. "When you're anxious, it's virtually impossible to focus, because there's too much static," says cardiologist Herbert Benson, chairman of the Mind/Body Medical Institute at Deaconess Hosptial and Harvard Medical School and coiner of the term relaxation response. "In the relaxation response, there's a quieting of the mind."

To induce the relaxation response, pick a word, sound, prayer or brief phrase that you like. Sit quietly in a comfortable position. Close your eyes, relax your muscles and breathe slowly and naturally, repeating the word silently with each exhalation. Assume a passive attitude. When thoughts intrude, gently dismiss them and return to your breathing. Continue breathing and repeating your word or phrase for 10 to 20 minutes, by which time you should be feeling an inner sense of calm. Practice once or twice daily. You can also induce the relaxation response while engaged in any activity that entails repetitive movement. Count armstrokes while swimming or footfalls while jogging, for example.

Dr. Benson claims that by itself the relaxation response counteracts the harmful effects of stress. But to harness the most energy, he says, you need a second step, which he terms the "maximum mind" principle. Once you've induced the relaxation response, expose yourself to positively reinforcing thoughts, images or readings related to the changes you want to make in your life, or turn immediately to a task you want to perform well. Research indicates, for example, that students who induce the relaxation response immediately before studying or taking exams perform better than those who practice it at other times, and that professionals who induce it immediately before brainstorming perform more creatively than those who don't.

discover you've only borrowed the energy—from yourself. "First comes the high, then the crash," says Ornish.

Surprisingly, cutting back on sleep to have more waking hours in which to get things done can also boost energy levels. During the later part of a normal night's sleep there's an increase in rapid eye movement, or REM, sleep. This is the dreaming stage, during which, it's theorized, we burn off excess "generalized drive"—psychological lingo for the basic energy that drives us. When we shorten REM sleep by getting up earlier, the theory goes, this energy accumulates. "We've shown that when you deprive laboratory animals of REM sleep, they become more active, more alert, more aggressive, less fearful of their environment and more willing to approach and explore novel things," says psychologist Robert Hicks of San Jose (Calif.) State University. Humans experience similar effects. "When people shorten sleep, one of the first things they notice is that rather than having less energy, they have more," he says. "And they may be less fearful and more aggressive in the way they approach their work."

But there's a trade-off. When tested on problem-solving ability, people who normally sleep six or fewer hours a night often come up short. "They tend to be more reactive than thoughtful, to act quickly and decisively within the range of things they know how to do," says Dr. Hicks. "But when a problem falls outside that range, they're less able to deal with it." What about people who claim to need only four hours of sleep a night? "Most 'short sleepers' take a lot of naps," he says. "They pile up sleep in other ways."

What about exercise? The paradox here is that you can get energy by expending energy. Because exercise makes you more oxygen efficient, you consume less oxygen when going about normal activities. "It's like improving the size of your engine," says Rippe. "If your engine is capable of doing 150 miles an hour, then when you're going 25 miles an hour, you're using less capacity." In addition, he says, people who exercise tend to carry less weight and hence to expend less energy carrying it. What's more, regular physical activity preserves lean muscle mass and strength and reduces stress. "One of the chief reasons exercise is such an energizer is that it makes us feel calm and at peace," says Rippe.

Nothing we don't already know, right? So why did a recent survey of men and women aged 40 and older find that, although almost all believed in the importance of exercise, 41% of the women and 33% of the men didn't exercise at all? Rippe thinks the problem is that many people mistakenly believe that exercise has to be punishing or that they have to exercise vigorously for at least 30 minutes in order to derive any health benefits from it. In fact, he says, you can get significant health benefits simply by incorporating a total of 30 minutes of moderate activity into your daily routine, such as brisk walking, gardening or climbing stairs. "This is a race won by the tortoise, not the hare," Rippe says.

Natural Light And Natural Settings

Better still if you exercise outdoors, where you can soak up some daylight. Psychiatrist Daniel Kripke of the University of California at San Diego has employed bright light—natural and artificial—as treatment for depression since 1981. "I don't want to make any recommendations until we've done more testing," he says. "But more testing will probably show that increased exposure to outdoor and bright interior light is good for health."

Other research suggests that being outdoors or even just gazing at certain natural settings may be good for health—and boost energy—for a different reason. Environmental psychologist Roger Ulrich of Texas A&M University in College Station believes that in more than a million years of evolution human beings may have learned to respond positively to certain types of natural settings—trees, open savannas and water—which our early ancestors found optimal for survival, and that being exposed to these settings may enhance functioning of the parasympathetic nervous system. This system helps restore energy following the fight-or-flight response to stress or threat.

"The parasympathetic nervous system is involved with physiological restoration in the sense of reducing energy consumption or even recharging energy," Dr. Ulrich says. "Blood pressure may go down, muscles may relax and brain electrical activity may alter in a way that suggests a more relaxed state." In one of Ulrich's studies, college students were shown an upsetting video about workplace accidents, followed either by a nature video or a video of man-made environments (streets and shopping malls). Ulrich found that the students shown the nature videos registered much more marked and rapid recovery from physiological stress than those who viewed the videos of man-made environments. "The effect occurred more quickly than we had anticipated—in about three minutes," says Ulrich.

Tapping Into the Power of the Mind

Even without exposure to natural settings, we can achieve an energizing state of relaxed wakefulness and apply it to improving our physical or mental performance wherever and whenever we choose, according to cardiologist Herbert Benson, chairman of the Mind/Body Medical Institute at Deaconess Hospital and Harvard Medical School. He originated the term relaxation response, which can be evoked by relaxation techniques including transcendental meditation and visualization, or guided imagery, the process by which some athletes improve their competitive performance by mentally rehearsing it beforehand (see "Relax for Energy?"). "It works for surgeons, artists, business executives—anyone trying to enhance performance," says psychologist Bruce Ogilvie of San Jose State University, who has trained Olympic athletes and other "high performance" men and women in this technique.

Much simplified, Dr. Ogilvie's training technique consists of guiding people through a relaxation exercise, then asking them to project themselves into a "beautiful, tranquil scene," vividly imagining it with all their senses—smell, sight, touch, taste, hearing. "I call that 'clearing the field,'" he says. Ogilvie then asks them to vividly recall or imagine a peak performance experience and describe it to him in detail, moment by moment, step by step, again employing all the senses. "That becomes the script," he says. "And we'll put that on tape as the person relates it to me." Clients then rehearse by reviewing this tape on their own.

Ogilvie also teaches them to quickly induce a state of relaxation immediately prior to their performance and to use self-affirming thoughts to attain "the highest level of poise and confidence," then to "let go" and let the mind and body give the performance they've been programmed to produce. "The essence is to lose your ego, defer judgment and evaluation and just be alive and receptive in pure form—to live in the moment, loving the process, deriving joy and pleasure from the experience," Ogilvie explains, adding, "It takes incredible self-discipline."

Time Management From the Inside Out

One characteristic Ogilvie's high-achieving men and women share is knowing where they want to go and what they want to accomplish. "These are people with high levels of aspiration," he says. "They have invariably written a script for themselves." In the lingo of the Covey Leadership Center in Provo, Utah, this is called "beginning with the end in mind." "It's important to have a direction and purpose," says A. Roger Merrill, vice president and cofounder of the center. "But there are two kinds of passion. One comes when we want something for ourselves. That's a selfish passion, which can create a great deal of heat but ultimately has a destructive element to it. The other is the passion to give, to contribute. That's a whole different kind of fire."

What if we don't have a clear sense of purpose? Merrill suggests trying the following exercise. Imagine it's your 80th birthday. Your friends and loved ones have gathered to honor you. One by one, they laud your accomplishments, your contributions, how you've touched their lives. What would you like to hear them say? Write down your fantasies. This is your "mission statement"—a list of your deepest and loftiest life goals, which will be made up of a number of subsidiary life goals, each pertaining to one of your life roles: as son or daughter, spouse, parent, friend, worker, neighbor, citizen.

Once you've completed your mission statement, you're ready to use it as a guide in organizing your time and your life. "We suggest weekly planning," says Merrill, "which gives you a better perspective on how you're using your time and prevents your getting lost in those urgent, important matters (crises, pressing problems, project deadlines) that we often allow to become so all-consuming that we neglect the nonurgent but important pursuits that make for a healthy, well-balanced life—exercising, furthering our education, tending to relationships, planning our economic future, allowing time for spiritual renewal, contributing to the common good. "The key isn't prioritizing your schedule," says Merrill. "It's scheduling your priorities."

Merrill cautions against squandering energy by letting other people's needs and demands dictate your life; spreading your energies too thin by taking on too many commitments; getting so caught up with urgent matters that you neglect the nonurgent but important pursuits; and scrambling madly up the ladder of success only to discover, once you've reached the top, that it's leaning against the wrong wall. "The deeper you connect with your most powerful motives, the more power you have to be strong in hard moments, to stay with something when the going gets tough," says Merrill. Even the drudge work that's part of working toward any goal may begin to feel less like drudgery. "It's that old story of two people laying bricks," he says. "One says to the other, 'What are you doing?' The other one says, 'Laying bricks. What are you doing?' The first one answers, 'Building a cathedral.'"

The Secrets of "Flow"

In the final analysis, according to Mihaly Csikszentmihalyi, the amount of energy we have may be less important than what we do with it. Take the once sickly, now high-energy, high-achieving elderly men and women he's been studying. "They invested their psychic energy in ways they felt were important," he says. "They forged a life that they felt in control of and that had purpose."

But what about those of us who aren't winning Nobel Prizes? How can we achieve the optimal-experience, boundless-energy state Csikszentmihalyi calls "flow"? One of the surest ways, he says, is by setting and pursuing challenging goals. "Without challenge, there's no growth. You can't experience yourself as an agent, and therefore your energies aren't being tapped."

"Activation energy is like priming the pump. Then things begin moving on their own."

One of the keys to achieving flow is matching challenge to skill by setting a goal that's difficult enough to force you to stretch but not so difficult as to be beyond your capabilities, which would only lead to anxiety and frustration. "You want to start by setting goals in areas of life where it's not so important what the goal is, so long as you have one," says Csikszentmihalyi. Begin, for example, by following a specific routine in the morning—getting up at a certain time, showering, brushing your teeth. The more successfully you meet such small goals, the more you'll begin to feel in control. From there you'll be able to go after larger goals, because you'll be starting with the feeling of security that comes from achieving the little things.

Learning to concentrate is also important; indeed, concentration to the point of losing all consciousness of yourself is a hallmark of flow. But it can be a difficult state to achieve if you don't find the task at hand interesting. The problem, says Csikszentmihalyi, is that you become distracted because you're not in flow, and you're not in flow because you're distracted. But you can break that vicious cycle by restructuring the task in a creative way. "You might say, 'All right, I have to do this report. Let's see if I can do it more quickly than last time.' Or, 'Let's see how many unnecessary sentences I can eliminate,'" suggests Csikszentmihalyi. "Set a small goal and then pay attention to whether you're achieving it. Then you'll get caught up in what you're doing."

Another tip: Make a list of the things you have to do, then do the least pleasant first. "If you can get rid of what you most hate doing, that will free up your energy," says Csikszentmihalyi. Remember also that no matter what the task, getting started is the hardest part. "In physics it's called activation energy," he says. "It's like priming the pump. It takes about 20 minutes, and then things begin moving on their own."

A common misconception is that high achievers don't have to struggle past this initial inertia. But they do. "To start cold on something is very difficult," says Csikszentmihalyi. "So people develop rituals as a way of getting into an almost self-hypnotic state in order to begin. The great philosopher Immanuel Kant used to gaze at the sunlight reflecting off a copper ball on a church spire before he started writing. Other people sharpen all their pencils and lay them out."

It's inevitable that as we grow and change, some of our goals will also change. But Csikszentmihalyi warns about abandoning goals or commitments too readily. "Certain goals are necessary to keep you from scattering your energies all over the place." he says. "If you're always asking, 'Should I give up on this?' that creates chaos. So you have to decide what things are really important to you—they may have to do with your job, with a relationship, with your beliefs—and decide that these are not negotiable."

This is not to say we should become rigid or take ourselves too seriously. That's an energy blocker too. "In our study of older people who've achieved great things, we're finding that at 80 and 90, these people are in some respects still like children—in their curiosity, their openness to what's going on around them, the way they don't prejudge things," says Csikszentmihalyi. "That open and playful attitude and willingness to change is what allows you to recognize possibilities and seize opportunities."

Out of the Blues

Walking regularly is turning out to be your best medicine for bad moods and bad days. Why? The answer is all in your head.

Kathleen McAuliffe

Kathleen McAuliffe is a freelance writer based in Miami. Her work has appeared in Omni, U.S. News & World Report, *and* The New York Times Magazine.

Laura G. had been feeling depressed, lonely, blah, so a psychiatrist suggested she try the antidepressant Prozac. After months of sessions and no luck with the wonder drug, she turned to another psychotherapist, Austin "Ozzie" Gontang. Therapy sessions were scheduled for sunrise. Almost miraculously, Laura's moods brightened; her lethargy went away.

What caused Laura to feel so much better? The catalyst wasn't a drug or talking about her childhood. Hardly. The cure was walking.

Surprisingly, perhaps, Laura's psychological experience isn't that far out. There's convincing clinical—and anecdotal—evidence that regular exercise improves self-esteem, reduces anxiety and hostility, and can even lift clinical depression.

How can something as simple as walking have such a profound effect on how you feel? Here's what researchers have to say.

Walk vs. Talk

Brisk walking ranks with the best talk therapies as a treatment for depression. Some studies even suggest that the long-term benefits of exercise may surpass the traditional tell-your-life-story cures.

In a landmark study conducted at the University of Wisconsin by psychiatrist John Greist, now at the Dean Foundation in Madison, exercise was compared to psychotherapy in the treatment of clinically depressed patients.

Although both groups were significantly improved by the end of the three-month study, they differed sharply a year later. A full 80% of the exercisers were symptom-free, whereas half of those who had received psychotherapy had returned for further treatment within the year.

TAKE TWO WALKS AND CALL ME

Scientists are finding out that walking affects your brain chemistry—and ultimately your moods—in two ways: by making you feel good and by keeping you from feeling bad.

An expert on this phenomenon is Keith Johnsgard, a clinical psychologist and professor at San Jose State University and the author of *The Exercise Prescription for Depression and Anxiety* (Plenum Press). According to Johnsgard, exercise is a mind-altering technique that brings about changes—sometimes for days at a time—in numerous chemical systems in the brain. There is ample evidence, for instance, that physical activity unleashes beta-endorphin, the natural opiate widely credited as the secret to "runner's high." But endorphin is only part of the story behind the psychological benefits of exercise—and perhaps only a small part at that.

Despite all the media hoopla surrounding endorphin, physical activity triggers a cascade of neuro-chemical events. Specifically, Johnsgard reports, researchers have found laboratory rats that exercise on a treadmill produce significantly higher levels of dopamine, norepinephrine, and serotonin. These, he notes, are the very brain compounds that antidepressant drugs are known to impact.

While most people report an immediate boost of spirit after working out, it usually takes three to five weeks of regular physical activity to lift a clinical depression. This is roughly the same amount of time it takes an antidepressant drug to begin to lift a clinical depression. Johnsgard believes this is more than a coincidence: He suspects that exercise mimics the neuro-chemical action of antidepressants.

Signs of Depression

Depression affects mood, thoughts, body, and behavior. The American Psychiatric Association recommends that you see your physician if you experience four or more of the following symptoms for more than two weeks:

- Significant loss or gain in weight
- Sleeping too much or too little
- Loss of interest in activities you once enjoyed
- Fatigue and loss of memory
- Inability to concentrate
- Recurring thoughts of death or suicide
- Overwhelming feelings of sadness or grief
- Headaches or stomach aches

In addition to juicing up our systems with all these "feel good" chemicals, regular exercise helps the body burn off stress hormones such as cortisol, which is found in abnormally high levels in stressed individuals.

In a recent survey, 98% of Walking *readers said that a primary reason for walking was to feel good afterward.*

"Regular exercise produces an antidote against stress even before it occurs," says University of Nebraska psychologist and exercise physiologist Wes Sime. He bases this claim on an ongoing study that compares how exercisers and non-exercisers react to a series of traumatic stimuli. Sime shows his subjects films of gruesome events such as the Holocaust and then gives them difficult cognitive tasks to perform in a hostile, competitive atmosphere. Early results appear to suggest that among the 50 people tested so far, regular exercisers who took part in the test produced less cortisol and other stress hormones than did their inactive counterparts.

"What this demonstrates is a conditioning effect," explains Sime. "The body uses the same system to deal with both physical and emotional stress. So, when we get ourselves in physical shape, it has a carryover effect in the mental realm."

AMERICA NEEDS TO WALK

Tonya C., a 24-year-old student, started walking briskly to help herself quit smoking. She kicked the habit—and much more. An unexpected benefit of her new exercise regimen is that her moods no longer control her life; she controls them. "People used to call me moody and ultra-sensitive. I was on an emotional roller coaster," she reports. "Now I don't have any more mood swings, and I'm a lot more confident around people."

Cathy L., a 26-year-old student from San Jose, Calif., experienced the same "mental transformation" when she started outrigger canoeing. "I was in therapy for a year and a half, but once I started paddling, I stopped going to therapy," she says. "I found the tool I needed to deal with my anxiety and confidence problems."

Why did three bright women—Laura, Tonya, Cathy—seek professional help to feel better? Why is the popularity of mood-lifting drugs increasing? Some say it's the curse of the couch potato. In our national effort to make life easy, we're making ourselves depressed and anxious.

According to the government's latest count, 12.6% of Americans are ridden with anxiety, and another 9.5% suffer from debilitating depression. Although we take this epidemic of malaise for granted today, Johnsgard insists that it is a comparatively new phenomenon that arose with the "good life"—arrival of automobiles, dishwashers, TVs, and all those other conveniences that have turned us into a nation of inert couch potatoes. As evidence, he cites several studies that show a gradual ten- to twentyfold increase in depression in the U.S. during this century—a trend that directly parallels the shift away from labor-intensive occupations to an increasingly mechanized, sedentary society.

"Americans," Johnsgard argues, "have become unnaturally depressed and anxious as a result of turning our backs on the active lifestyle which characterized all but our most recent past."

USE IT OR LOSE IT

To experience the mood-elevating impact of exercise, experts now believe that the frequency—rather than the type—of activ-

Therapy on the Move

"Talking it out" is now being paired with "walking it out" by a handful of energetic psychotherapists such as Ozzie Gontang and Keith Johnsgard, who practice therapy during walks or runs with their clients. Stress management and improvement of the self-concept of their clients are common goals cited by these pioneers. Also, they find that exercise is cathartic. "Feelings and creative thoughts come to mind a lot more easily while participating in exercise involving rhythmic flow of the body," reports University of Nebraska psychologist and exercise physiologist Wes Sime, who takes clients on a walk for a "good portion of the clinical hour, weather permitting."

Kate Hays, a clinical psychologist in private practice specializing in sports psychology in Concord, N.H., concurs: "Individuals who are extremely agitated or withdrawn will often open up while walking."

Your local hospital or athletic clinic may know of a walking therapist in your area.

ity is the most important factor. As little as 40 minutes of exercise three times a week has been demonstrated to lift depression.

But don't expect to maintain the gain for long if you revert back to your sedentary ways. A study by Sime at the University of Nebraska tracked patients whose depression had been alleviated through exercise almost a year earlier. Only those who remained active were still free of symptoms.

Those who make the effort to fit exercise into their schedule may find it a small price to pay for peace of mind. Indeed, exercise compares favorably with traditional therapy or drugs when you consider cost, convenience, and the exhilarating process of mastering a sport, which leaves little room for the feelings of helplessness and hopelessness that breed depression. As Johnsgard emphasizes, "Strenuous exercise is not something you can purchase and not something an expert does to you, for you, or with you. It is your very own virtually cost-free, self-administered, guaranteed intervention."

WORKING IT OUT

Even extreme phobic reactions may yield to exercise if it is creatively combined with other behavior-modification techniques. Johnsgard tells the dramatic story of a female patient who was debilitated by panic attacks that first struck when she was in a shopping mall and eventually confined her to her home. Her treatment consisted of running across a huge parking lot toward the entrance of the mall until she was completely breathless. The physical exhaustion she felt upon arrival at the feared target—no doubt coupled with the sedative effects of endorphin—made it impossible for her to experience a panic attack. This strategy also enabled her to reinterpret symptoms normally associated with a panic attack in a more positive light. Her elevated heart rate and strained breathing, for example, could now be attributed to the healthful effects of running. By repeating this routine over a number of days, she ultimately gained the confidence to return to public places unescorted.

Johnsgard credits the British psychologist Arnold Orwin with pioneering this approach, and notes that Orwin has used variations of it to successfully treat more than 100 patients hospitalized with agoraphobia (fear of open spaces) and other disorders.

To be sure, some phobias and depressions are so severe that exercise alone will not be sufficient to bring relief. In such intractable cases, Johnsgard would be the first to admit that all the tools of modern medicine may need to be brought to bear. But for most of us, walking may be enough to ward off the periodic stresses and strains of life. "To be blessed," says Johnsgard, "all we have to do is behave the way we were designed to work the best."

Depression

Way Beyond the Blues

Sandra Arbetter

Maria hasn't smiled in a month. Not even when her terrier rushes around in circles trying to bite his tail. Not even when her boyfriend lip-synchs to the Spin Doctors. Either of those things used to set her to howling, but lately she just wants to stay in her room and sleep, and it's a struggle for her to get up in the morning and go to school.

Andy, on the other hand, is always smiling. He talks nonstop, and his energy is endless. He jumps into things without a second thought—he drives too fast, drinks alcohol, and can't wait to bungee jump. At night his mind races over the next day's activities, until he finally falls into a restless sleep.

Which of these two may be depressed? If you say Maria, you're right. And if you say Andy, you're right, too. Even though they act very differently, they both are in the midst of a long period of depression. If you say that's confusing, you're right again. Depression is a murky pool of feelings and actions that scientists have been trying to plumb since the days of Hippocrates, who called it a "black bile."

To further muddy the waters, feelings of depression come and go in most of us from time to time. But short periods of sadness or hyperactivity don't mean clinical depression.

Clinical depression is severe enough to require treatment. It lasts a longer time than the blues—at least two weeks—and it interferes with daily life—school, friends, family. It's considered a medical disorder and can affect thoughts, feelings, physical health, and behaviors. Here's what it's not: It's NOT a personality weakness or a moral lapse. And it's NOT the fault of the person who is depressed.

Diagnosing depression in a teenager is not easy, says Dr. Richard Marohn, past president of the American Society of Adolescent Psychiatry. That's because it's normal for teens to have mood swings—within limits.

It's a confusing time of life, says Marohn. For one thing, the teen's body is changing. Teenagers have little control over those changes. Secondly, their relationship with parents is changing, and teens are pulled between

Science Whips Up a Moral Dilemma

Ron was a pleasant, quiet boy who liked to spend time by himself, mostly with his computer. His mother said he "moved at his own pace," which was a bit slower than the rest of the family.

When Ron was 17, he withdrew further from others, stopped showering and shampooing, and even lost his interest in computers. His parents arranged for him to see a psychiatrist, who prescribed an antidepressant medication.

To say he responded well would be an understatement. He was peppier than ever before, moved faster, laughed more readily, liked being with people, went from being a B to an A student, and got a girlfriend.

His doctor was pleased—but puzzled. Now that Ron was no longer depressed, should he go off medication and return to his former quiet self? Or should he stay on medication and retain his livelier, more confident personality? Did the medication uncover the "real" Ron who had lived a lifetime beneath a cover of chronic, mild depression? Or did it create a false self?

Antidepressants are designed to relieve the symptoms of depression. But is it OK to use them as what one doctor called "mood brighteners"? That's the question posed by author Peter Kramer, M.D.

Mental health experts express the concern that we will look to a pill to make us feel better and we'll ignore the external problems in our world. Some fear that antidepressants interfere with reality by making things look more positive. Or could it be that depression distorts reality by making things look more grim?

the security of home and the challenge of testing out their own beliefs.

So how do you tell if it's depression? Time tells, says Marohn. If your feelings affect your schoolwork, your activities, your relationship with family and friends, then it's beyond normal.

Suicidal urges and plans are also a warning sign. But even that's not surefire, because lots of teens have transient thoughts of suicide.

Finally, adolescent depression is difficult to diagnose because adolescents don't necessarily look sad and depressed. To be a teen means to externalize feelings and deal with the world through action. So depression may show up as truancy, running away, violent behavior, or substance abuse. Teens may self-medicate with alcohol or other drugs to try to feel better.

WHAT IS DEPRESSION?

Lots of people assume they know what depression is because they've had at least a touch of it. It's natural to feel sad when you're hit by one of life's inevitable losses. It's a loss when you start kindergarten and give up the safety of home. It's a loss when you move to a new house and leave the old one behind. It's a loss to break up with a boyfriend or girlfriend, and it's even worse when he or she is doing the breaking up.

The sadness that comes with events like these can be intense at first, but usually mellows in a short while. If you get back to a relatively normal state in a week or so, there's nothing to worry about. But if feelings of great sadness or agitation last for much more than two weeks, it may be depression.

Depressed feelings after a major loss, such as the death of a loved one, last much longer, and no one expects recovery in a week or two. Experts won't make a diagnosis of depression (at least, not right away) if a person has had a recent major loss. They'll also hold off if a person is taking certain medications or has certain illnesses that bring on depression-like symptoms.

How Antidepressants Work

Antidepressants help people feel better by affecting neurotransmitters and, in turn, brain function. Neurotransmitters are brain chemicals that help nerve cells communicate with each other. Certain ones are thought to control feelings of security and alertness.

Although the specific effects have not been worked out, it is though that antidepressants work by helping to regulate the dysfunction in the brain that is causing a person to feel depressed.

CHECK THESE SYMPTOMS

Changes in habits and personality are clues to depression. Here are some specifics:

1. There's no interest in school and grades fall.
2. Being with friends holds absolutely no appeal.
3. Sleep problems are common—either not being able to fall asleep at night or wanting to sleep all day.
4. Appetite is out of whack. There's either no desire for food, or the person seems to be eating all the time.
5. The person is obsessed with thoughts of death, maybe suicide. It's estimated that 15 percent of people with major depression commit suicide, and many more attempt it. There are 6,000 suicides by adolescents each year, and depression is the biggest risk factor.
6. Everything seems hopeless, and there's the feeling it will never get better.
7. Headaches, stomachaches, or other aches and pains appear.
8. It's impossible to concentrate or make a decision.

WHAT IT FEELS LIKE

Anyone who's ever felt sad has only the barest clue as to what major depression is like, according to one 16-year-old who recently spent three weeks in a hospital after taking an overdose of pills.

"I had this buzzing in my head all the time," says Emmy, a small, dark-haired girl with large brown eyes. "And I felt tired. I didn't want to do anything except lie on my bed and listen to tapes. When my friends called, I didn't feel like talking to them. I knew they were getting mad, and sometimes I'd try to talk on the phone, but I couldn't push the words up out of my throat."

Emmy had always been a good student and had managed a B+ average while holding a job at a discount store and swimming in competition. Her father was a building contractor, and her mother was a secretary.

"My mother never liked her job, and she kept telling me that I needed to get into a good college so I could be a lawyer and have a happier life than she had. I know now that she was struggling with her own problems, but I used to worry all the time that I was disappointing her. I wanted so badly to be an A student, but no matter how hard I studied, I couldn't pull it off.

"Then I just started not caring. Nothing special happened; I just shut down. I felt so alone, like I was living in a bubble and couldn't punch my way out. I felt like screaming so someone would notice me.

"And I was so tired all the time. Nobody can understand that. I wasn't tired physically like after a swim meet or staying up late. I was tired in every cell of my body, so that I couldn't think straight, and it was too much of an effort to eat. Finally, one day I decided it was too much of an effort to live. That's when I took the pills."

The doctor prescribed an antidepressant drug for Emmy for about six months, and she and her parents were in family therapy for more than a year. She's a junior now and planning to go to college to study environmental sciences. Her mother is in law school.

DEPRESSION IS A MIXED BAG

For a long time, people who were feeling depressed were told to "snap out of it," and, if they didn't, people said they had a flaw in their personality. That's simply not true and only added guilt to the heavy burden these people were already carrying.

Research in the last decade or two has shown, first of all, that there are several kinds of depression and a multitude of causes.

•Major depression: More than one episode of clinical depression is considered major depression, an illness marked by hopeless feelings, inability to feel pleasure, physical changes or complaints, thoughts of death and suicide. The Public Health Service estimates that 11 million people in this country have episodes of major depression, women outnumbering men more than 2 to 1.

•Bipolar disorder (also known as manic-depressive disorder): A person with this illness alternates between periods of high activity, or mania, and periods of hopelessness or depression.

In the manic phase, people may talk a lot—and fast. They have feelings of greatness and think nothing is beyond them. They've been known to go days without sleeping. They've got lots of thoughts racing through their mind at once. They often act on these thoughts and get into trouble because of their behaviors. So, if you have a friend who is in the manic phase of this illness, don't be surprised if you get a call at three in the morning about his or her plans to save the earth.

Bipolar disorder occurs in about 1 percent of the population, or about 2 million people, equally in men and women. Bipolar disorder can take years to develop into its classic form. When a bipolar disorder emerges during adolescence, it's sometimes hard to distinguish it from the normal emotional ups and downs associated with that age.

•Seasonal Affective Disorder, or SAD: It's not exactly a news flash that most people feel better when the weather is sunny and bright than when it's gloomy. But for some people, wintry weather brings on feelings of depression. Here's one explanation: Many of the body's functions operate on circadian cycles, which are about 24 hours in length. Lack of light puts these cycles out of whack. One treatment is to have patients sit under bright lights for a few hours each day.

•Dysthymia: This is low-level chronic depression. It's usually not severe enough to put someone in the hospital, or to prompt suicide, but it robs a person of the capacity to take pleasure in living.

WHY, OH, WHY?

Experts don't completely understand the causes of depression, but there seems to be an important interplay of two factors: environmental and biological.

Environmental factors include such events as death of a parent, parents' divorce, physical or emotional abuse, family violence, and other difficult family relationships. A depressive episode can be triggered by moving, graduating, losing a job, winning an award, or a hundred other life changes. It can be related to emotional conflicts within the person, such as a past experience that was not resolved. It's been described as "anger turned inward." Or it can come on for no apparent reason.

Biological factors, primarily changes in brain function, are an important aspect of depression. It is not known whether the observed changes in the function cause depression, or whether depression from some other cause accounts for the changes in brain function.

There seems to be a genetic factor involved, too. A child whose parent has suffered from depression has a greater chance of developing the illness than a child with no family history of depression.

TREATMENT

Major approaches to helping depression are medication and psychotherapy, or counseling. Experts say upward of 80 percent of people with depression can be helped.

Medications affect brain function and reduce the symptoms of depression but do not provide a cure. All antidepressants have side effects. Experts worry that people will think of them as magic potions and not accept responsibility for their own behaviors. (See "Science Whips Up a Moral Dilemma".) Finally, parents are cautious about allowing medications for their children.

Psychiatrist Richard Marohn says that many experts view adolescent depression as short-lived and say treatment should deal with underlying issues rather than the symptoms themselves. Therefore, "talk therapy" is preferable and "most of us working with adolescents tend to stay away from medication." Exceptions are suicidal behaviors and depression that's been going on since childhood.

Dr. Marohn says he is concerned about the increasing lack of mental health services. "Kids wind up in prison," he says, rather than in hospitals where treatment is available and they may get some help.

TALKING IT OUT

Some experts say the most effective treatment for severe depression is a combination of medication and counseling. Counseling can help by making people aware of negative thought patterns, such as: "If I'm not perfect, people will think less of me." Or, "If I fail this test, it means I'll always be a failure." It can improve a person's ability to get along with others and to understand him- or herself better. It can bolster self-esteem.

What's more, there are lots of things people can do on their own to help themselves feel better. Michael Maloney and Rachel Kranz, authors of *Straight Talk About Anxiety and Depression,* suggest these:

•Try to focus on the positives about yourself rather than the negatives.
•Accept the fact that others aren't perfect. Then you won't be disappointed when they act human.
•Accept that you aren't perfect, either.
•Enjoy the present moment. Stop regretting the past and worrying about the future.
•Take care of yourself physically. Eat well, exercise, get plenty of sleep.
•Do something nice for yourself.
•Improve your surroundings. Clean your closet. Get a new poster. Surround yourself with things you like to look at.
• Talk to someone. Call up a friend you trust, or start a conversation with a neighbor to prove you *can* connect.
•Indulge your feelings. Let yourself cry and wallow in sad songs. But only for a little while.

Depression is one of the most common mental illnesses of our era and responds well to treatment. So while people don't do anything to make themselves feel bad, they *can* do something to make themselves feel better. A generation ago, there was a comic strip character named Arthur, who walked everywhere with a cloud over his head. If he knew then what you know now, he'd reach up and pull out a silver lining.

How to Help a Friend Who Is Depressed

Sometimes it's more difficult to help others than to help yourself. But here are some things to think about if a friend seems depressed.

1. Make an effort to be with your friend, even though it might not be easy. Depressed people tend to feel isolated.
2. Don't use false cheerfulness. Your friend may feel you aren't taking the problem seriously.
3. Don't blame. Depression is no one's fault.
4. Don't get angry. It's nothing personal if your friend doesn't respond to your help.
5. Express your own feelings. If you don't want to listen to your friend's woes again, just say so. Go out and have fun and don't feel guilty.
6. Get adult help. If your friend talks about suicide, or you're worried for any other reason, talk to your parents, your friend's parents, your school counselor. It's not a breach of loyalty to save a friend's life.

FOR MORE INFORMATION

American Psychiatric Association
1400 K St. NW
Washington, DC 20005
Pamphlets: "Depression," Manic-Depressive Disorder," "Teen Suicide," single copy of each free. Booklet: "Let's Talk About It," $1 per copy. Also available in Spanish.

S. James
Consumer Information Center-3C
P.O. Box 100
Pueblo, CO 81002
Pamphlets: #564z "What To Do When A Friend Is Depressed—A Guide For Teenagers," #566z "You Are Not Alone," single copy of each free.

National Mental Health Association
1021 Prince St.
Alexandria, VA 22314-2971
Pamphlets: "Adolescent Depression," "Adolescent Suicide," single copy of each free with self-addressed, stamped business-size envelope.

American Academy of Pediatrics
Dept. C-Depression
P.O. Box 927
Elk Grove Village, IL 60009-0927
Pamphlet: "Surviving: Coping With Adolescent Depression/Suicide," single copy free with self-addressed, stamped business-size envelope.

Drugs and Health

As a culture, Americans have come to rely on drugs not only as a treatment for disease, but as an aid for living normal, productive lives. This view of drugs has fostered both a casual attitude regarding their use and a tremendous drug abuse problem. The term "drug abuse" conjures up visions of derelicts, dark alleys, and wasted lives. In reality, this description is accurate for only a small minority of drug users. This is not to say that drugs are not responsible for destroying many lives, but rather that drug abuse has become so widespread that there is no way to describe the typical drug abuser, except to say that he or she could be anyone. What constitutes abuse varies, depending on the drug used and the circumstances in which it is used. Based on current trends, it seems likely that the problems of drug abuse will remain as long as attitudes toward drugs remain so casual.

What accounts for this casual attitude toward drug usage? There is no simple explanation for why America has become a drug-taking culture, but there is certainly evidence to suggest some of the factors that have contributed to this development. From the time that we are children, we are constantly bombarded by advertisements about how certain drugs can make us feel and look better. While most of these ads deal with proprietary drugs, the belief is created that drugs are a legitimate and effective way to help us cope with everyday problems. Growing up, most of us probably had a medicine cabinet full of over-the-counter (OTC) drugs, freely dispensed to family members to treat a variety of ailments. This familiarity with OTC drugs, coupled with rising health care costs, has prompted many people to diagnose and medicate themselves with OTC medications without sufficient knowledge of their possible side effects. "OTC Drugs: Prescription for Danger?" discusses the hazards associated with using OTC drugs.

Over the last few years, the Food and Drug Administration (FDA) has come under increasing pressure to expedite its drug approval process so that experimental drugs used to treat conditions such as AIDS, Alzheimer's disease, and cancer can be made available to U.S. citizens much sooner than the typical 12-year waiting period. The FDA has responded by initiating the investigational new drug program (IND) that makes experimental drugs available to desperately ill patients. This change in policy on the part of the FDA may help save some lives, but it will most certainly raise many new questions regarding how new drugs are to be evaluated. The evaluation process is confounded even further when one considers recent findings concerning the placebo effect. Recent investigations concerning the placebo effect have turned up new evidence that suggests that the placebo effect is twice as powerful as was previously thought. These findings have prompted some researchers to call for stricter standards for testing new medications. How these findings will influence the FDA's approval process is unclear, but it will certainly be interesting to watch. Daniel Goleman's article "Placebo Effect Is Shown to Be Twice as Powerful as Expected" raises some interesting questions regarding the nature of drug testing and suggests that in certain instances, the placebo effect may be an important tool for bolstering the body's own healing powers.

Of the drug problems facing this nation, alcohol use is clearly one of the most complex. This complexity stems from the ambivalence we feel regarding its use. While we deplore alcohol for the countless deaths and disabilities it accounts for each year, we openly sanction moderate use of alcohol in a variety of social situations. This ambivalence regarding alcohol use even permeates the scientific community. While it is clear that heavy alcohol use results in significant damage to a variety of organ systems, the same cannot be said of moderate use. In fact, the scientific community is currently wrestling with this issue regarding cancer and coronary artery disease. Several recent studies have reported that moderate alcohol use increases a woman's risk of breast cancer, and, at the same time, several studies have suggested that moderate alcohol use may help prevent coronary artery disease. What is the public to think in response to reports such as these? "Does Moderate Alcohol Consumption Prolong Life?" examines the controversy and concludes that while the research appears to demonstrate a positive correlation between moderate alcohol use and longevity, the personal and societal costs associated with alcohol abuse must be factored into the equation. The article "Alcohol in Perspective" discusses how our ambivalence toward alcohol contributes to the problem of alcohol misuse and abuse. This article also examines the physiological effects of alcohol and concludes that physiological differences between men and women may explain why excessive drinking appears to have more serious long-term consequences for women.

Few people today continue to harbor any misconceptions about the health hazards caused by the prolonged use of tobacco. Most realize that this drug is associated with emphysema, lung cancer, strokes, and heart disease, but they may not be aware that smoking can cause retinal damage, impotence, cold fingers, and low back pains. Kristine Napier's article "Alcohol and Tobacco: A Deadly Duo" is particularly interesting because, in addition to presenting the health hazards of this dual addiction, it discusses why drinkers are heavier smokers. Given the amount of bad press that tobacco has had over the last few years, why is it that so many Americans continue to smoke? Perhaps the answer is nicotine. Recent studies indicate that nicotine is as addictive as heroin; thus, smoking is an addiction rather than merely a habit. "Kicking Butts" by Carl Sherman discusses the process of quitting smoking and suggests that for many smokers, the drug nicotine not only gives pleasure, but it eases pain.

Unit 4

One of the unique characteristics of smoking cigarettes is that the smoker has precise fingertip control over the dosage that is taken. This factor coupled with the mood elevation that is associated with nicotine make it particularly difficult for a smoker to quit. The addiction to nicotine by some smokers is so strong that even if they do stop smoking they will always need to get nicotine from somewhere just to feel normal. Another area of concern regarding tobacco use has to do with a form of smokeless tobacco called snuff. The popularity of snuff is largely due to the fact that many famous professional athletes use it, leading their admiring young fans to believe that it is relatively harmless. The sad truth is that smokeless tobacco also poses a real health threat to the user.

Prozac, a drug that has stirred considerable controversy since its introduction, may have touched off a pharmacological revolution. Initially Prozac, an antidepressant, was developed and approved as a psychotherapeutic drug for treating clinical depression. Today Prozac is being prescribed by general practitioners not for the treatment of mental illness, but as an aid to healthy people to make them feel more cheerful and mellow. The success of Prozac has stirred the pharmaceutical industry to investigate the possibility of manufacturing various drugs that could be used by healthy individuals to enhance their enjoyment of life. Some researchers have even suggested that it may one day be possible to purchase drugs capable of modifying one's personality. "One Pill Makes You Larger, and One Pill Makes You Small . . ." by Sharon Begley discusses how Prozac is changing the way the medical and pharmaceutical community views drugs. Prozac is the first drug, other than the birth control pill, that is being prescribed for healthy people. Begley argues that even if the pharmaceutical industry is capable of producing drugs that can modify specific personality traits, that does not necessarily make it the right thing to do.

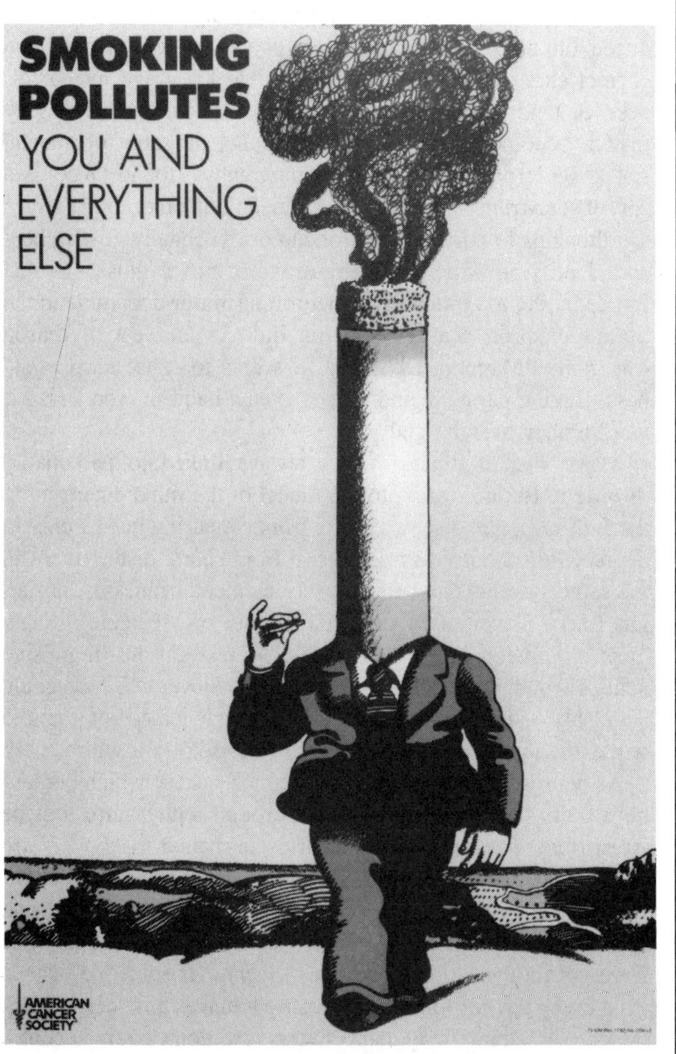

For years we have heard our political leaders declare that we are in the midst of a drug war, but who is the enemy in this war? As a culture, we have grown up believing that there is, or should be, a drug to treat any malady or discomfort that befalls us. The pharmaceutical industry, driven by profits, has responded to this demand as have the illicit drug dealers. Would we have a drug problem if there was no demand for drugs? We have seen the enemy and it is us!

Looking Ahead: Challenge Questions

Do you think America has a drug problem? Why or why not?

How do you feel about drug companies manufacturing drugs that you could use to modify your personality?

How might a person decide when drug use has become drug abuse?

What responsibility does the U.S. government have in the area of drug abuse?

What responsibility do communities have in the area of drug abuse?

Should insurance companies pay medical costs incurred as a result of drug abuse?

Given societies ambivalence toward alcohol, how can we best curb the problem of alcohol abuse?

What restrictions, if any, should be placed on the use of tobacco products?

Recently the mass media has been charged with contributing to the growing drug problem by portraying drugs in an appealing manner. Do you feel this charge is justified? Why or why not?

Some states are considering passing laws that would make it a crime to abuse drugs during pregnancy. How do you feel about this?

One pill makes you larger, And one pill makes you small . . .

BEYOND PROZAC: Scientific insights into the brain are raising the prospect of made-to-order, off-the-shelf personalities

Sharon Begley

. . . That was 1960s pharmacology. In that turned-on, tuned-out decade, the pharmacopeia of mind-altering drugs was about as subtle as a sledgehammer—uppers replaced sleep, downers offered calm, hallucinogens projected visions of marmalade skies into the brain. Many of them were illegal, and all of them threatened to stop the heart, blow out neurons or cause permanent addiction. This is 1990s pharmacology: suffering stage fright before delivcring a speech? Pop a little orange pill. Moping around in the winter doldrums? Try a white one. Want to boost your self-esteem, focus better on your work, tame the impulse to shop till you drop, shrug off your spouse's habit of littering the floor with underwear, overcome your shyness or keep yourself from blurting out your deepest secrets to the first stranger who comes along? Science has, or soon will have, just the legal, doctor-prescribed pill for you.

It's gone beyond Prozac. That antidepressant has spawned a culture of pill poppers: people who do not suffer from severe depression (for which the Food and Drug Administration approved Prozac in 1987) but who find that the little green and white capsule makes them more cheerful, more mellow, more self-assured. Now the same scientific insights into the brain that led to the development of Prozac are raising the prospect of nothing less than made-to-order, off-the-shelf personalities. For good or ill, research that once mapped the frontiers of disease—indentifying the brain chemistry involved in depression, paranoia and schizophrenia—is today closing in on the chemistry of normal personality. As a result, researchers are on the verge of "chemical attempts to modify character," writes neuropsychiatrist Richard Restak in the soon-to-be-published "Receptors." Most of the new drugs will be aimed not so much at 'patients' as at people who are already functioning on a high level . . . enriching [their] memory, enhancing intelligence, heightening concentration, and altering for the good people's internal moods."

That prospect has brought psychopharmacology—the science of drugs that affect the mind—to "the brink of revolution," as psychiatrist Stuart Yudofsky of Baylor University puts it. It is a revolution propelled by three advances. First came the theory that every memory, every emotion, every aspect of temperament originates in molecules called neurotransmitters. These chemical signals course through specialized circuits in the brain. Research on brain chemistry starting in the 1940s produced lithium, Valium and other psychoactive drugs, which correct chemical imbalances responsible for grave mental illness. Second, "brain mapping" pinpoints which areas of gray matter become active during particular thoughts or mental states. PET (positron emission tomography), for instance, is a sort of sonogram of the brain that can, among other things, trace sad thoughts to parts of the frontal cortex. Finally, researchers are identifying which neurotransmitters travel those circuits. For example, too much of the neurotransmitter dopamine in the brain's emotion centers, and too little in the seat of reason (diagram, "Mapping the Mind"), seems to cause suspiciousness—raving paranoia and maybe even a habit of wondering if the plumber overcharged you.

Major mental illness wasn't always linked to personality disorders. But according to the model of the mind emerging in the 1990s, mental disease differs from endearing quirks only in degree. Personality disorders arise from *subtle* disturbances in the same systems that produce serious mental illnesses, argues Dr. Larry Siever of Mount Sinai School of Medicine in New York. "Someone just barely able to restrain his impulsive actions wouldn't [seem] psychotic," says Siever. "But he could act rashly"—habitually ducking into a movie instead of going to work, or buying unseen property in Florida on a whim.

As neuroscientists learn what chemicals cause which personality traits, the temptation to fool around with nature will be irresistible. The drugs that perform the mental makeovers are supposed to have no serious side effects and not cause addiction. But more than 40 years of psychoactive drugs has proved that nothing is without hazard (at first, Valium, cocaine, and nicotine were not thought to be addictive, either). "If someone takes a drug every day for four years because it makes him feel or work better, something may happen that we don't know about," warns psychiatrist Solomon Snyder of Johns Hopkins University. That caution, however, has a difficult time standing up against the Faustian power of the new drugs. "For the first time in human history," says Restak, "we will be in a position to design our own brain." Some of the targets:

SHYNESS AND HYPERSENSITIVITY

Of all the traits that bedevil humans, shyness may be the most hard-wired into the brain. About 20 percent of people start life with neurochemistry that predisposes them to be shy, concludes Harvard University psychologist Jerome Kagan; the other 80 percent become shy or outgoing because of life's experiences. Now scientists may have figured out how biology becomes destiny. An inhibited child seems to be born with what amounts to a hairtrigger brain circuit: compared with other children, it takes much less to stimulate his amygdala, a small cashew-shaped structure deep in the brain that helps control heart rate and perspiration. No wonder shy infants squirm and cry: even mild stress makes their hearts pound and their palms sweat. In addition, inhibited children may have excessive levels of the neurotransmitter norepinephrine, a cousin of the fight-or-flight chemical adrenaline: just walking into kindergarten for the first time produces as much stress as a gladiator's facing the lions. "I think the time will come when we will know exactly the chemical profile of the temperamentally fearful child," says Kagan. "Then pharmacologists could work on very specific cures."

In some people, shyness is not a primary trait but instead a means of coping. "So much of social interaction is based on unspoken rhythms and pacing," says Mount Sinai's Siever, "that people who don't get those beats often feel left out and alienated"—like the woman who can't tell from body language that the man she's chatting with wants to flee. Society perceives her as slightly strange; she responds by withdrawing. Siever suspects that suspiciousness and an inability to process the information contained in the rhythms and cues of social interactions arise from an oversupply of dopamine in the brain's emotion-control room and a shortage in the more rational cortex.

One jobless, fiftyish man seemed to fit this description perfectly. He lived alone, filled his days with crossword puzzles and TV, and "worried that others were making fun of him,"

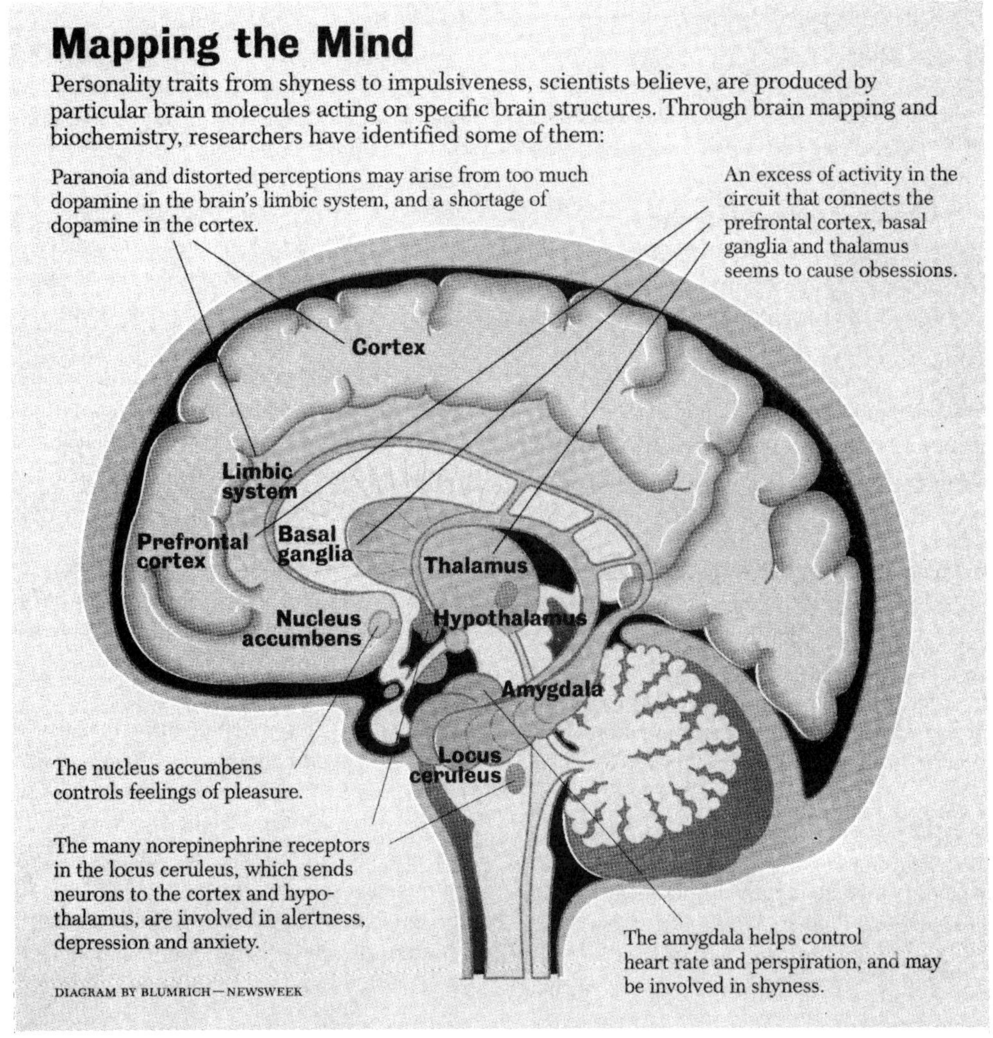

says Siever. Like all of Siever's patients, he was seriously ill. Siever suspected, based on biochemical tests, that the man's inability to understand social cues stemmed from a dopamine imbalance. The antidepressant Wellbutrin, which stokes the cortex with dopamine, seemed to help: the man felt sharper and "more activated" (though a back disability kept him from working). Still, scientists caution that what works on the seriously ill might have no effect on someone who decides to cure her lack of social grace with a pill when all she needs is a crash course in etiquette.

Shyness can also grow in the shadow of hypersensitivity, the tendency to fall into a deep funk over even an innocuous rejection. For years, psychiatrist Donald Klein of Columbia-Presbyterian Medical Center in New York had noticed something strange about this funk: it closely resembled the reaction of an amphetamine user suffering withdrawal symptoms. That sparked a bold theory. "The brain is normally making its own stimulant," which keeps people on an even keel, and even makes them outgoing, says Klein. Some people who embarrass easily and cower at the very thought of rejection may do so because their brain does not pump out enough stimulants. They become physically pained by rejection just as a speed freak is physically pained by going cold turkey. "Recently we have shown that we can treat this by preserving the balance of stimulants in the brain and so blocking the withdrawal symptoms," says Klein. He and Columbia's Michael Liebowitz give hypersensitive patients Nardil, the trade name for a substance that blocks the destruction of the brain's natural uppers. As a result, it restores a healthy chemical balance in the hypersensitive mind. "With pills twice a day you usually see results in six weeks," says Klein.

IMPULSIVENESS AND OBSESSION

Just about everyone has, at one time or another, succumbed to the impulse to buy those goodies at the supermarket checkout. In more severe forms, such impulsive behavior expresses itself as kleptomania and other mental illnesses whose sufferers act first and think second. But mild or severe, impulsivity may arise from the inability to learn that behaviors have consequences, like punishment, and so must be controlled or modified.

Depending on where the impulsivity comes from, psychopharmacologists may soon know how to stifle it. As a teenager, did you repeatedly stay out until dawn despite getting grounded for it every time? Are you prone to doing what gets you fired? The problem may stem from too little serotonin, the chemical whose job it is to censor behavior that previously led to punishment, says Siever. Shortages of serotonin in the frontal lobes and in the brain's limbic system, where emotions come from, also seem to lift the lid off impulses. In this case, the dearth of serotonin seems to have the same effect as a shortage of ink in which to write life's lessons: the person is unable to connect disagreeable consequences with what provoked them. Or the problem may simply be an inept working memory. (*But Mom, I forgot you wanted me home!*) Working memory stores information while the mind considers whether it is worth keeping and how to file it. Working memory falters without enough dopamine.

There's a final suspect in impulsivity. Noticing everything can be as debilitating as noticing nothing. Norepinephrine tells the mind what's important by, in effect, putting a chemical red flag on it to say, "Look at this!" In normal people that system kicks in when, for instance, a lion is charging. But in people with too much norepinephrine *everything* gets pumped up. Every perceived slight from a co-worker demands a response, every twinge of desire becomes an irresistible urge to buy.

If impulsives think about their actions too little, obsessives think about them too much. When Mother double-checks that the sleeping children are indeed breathing, and when she's a stickler about dirt on the carpets or grime in the kitchen, she is being mildly compulsive; when she checks 100 times, vacuums 20 times a day and goes through Fantastik like an alcoholic through rotgut, she is manifesting obsessive-compulsive disorder. Sufferers seem unable to get a sense of completeness from any action, like scrubbing the bathtub a mere once. Brain imaging is now showing such obsession in living color. PET scans of a patient touched with a dirty rag—cleanliness is a typical obsession—show a response like a broken record. Signals travel between three structures in the brain stem—the prefrontal cortex, the basal ganglia and the thalamus—endlessly. In normal people, the signal stops after one orbit thanks to a new message, screaming, "*The floor is clean already!*" "Lots of people have milder variants of this," says neuroscientist Lewis Baxter of the University of California, Los Angeles. "They check the stove two times, though not 102. They say that intellectually they know the stove is OK, but they can't get the *emotional* boost that says, 'Hey, it's working'." Baxter believes that even mild compulsiveness might succumb to drugs that change the brain's regulation of serotonin. In fact, Prozac is about to be approved for use against obsessive-compulsive behavior. The great unknown is whether Prozac and other powerful drugs will work on milder forms of severe disorders.

ANXIETY AND CONCENTRATION

The neural pathways to anxiety exist because early humans who got a little nervous at the sight of, say, a crouching saber tooth had a survival edge over more laid-back tribesmen. Now, in the age of anxiety, many people would just as soon give back this legacy of natural selection. At the National Institute of Mental Health, Philip Gold is figuring out how. He traces stress to the circuit responsible for the fight-or-flight response. In the chronically anxious, he says, "it turns on, but it doesn't turn off." Antidepressants called tricyclics, which throttle back levels of the fight-or-flight norepinephrine, seem to still the perpetual arousal in the circuit.

A *shortage* of norepinephrine seems to rob people of the ability to pay attention to what's important, and only to what's important. Sally Jackson, the fortysomething owner of a Boston public-relations firm, knows the problem well. She had often felt unfocused, so last winter she began taking Ritalin, a stimulant that increases the availability of norepinephrine. Although Ritalin is best known as the controversial medication for children diagnosed with attention-deficit disorder (ADD, alias hyperactivity), adults are now taking the yellow pills to improve their concentration. "Without it, I would sit at my desk for hours and get nothing done," says Jackson, who believes she has ADD. "But once I started Ritalin, every proposal I wrote, we won the account. I'm better on deadline and it keeps me focused on one task at a time." She swallows one pill in the morning and another if she hits a 3 p.m. lull.

I MEDICATE, THEREFORE WHO AM I?

Prozac to cheer you up and Ritalin to focus are merely the most prominent new mind drugs. Anticonvulsants such as Dilantin, prescribed for epileptics, turn out to reduce stress in some people. Beta blockers are heart drugs: they lower blood pressure and heart rate. But doctors figured out an entirely new use for them: combating stage fright. The drugs block receptors for norepinephrine; with less adrenaline igniting their brain circuits, people like oboist Stuart Dunkel, who plays for the Boston Opera, have no trouble calming performance anxiety. Before, complicated solos would make Dunkel's heart beat like a jackhammer and his breathing so shallow he couldn't sustain notes. With beta blockers, "there's a psychological release," he says. The drugs are not addictive, and Dunkel reports no side effects.

Other mind drugs are in the pipeline. One, with the tongue-tying name dexfenfluramine, seems to smooth out mood swings, especially those caused by winter doldrums and premenstrual syndrome. Naturally, it targets neurotransmitters: it keeps brain neurons bathed in serotonin longer than otherwise, explains Judith Wurtman of the Massachusetts Institute of Technology. Already used in Europe and South America as an anti-obesity drug (mood swings often trigger eating binges), dexfenfluramine has been submitted to the FDA for approval. A few weeks ago researchers at UC Irvine announced the discovery of the first drug that seems to improve working memory. The discovery sprang from work on neurotransmitters and their receptors, the shapely molecules that neurotransmitters fit like keys in locks. Researchers led by Gary Lynch found that in rats, the drug BDP binds to receptors for the neurotransmitter glutamate, which triggers neuronal changes that constitute memory. As a result, it acts like the father who lowers the basketball net for his vertically challenged child, reducing the amount of stimulation neurons require to form memories. If BDP works in people, the history lesson that once took hours to learn would take mere minutes. An Irvine-based start-up, Cortex Pharmaceuticals, Inc., plans to test BDP's safety.

Who could criticize a drug that stamps the rules for long division into your child's head after a single lesson? As psychiatrist Daniel Luchins of the University of Chicago points out, society accepts plastic surgery (albeit with some jokes): "If we have something that made people unshy, are they obliged to stay shy because of some ethical concern? What's the difference between 'I'm unhappy because I don't like my looks' and 'I'm unhappy because I'm shy?' "

For openers, one's core being is defined more by character traits than by the shape of one's nose. Just ask Cyrano. And not everything we feel, let alone everything we are, is shaped by too much or too little of some polysyllabic brain chemical. Yet as society moves ever closer to minds-made-to-order, the pressure on those who cannot, or choose not to, give their brain a makeover becomes intense. Some colleagues, and competitors, of Ritalin-popping executives feel themselves at a disadvantage, like rules-respecting sprinters facing a steroid user. Will guidance counselors urge parents to give their kids memory pills before the SATs? Will supervisors "suggest" workers take a little something to sharpen their concentration? The prospect of pills to make the dour cheery, and the tense mellow, calls into question the very notion of the self—is it truly the "self" in any meaningful sense if it is as easy to change as a bust measurement? "The brain is where our soul and spirit lie," says Harvard's Kagan. "People are very threatened by this."

Perhaps most worrisome is the idea of sandpapering away personality traits that not only make us individuals, but which evolved for a good reason. Anxiety, for instance, "probably evolved in tandem with the evolution of the human brain," writes Restak. Blunting that edge has a price. And just as physical pain keeps us from burning our flesh, perhaps mental pain, like that brought on by the death of a child, serves a purpose—one that is defeated by a pill that soothes when one should instead be raging. Shyness has also served civilization well. Some of history's great thinkers and creators—T. S. Eliot, Emily Dickinson, Anton Bruckner—were shy. "Inhibited children tend to wander off into vocations like music, literature and philosophy," says Kagan. A society that uses drugs to induce conformity does so at its peril.

With Debra Rosenberg in Boston, Joshua Cooper Ramo in New York and Mary Hager in Washington

OTC DRUGS: PRESCRIPTION FOR DANGER?

Soothing. Strong. Trustworthy." According to the maker of the new over-the-counter pain reliever *Aleve*, that's the message conveyed by the product's white and blue colors. But anti-inflammatory pain relievers like *Aleve* and aspirin are not so soothing to the stomach: Prolonged use of such drugs is one of the main causes of ulcers.

Indeed, nonprescription drugs can cause serious harm if you don't know—or don't follow—the appropriate precautions, not all of which are listed on the label. Taking these medications too often or in high doses can produce severe side effects, worsen the very symptoms you're trying to treat, or delay diagnosis of major diseases. Taking them with the wrong foods, drinks, or medications can spark dangerous reactions.

You can now buy some 450 over-the-counter drugs that would have required a prescription just 15 years ago. Naproxen (*Aleve*) is the latest to make the switch. That trend increases your ability to manage your own health—but it also increases the potential for overuse and misuse. Moreover, it means that people will now be getting much of their information about drugs from advertisements, such as an ad for the yeast-fighting drug *Monistat 7*, which printed a crucial warning in such tiny type that you could easily mistake it for a smudge at the bottom of the page. (That warning cautioned women not to treat an apparent yeast infection on their own unless their doctor had diagnosed the same kind of infection in the past.)

This report describes the kinds of trouble that nonprescription drugs can cause, lists the specific risks of the most common drugs (see table), and tells you how to get the information you need to use over-the-counter drugs safely.

A grab bag of risks

Although over-the-counter drugs taken at the recommended doses rarely cause dangerous side effects in healthy people, they can cause a number of unpleasant symptoms. Those include insomnia and irritability from oral decongestants, constipation from aluminum-containing antacids, diarrhea from magnesium-containing antacids, and indigestion from all pain relievers except acetaminophen (*Tylenol*). One common side effect—drowsiness from antihistamines, which are contained in all allergy drugs and some cold medications—could be more hazardous. In fact, the maximum recommended dose of some antihistamines can slow reaction time more than the amount of alcohol that would make driving illegal in most states.

The risk of side effects from over-the-counter drugs increases sharply when people take more than they should. For example, swallowing just three times more than the maximum recommended dose of phenylpropanolamine—contained in the oral decongestant *Propagest*, many cold remedies, and all diet pills—can cause severe and even life-threatening rises in blood pressure. Taking a drug continually without consulting a doctor also multiplies the risk of side effects, such as anemia from chronic use of aspirin or potassium depletion and bowel damage from excessive use of the laxative bisacodyl (*Carter's Little Pills, Dulcolax, Fleet Bisacodyl*).

Further, overuse of certain nonprescription drugs can lead to an insidious form of dependency. People who keep taking drugs to relieve headaches or nasal congestion will often get "rebound" symptoms—headaches or congestion worse than the original symptoms—as soon as the drug starts wearing off. That may lead to a vicious cycle of increasingly frequent use of the drug and worsening rebound. Similarly, prolonged use of laxatives can weaken the bowel muscles, causing renewed constipation as soon as the drug is discontinued.

The gravest danger from sustained use of over-the-counter medications is that you might be controlling symptoms while allowing an underlying disease to go untreated. For example, people with stomach pain sometimes take over-the-counter antacids or pain relievers for months without seeing a doctor. Those people may have ulcers or inflammation of the stomach, which can cause serious bleeding; or they may even have stomach cancer.

Just because you can buy them without a doctor's okay doesn't mean they can't harm you.

Drug interactions

Over-the-counter drugs can become more dangerous when they're taken with other medications—an all-too-common practice. According to a recent survey, one out of three people who take antihistamines for allergies take other drugs at the same time. But many common medications can make antihistamines even more sedating than they are when taken alone. The alcohol in a cough syrup such as *Comtrex Liquid*, *Tylenol Cough with Decongestant Liquid*, or *Vicks Formula 44 Multi-Symptom Cough Medicine* can combine with antihistamines to cause excessive drowsiness. In addition, you can get an unexpected double dose of antihistamines by taking an allergy drug along with a cold remedy such as *Alka-Seltzer Plus Cold* or *Contac Severe Cold Formula* or with a sleep aid such as *Nytol* or *Sominex*, all of which contain antihistamines.

Nonprescription drugs can also change the way other, more vital medications are supposed to work. Taking an antacid to prevent an antibiotic from upsetting your stomach may also prevent your body from absorbing the medicine, so it never reaches the infection. Conversely, taking a stool-softening laxative may ease constipation caused by the antihypertensive drug verapamil (*Isoptin, Calan*)—but it may also increase absorption of the drug, leading to an excessive reduction in blood pressure and, in turn, possibly to fainting.

Even ordinary foods can turn a seemingly innocuous drug into a hazardous one. For example, trying to calm your stomach by drinking large quantities of milk and taking antacids containing either calcium, magnesium, or sodium bicarbonate can eventually cause kidney failure.

People with certain chronic diseases are particularly vulnerable to the adverse effects of over-the-counter medications. But by far the most common condition that increases such vulnerability is simply old age.

Older people have more diseases and take more drugs than younger people, which increases all drug-related risks. In addition, the body becomes less efficient at breaking down and eliminating drugs as it ages. As a result, drugs may reach higher levels in the bloodstream and remain there longer. Even at normal levels, many medications have more pronounced effects on the brain and other parts of the aging body. Unfortunately, researchers rarely test new drugs on older people, so the recommended doses are often set too high for them.

The limits of labels

Labels for over-the-counter drugs do print certain crucial directions and precautions. Some packages also contain an insert, which may give more complete information. But neither labels nor inserts tell you everything you need to know about using these drugs, in part because the manufacturers don't want to scare people away.

The label or insert usually specifies how long you can safely use the medication—but it doesn't always. Some labels or inserts say nothing about possible side effects, interactions with food or other medications, or conditions that might make using the drug risky; those that do list such risks omit a good deal of potentially significant information. For example, neither the label nor the insert for *Aleve* mentions two relatively common side effects, dizziness and gastrointestinal bleeding. And neither label nor insert warns that the drug can harm people who have liver or kidney disease, or that it can neutralize the effect of antihypertensive medications.

Here's how to get more complete information about drugs than the manufacturer provides.

Ask the pharmacist

If you buy all your prescription and over-the-counter medications at one neighborhood pharmacy, rather than price shopping, make sure the pharmacist enters those medications—as well as any drug allergies you may have—in the pharmacy's computerized drug record. The computer will automatically alert the pharmacist to potential drug interactions and allergic reactions. If you're allergic to aspirin, for example, you might not realize that *Alka Seltzer Plus Nighttime Cold* contains aspirin, or that ibuprofen (*Advil, Motrin-IB*) and naproxen (*Aleve*) may each trigger similar reactions in aspirin-sensitive individuals. Even mail-order pharmacies typically provide a toll-free hotline staffed by pharmacists who will answer customer questions.

Read the package insert or label before you leave the store—or after you receive the drug in the mail—so you can ask the pharmacist to clarify anything that you don't understand or that the packaging doesn't specify, such as the following:

- What's the maximum length of time you should take the medication on your own without consulting your doctor?
- Does the drug interact with any of the other medications you might be taking or with any food or beverage?
- Are there any unlisted side effects you should know about?
- Should you take the drug with meals or on an empty stomach?
- Should you take the drug at bedtime?
- Can anything help you minimize minor side effects such as an upset stomach?
- How should you store the drug?

In addition to those questions, older people may want to ask the pharmacist whether the medication poses any increased risk for them.

Ask the doctor

Call your doctor before starting to take an over-the-counter drug if:

You have an unfamiliar symptom. It's safe to treat yourself with medication temporarily only if you have commonplace symptoms such as a runny nose, cough, headache, or upset stomach, or if your physician has diagnosed the same problem, such as an asthma attack or a vaginal yeast infection, on an earlier occasion.

- You have any chronic disorder.
- You are pregnant or nursing.
- The pharmacist says the drug may pose an increased risk for you. If so, your doctor can suggest solutions, such as reducing the dosage or trying a different medication.

Keep your doctor up to date on all the over-the-counter medications you're taking, including vitamins, minerals, or other supplements. If you're experiencing symptoms, those drugs or supplements may actually be the cause of the problem; or they may interact with prescribed medications or skew the results of laboratory tests. Even better, throw all your medications in a bag and bring them with you on your next office visit, so your physician can review your entire drug regimen.

In addition to talking with a pharmacist or doctor, consult a consumer drug-information book such as The Complete Drug Reference, available in most libraries or from Consumer Reports Books. (Send $39.95 to Box 10637, Des Moines, Iowa, 50336. Or call 515-237-4903.)

RISKS OF SOME COMMON OVER-THE-COUNTER DRUGS

Drug	Side effects	High-risk groups [1]	Interactions
PAIN RELIEVERS			
Aspirin *Bayer* *Empirin* *Norwich*	Common: Stomach upset [2], heartburn, gastrointestinal bleeding, nausea, vomiting, decreased clotting. Less common or rare: Bloody or tarry stools, bloody urine, ringing in the ears, loss of hearing, allergic reaction (skin rash, hives, itching, tightness in chest). Signs of overdose: Confusion, severe diarrhea, fast or deep breathing, severe drowsiness, convulsions.	People with allergies to aspirin or other nonsteroidal anti-inflammatory drugs, ulcers, anemia, bleeding disorders, overactive thyroid, asthma, high blood pressure, kidney or liver disease; children or teenagers with flu or chicken pox.	Can increase effect of anticoagulants. Can alter urine-sugar tests for diabetics.
Acetaminophen *Actamin* *Tylenol* *Valadol*	Common: None. Rare: Bloody or decreased urination, allergic reaction (skin rash, hives, itching, tightness in chest). Signs of overdose: Diarrhea, increased sweating, loss of appetite, nausea, vomiting, or stomach pain.	People with kidney or liver disease; active alcoholics.	Can alter urine-sugar tests for diabetics.
Ibuprofen *Advil* *Motrin-IB* *Nuprin*	Common: Stomach upset [2], gastrointestinal bleeding, heartburn, nausea, vomiting, dizziness, drowsiness, lightheadedness, headache. Less common or rare: Bitter taste, gas, constipation, loss of appetite, allergic reaction (skin rash, hives, itching, tightness in chest). Signs of overdose: Lethargy, low blood pressure, irregular heartbeat, difficulty breathing.	People with diabetes, asthma, kidney or liver disease, colitis, ulcers, congestive heart failure, high blood pressure, epilepsy.	Can increase effect of anticoagulants. Side effects increase when taken with aspirin. Can decrease effect of antihypertensive drugs.
Naproxen *Aleve*	Generally same as ibuprofen. [2]	Generally same as ibuprofen. [3]	Same as ibuprofen.
ANTIHISTAMINES [4]			
Brompheniramine *Dimetane* **Chlorpheniramine** *Aller-Chlor* *Chlor-Trimeton* *Pfeiffer's Allergy* **Clemastine** *Tavist-1* **Diphenhydramine** *Benadryl 25* *Benylin Cough* *Sominex*	Common: Drowsiness, thickening of mucus. Less common or rare: Blurred vision, confusion, difficulty urinating, dizziness, dryness of mouth, nose, or throat, loss of appetite, nervousness, restlessness, irritability. Signs of overdose: Clumsiness or unsteadiness, facial flushing, difficulty breathing, severe drowsiness, seizures.	People with glaucoma, liver disease, enlarged prostate, difficulty urinating.	Increases sedative effect if taken with alcohol, narcotics, sleeping medications, or tranquilizers. Can cause increased drowsiness or dry mouth if taken with or up to two weeks after a monoamine oxidase inhibitor (antidepressant drugs). Can cause dry mouth if taken with anticholinergics (drugs for stomach cramps).
ORAL DECONGESTANTS			
Pseudoephedrine *Efidac/24* *Halofed* *Sudafed* **Phenylpropanolamine** [5] *Propagest*	Common: Insomnia, nervousness, restlessness, irritability. Less common or rare: Difficulty urinating, dizziness, fast, slow, or irregular heartbeat, headache, sweating, nausea, vomiting. Signs of overdose: Convulsions, fast breathing, hallucinations, increase in blood pressure, irregular heartbeat, difficulty breathing.	People with diabetes, enlarged prostate, heart disease, high blood pressure, or overactive thyroid.	Can reduce effect of beta blockers. Can cause high blood pressure, fever, or seizures if taken with or up to two weeks after a monoamine oxidase inhibitor (antidepressant drugs). Can cause insomnia, irritability, irregular heartbeats, or seizures if taken with asthma medications, caffeine, or amphetamines.
TOPICAL DECONGESTANTS [6]			
Oxymetazoline *Afrin 12-Hour* *Dristan 12-Hour* *Duration 12-Hour* **Phenylephrine** *Alconefrin* *Neo-Synephrine* *Vicks Sinex*	Common: Prolonged use may cause rebound congestion. Less common or rare: Rapid heartbeat, lightheadedness, trembling, insomnia, nervousness.	People with diabetes, heart disease, high blood pressure, or overactive thyroid.	May increase risk of serious side effects if taken with or up to two weeks after a monoamine oxidase inhibitor (antidepressant drugs).

[1] People with these conditions should avoid drug or check with doctor.

[2] Aspirin causes the most stomach upset; naproxen causes somewhat less, but more than ibuprofen.

[3] People over age 65 must follow lower dosage instructions.

[4] Antihistamines vary in their sedative effects: Diphenhydramine is highly sedating, clemastine moderately sedating, and the others mildly sedating.

[5] More likely than pseudoephedrine to increase blood pressure sharply. Phenylpropanolamine is also found in all over-the-counter diet pills and in many cold medicines.

[6] Available in drops or sprays.

Placebo Effect Is Shown to Be Twice as Powerful as Expected

Daniel Goleman

"Hurry, Hurry—use the new drugs while they still work!" a 19th-century French physician urged his colleagues. He may not have known why faddish drugs work on credulous patients, but the fact that they do has been borne out by scientists studying the power of the placebo to cure.

New findings show that the placebo effect—in which patients given an inactive treatment believe it can cure them—is most powerful when a trusted physician enthusiastically offers a patient a new therapy. In a study of more than 6,000 patients being given experimental treatments for asthma, duodenal ulcer and herpes, two-thirds improved, at least temporarily, even though rigorous tests later found the treatments medically useless. They were then abandoned.

Some argue that the placebo effect should be exploited to help the patient.

The old rule of thumb among medical researchers was that only about one-third of patients will show some improvement when given a placebo. The results of the new studies reveal the effect to be twice as powerful as was thought.

These and other findings that the placebo effect can be far stronger than had been widely assumed are leading some researchers to call for stricter standards for testing new medications. Others are proposing that physicians try to capitalize on the placebo effect in treating their patients in order to marshall the body's own healing powers.

"I argue that instead of just trying to control for placebo, we should try to maximize it," said Dr. Frederick Evans, a psychologist at the Robert Wood Johnson School of Medicine in New Brunswick, N.J. "If a doctor believes in what he's doing and lets the patient know that, that's good medicine."

While many people think a "placebo" is simply a sugar pill or other medicine with no active ingredients, the term has a broader meaning. The "placebo effect" includes any improvements in a patient not specifically due to a particular ingredient in a treatment,like a drug or surgical procedure. These "nonspecific," or placebo, effects, may be due to causes ranging from a patient reporting relief from symptoms in an unconscious effort to please a well-liked physician, to actual biological improvement.

TESTING THE PLACEBO EFFECT

To assess the potency of the placebo effect during the burst of enthusiasm for a new medical treatment, researchers reexamined data from initial clinical trials of five procedures which had at first seemed highly promising, and then later were shown to be useless. The procedures included surgical removal of the glomus, a structure near the carotid arteries in the neck, to treat asthma; and gastric freezing for duodenal ulcers. They also included three treatments for herpes simplex virus—the drug levamisole, organic solvents like ether and exposure of dyed herpes lesions to fluorescent light.

"In these studies, the doctors treating were also those evaluating the symptoms, which is what happens in a typical physician's office," said Dr. Alan H. Roberts, a psychologist at the Scripps Clinic and Research Foundation in La Jolla, Calif., who led the research. The results were published in the current issue of Clinical Psychology Review.

The physicians, who offered the treatments as part of an early clinical trial and believed in their efficacy, told their patients the various approaches were new and promising. With both physicians and patients having high hopes for a cure, the resulting placebo effect was potent. Because these were very early trials of new drugs, no control groups were used.

Of a total of 6,931 patients receiving one or another of the five treatments, 40 percent were reported to have excellent results, another 30 percent had good outcomes and only 30 percent were reported to have "poor" results, Dr. Roberts and his colleagues found.

Yet in later trials, when patients who received the treatments were methodically compared with control groups of patients who received placebos or nothing at all, "the effectiveness disappeared," said Dr. Roberts.

Dr. Roberts believes that for relatively mild medical problems, under the best conditions the placebo effect will produce positive results in roughly two-thirds of patients. The effects would not be nearly as strong for serious diseases such as AIDS or cancer, he said: "In the more severe disorders, the placebo effects would be mainly in terms of patient's subjective complaints, not their physical symptoms."

PSYCHOLOGICAL FACTORS

In Dr. Robert's view, the improvements associated with placebos are caused by factors like patients unconsciously exaggerating improvements of their symptoms in order to please their doctors, and doctors who hope for positive results skewing their evaluations of symptoms favorably.

The notion that the placebo effect is due to biological changes from patients' hopes being raised is met with skepticism by Dr. Roberts. But other researchers disagree.

"Could an enthusiastic physician and a believing patient create a clinical improvement in a patient?" said Dr. Ronald Glaser, a virologist at Ohio State University Medical School. "That question has haunted drug studies. But there may well be a psychological effect with a significant biological outcome, if you extrapolate from data showing that psychological factors like stress can affect viruses like herpes. It's definitely one possible explanation."

The herpes virus is one of Dr. Glaser's specialties; with his wife, Janice Kiecolt-Glaser, a psychologist, he has studied the effects of people's emotional swings on the replication of herpes virus.

"We've found herpes viruses are responsive to stress, improving or worsening depending on a patient's emotional state," said Dr. Kiecolt-Glaser. "Since herpes virus is quite responsive to psychological influences, the first wave of physicians' enthusiasm could well have a beneficial medical effect."

Dr. Roberts is not the first researcher to find that the placebo effect can account for improvements in more than one-third of patients, a ratio proposed in the 1950's by Dr. Henry Beecher, one of the first to do research on the placebo.

PATIENTS MOST LIKELY TO BENEFIT

"The range for placebo recovery I've seen varies from zero to 100 percent," said Dr. Arthur K. Shapiro, a psychiatrist at Mt. Sinai Medical Center in Manhattan. "Different factors combine to produce the magnitude of a placebo. For example, in my own research with 1,000 patients, those who like their physician most and who were most anxious showed the greatest improvement from placebo."

Such findings on the power of the placebo are bringing calls for revising the way in which new treatments are tested. In order to be sure the benefits attributed to experimental treatments are not simply due to placebo, tests of new medications now use a "double-blind" design, in which neither the physician nor the patient knows what medicine is being given, and some patients are given a nonactive treatment.

"There is a false sense of security about the scientific tests of drugs, particularly psychiatric drugs," said Dr. Roger Greenberg, a psychologist at the State University of New York Health Science Center at Syracuse.

One of the main problems with the standard double-blind test, said Dr. Greenberg, is that patients and physicians alike can very often tell who is getting the active medication and who is getting the placebo, because only the true medication has side effects. This can lead to placebo enhancement of the seeming effectiveness of the medication being tested.

"In instances when researchers have asked patients and physicians to guess whether they were using the active medication or the placebo, the results are sobering—in one such study, 78 percent of patients and 87 percent of their physicians could tell," said Dr. Greenberg. "That means the so-called 'double-blind' is not really blind."

For that reason, Dr. Greenberg proposes that in addition to the medication being tested and the usual inert placebo, tests of new drugs should include an "active" placebo which produces side effects but has no medical consequence. And, in the most rigorous test, a physician other than the one giving the medicines would make the evaluations of improvement.

In a meta-analysis of 22 studies of antidepressants, Dr. Greenberg and colleagues found that if, in addition to the new drug being tested, some patients were given an older antidepressant as a control, the new drug was only one-quarter to one-half as powerful as was reported in studies without the comparison drug, in which the new drug was pitted only against an inert placebo.

The research finding, published last year in the Journal of Consulting and Clinical Psychology by Dr. Greenberg and colleagues, concludes that current standard practices for drug testing often exaggerate the potency of new medicine.

"In general," said Dr. Greenberg, "the better a study is controlled, the blinder it becomes and the smaller the difference becomes between the real drug and the placebo."

KICKING BUTTS

Nicotine is more powerfully addictive than most people realize. It will probably take several tries before you learn enough tricks to stay cigarette-free for good.

Carl Sherman

Carl Sherman writes on health, medicine, and psychology for national magazines and medical newspapers. He lives in New York City. He last wrote for Psychology Today *about sexual abuse in psychotherapy. He is the coauthor of a book on psychological aspects of skin disorders and his writings are anthologized in many collections.*

It may not be a "sin" anymore, but few would dispute that smoking is the devil to give up. Of the 46 million Americans who smoke—26 percent of the adult population—an estimated 80 percent would like to stop and one-third try each year. Two to 3 percent of them succeed. "There's an extraordinarily high rate of relapse among people who want to quit," says Michael Fiore, M.D., M.P.H., director of the Center for Tobacco Research and Intervention at the University of Wisconsin.

The tenacity of its grip can be matched by few other behaviors, most of which, like snorting cocaine and shooting up heroin, are illegal. Since 1988, nicotine dependence and withdrawal have been recognized as disorders by the American Psychiatric Association, legitimizing the experience of the millions who have tried, successfully and otherwise, to put smoking behind them while kibitzers told them to use more willpower.

It's not just a habit, the medical and scientific communities now fully agree, but an addiction, comparable in strength to hard drugs and alcohol.

In fact, the odds of "graduating" from experimentation to true dependence are far worse for cigarettes than for illicit drugs, which testifies to tobacco's one-two punch of addictiveness and availability: Crack and heroin aren't sold in vending machines and hawked from billboards. Alcohol is as legal and available as cigarettes are, and as big a business, but apparently easier to take or leave alone. The majority of people who drink are not dependent on alcohol, while as many as 90 percent of smokers are addicted.

If nothing else, the persistence of smoking in the face of a devastating rogue's gallery of bodily damage, little of which has been kept secret, attests to the fact that this is no rational lifestyle decision. "Take all the deaths in America caused by alcohol, illicit drugs, fires, car accidents, homicide, and suicide. Throw in AIDS. It's still only half the deaths every year from cigarettes," says Fiore.

The news, however, isn't all bad. For the last 20 years, the proportion of Americans who smoke has dropped continuously, for the first time in our history. In America today, there are nearly 45 million ex-smokers, about as many as are still puffing away.

These quitters, perhaps surprisingly, are for the most part the same folk who tried and failed before. The average person who successfully gives up smoking does so after five or six futile attempts, says Fiore. "It appears that many smokers need to go through a process of quitting and relapsing a number of times

TIPS FOR QUITTERS

- Nicotine addiction is powerful. Expect to struggle for a couple of months. It's an up-and down course.
- Don't despair. It may take six tries to learn enough skills to beat this addiction.
- Aim for absolute abstinence—even a single puff leads to relapse.
- Inventory those things that make you feel good and treat yourself to them—exercising, kissing, reading, taking a nap—instead of a smoke.
- Watch your coffee intake. Not only is it a trigger to smoke, your sensitivity to caffeine increases, mimicking nicotine-withdrawal symptoms.
- Change routines associated with smoking. Take a walk before your morning coffee. Drive to work a different way.
- Although most quitters succeed (eventually) on their own, programs that involve counseling improve the odds, especially for the depressed or anxious.
- Don't dismiss nicotine replacement with patch or gum. Gum allows you control over your blood nicotine level.
- Keep your guard up. Most lapses occur three or four weeks out, when you're feeling better.
- In the first weeks, avoid, or severely limit, alcohol.

before he or she can learn enough skills or maintain enough control to overcome this addiction."

'Evidence has mounted that a substantial number of smokers use cigarettes to regulate emotional states, particularly to reduce anxiety, sadness, or boredom.'

Never underestimate the power of your enemy. Although nicotine may not give the taste of Nirvana that more notorious drugs do, its effects on the nervous system are profound and hard to resist. It increases levels of acetylcholine and norepinephrine, brain chemicals that regulate mood, attention, and memory. It also appears to stimulate the release of dopamine in the reward center of the brain, as opiates, cocaine, and alcohol do.

Addiction research has clearly established that drugs with a rapid onset—that hit the brain quickly—have the most potent psychological impact and are the most addictive. "With cigarettes, the smoker gets virtually immediate onset," says Jack Henningfield, Ph.D., chief of clinical pharmacology research for the National Institute on Drug Abuse. "The cigarette is the crack-cocaine of nicotine delivery."

Physiologically, smoking a drug, be it cocaine or nicotine, is the next best thing to injecting it. In fact, it's pretty much the same thing, says Henningfield. "Whether you inhale a drug in 15 seconds, which is pretty slow for an average smoker, or inject it in 15 seconds, the effects are identical in key respects," he says. The blood extracts nicotine from inhaled air just as efficiently as oxygen, and delivers it, within seconds, to the brain.

The cigarette also gives the smoker "something remarkable: the ability to get precise, fingertip dose control," says Henningfield. Achieving just the right blood level is a key to virtually all drug-induced gratification, and the seasoned smoker does this adeptly, by adjusting how rapidly and deeply he or she puffs. "If you get the dose just right after going without cigarettes for an hour or two, there's nothing like it," he says.

The impetus to smoke is indeed, as the tobacco companies put it, for pleasure. "But there's no evidence that smoke in the mouth provides much pleasure," says Henningfield. "We do know that nicotine in the brain does."

For many, nicotine not only gives pleasure, it eases pain. Evidence has mounted that a substantial number of smokers use cigarettes to regulate emotional states, particularly to reduce negative affect like anxiety, sadness, or boredom.

"People expect that having a cigarette will reduce bad feelings," says Thomas Brandon, Ph.D., assistant professor of psychology at the State University of New York at Binghamton. His research found this, in fact, to be one of the principal motivations for daily smokers.

Negative affect runs the gamut from the transitory down times we all have several times a day, to clinical depression. Smokers are about twice as likely to be depressed as nonsmokers, and people with a history of major depression are nearly 50 percent more likely than others to also have a history of smoking, according to Brandon.

Sadly, but not surprisingly, depression appears to cut your chance of quitting by as much as one-half, and the same apparently applies, to a lesser extent, to people who just have symptoms of depression.

According to Alexander Glassman, M.D., professor of psychiatry at the Columbia University College of Physicians and Surgeons, the act of quitting can trigger severe depression in some people. In one study, nine smokers in a group of 300 in a cessation program became so depressed—two were frankly suicidal—that the researchers advised them to give up the effort and try again later. All but one had a history of major depression.

"These weren't average smokers," Glassman points out. All were heavily dependent on nicotine, they smoked at least a pack and a half daily, had their first cigarette within a half hour of awakening, and had tried to quit, on average, five times before. It is possible, he suggests, that nicotine has an antidepressant effect on some.

More generally, suggests Brandon, the very effectiveness of cigarettes in improving affect is one thing that makes it so hard to quit. Not only does a dose of nicotine quell the symptoms of withdrawal (much more on this later), the neurotransmitters it releases in the brain are exactly those most likely to elevate mood.

For a person who often feels sad, anxious, or bored, smoking can easily become a dependable coping mechanism to be given up only with great difficulty. "Once people learn to use nicotine to regulate moods" says Brandon, "if you take it away without providing alternatives, they'll be much more vulnerable to negative affect states. To alleviate them, they'll be tempted to go back to what worked in the past."

In fact, negative affect is what precipitates relapse among would-be quitters 70 percent of the time, according to Saul Shiffman, Ph.D., professor of psychology at the University of Pittsburgh. "We invited people to call a relapse-prevention hot line, to find out what moments of crises were like; what was striking was how often they were in the grip of negative emotions just before relapses, strong temptations, and close calls." A more precise study using palm-top computers to track the state of mind of participants is getting similar results, Shiffman says.

Most relapses occur soon after quitting, some 50 percent within the first two weeks, and the vast majority by six months. But everyone knows of people who had a slip a year, two, or five after quitting, and were soon back to full-time puffing. And for each of them, there are countless others who have had to fight the occasional urge, desire, or outright craving months, even years after the habit has been, for all intents and purposes, left behind.

Acute withdrawal is over within four to six weeks for virtually all smokers. But the addiction is by no means *all* over. Like those who have been addicted to other drugs, ex-smokers apparently remain susceptible to "cues," suggests Brandon: Just as seeing a pile of sugar can arouse craving in the former cocaine user, being at a party or a club, particularly around smokers, can rekindle the lure of nicotine intensely. The same process may include "internal cues," says Brandon. "If you smoked in the past when under stress or depressed, the act of being depressed can serve as a cue to trigger the urge to smoke."

Like users of other drugs, Henningfield points out, addicted smokers don't just consume the offending substance to feel good (or not bad), but to feel "right." "The cigarette smoker's daily function becomes dependent on continued nicotine dosing: Not just mood, but the ability to maintain attention and concentration deteriorates very quickly in nicotine withdrawal."

Henningfield's studies have shown that in an addicted smoker, attention, memory, and reasoning ability start to decline measurably just four hours after the last cigarette. This reflects a real physiological impairment: a change in the electrical activity of the brain. Nine days after quitting, when some withdrawal symptoms, at least, have begun to ease, there has been no recovery in brain function.

How long does the impairment persist? No long-term studies have been done, but cravings and difficulties in cognitive function have been documented for as long as nine years in some ex-smokers. "There are clinical reports of people who have said that they still aren't functioning right, and eventually make the 'rational decision' to go back to smoking," Henningfield says.

The conclusion is inescapable that smoking causes changes in the nervous system that endure long after the physical addiction is history, and in some smokers, may never normalize.

The wealth of recent knowledge about smoking clarifies why it's hard to quit. But can it make it easier? If nothing else, it should help people take it seriously enough to gear up for the effort. "People think of quitting as something short term, but they should expect to struggle for a couple of months," says Shiffman.

What works? About 90 percent of people who give up smoking do so on their own, says Fiore. But the odds for success can be improved: Programs that involve counseling typically get better rates, and nicotine replacement can be a potent ally in whatever method you use.

In a metaanalysis of 17 placebo-controlled trials involving more than 5,000 people, Fiore found that the patch consistently doubled the success of quit attempts, whether or not antismoking counseling was used. After six months, 22 percent of the people who used the patch remained off cigarettes, compared to 9 percent who had a placebo. Of those who had the patch and a relatively intense counseling or support program, 27 percent were smoke-free.

More than 4 million Americans have tried the patch, which replaces the nicotine on which the smoker has become dependent, to ease such withdrawal symptoms as irritability, insomnia, inability to concentrate, and physical cravings that drive many back to tobacco.

'Smoking causes nervous system changes that endure after the physical addiction is history. Some people may never normalize.'

You're likely to profit from the patch if you have a real physical dependence on nicotine: that is, if you have your first cigarette within 30 minutes of waking up; smoke 20 or more a day; or experienced severe withdrawal symptoms during previous quit attempts.

Standard directions call for using the patches in decreasing doses for two to three months. Some researchers, however,

BORN TO SMOKE

Although the difference between smokers and nonsmokers appears to reflect complex environmental and social factors, genetics apparently plays a role comparable to that observed in alcoholism, responsible for about 30 percent of the propensity.

In particular, shared genetics appears to account for the link between smoking and depression, according to data collected on nearly 1,500 pairs of female twins. "The twin data show that whatever gene puts you at risk for depression, the same gene puts you at risk for smoking," says Alexander Glassman.

Further evidence for this conclusion comes from a prospective epidemiological study, in which 1,200 people in their twenties were surveyed twice, 18 months to two years apart. Nonsmokers who were depressed at the first interview were more likely to be smoking at the time of the second, while nondepressed smokers were more likely to have become depressed by then.

Genetics may even play a role in *how* you smoke. Shiffman studied a group of people who had smoked regularly but lightly, five cigarettes or less, four days or more a week, for several years at least. Says Saul Shiffman: "They had ample opportunity to become addicted—on average, they'd smoked 46,000 cigarettes, but we found not the slightest evidence of dependence: they showed no signs of withdrawal when abstinent. They really could casually take smoking or leave it."

Such nonaddicted users—"chippers," in drug culture parlance—are also seen among consumers of hard drugs. "We didn't delve deeply into what made these smokers different," says Shiffman. "But we did find evidence that they also had relatives who smoked with little dependence, who followed the same pattern. This makes it plausible, although it doesn't prove that these folks are biologically different." With rare exceptions, chippers have always smoked that way, he points out. For a once-addicted smoker to try to become a chipper is "a risky business" that's probably doomed to failure.—C.S.

suggest that for certain smokers, the patch may be necessary for years, or indefinitely.

"It's already happening," says Henningfield. "Some doctors have come to the conclusion that some patients are best able to get on with their life with nicotine maintenance." One such physician is David Peter Sachs, M.D., director of the Palo Alto Center for Pulmonary Disease Prevention. "I realized that with some of my patients, no matter how slowly I tried to taper them off nicotine replacement, they couldn't do it," says Sachs. "They were literally using it for years. Before you start tapering the dose, you should be cigarette-free for at least 30 days."

His clinical experience leads him to believe that 10 to 20 percent of smokers are *so* dependent that they may always need to get nicotine from somewhere. One study of people using the gum found that two years later, 20 percent of those who had successfully remained cigarette-free were still chewing. The idea of indefinite, even lifetime, nicotine maintenance sounds offensive to some. "Clearly, the goal to aim for is to be nicotine-free," says Sachs. "But if that can't be reached, being tobacco-free still represents a substantial gain for the patient, and for society." And getting nicotine via a patch or gum source means a far lower dose than you'd get from a cigarette. Plus, you're getting just nicotine, and not the 42 carcinogens in tobacco smoke.

Although the once-a-day patch has largely supplanted the gum first used in nicotine replacement, Sachs thinks that for some, the most effective treatment could involve one or both. The patch may be easier to use, but the gum is the only product that allows you control over blood nicotine level. Some people know they'll do better if they stay in control. And would-be quitters who do fine on the patch until they run into a stressful business meeting may stifle that urge to bum a cigarette if they boost their nicotine level in advance with a piece of gum, Sachs says.

However, nicotine replacement "is not a magic bullet," says Fiore. "It will take the edge off the tobacco-withdrawal syndrome, but it won't automatically transform any smoker into a nonsmoker." Other requisite needs vary from person to person. A standard approach teaches behavioral "coping skills," simple things like eating, chewing gum, or knitting to keep mouth or hands occupied, or leaving tempting situations. Ways people cope cognitively are as important as what they do, says Shiffman.

He advises would-be quitters at times of temptation to remind themselves just why they're quitting: "My children will be so proud of me," or "I want to live to see my grandchildren," for example. Think of a relaxing scene. Imagine how you'll feel tomorrow if you pass this crisis without smoking. Or simply tell yourself, "NO" or "Smoking is not an option."

Coping skills, however, are conspicuously unsuccessful for people who are high in negative affect. Supportive counseling works better. Depression or anxiety may interfere with the ability to use cognitive skills.

One exercise that Brandon teaches patients asks them to inventory—and treat themselves to—things that make them feel good, a substitute for the mood-elevating effect of a cigarette. These might include exercising, being with friends, going to concerts, reading, or taking a nap. "Positive life-style changes that improve mood level" are particularly useful if you use cigarettes to deal with negative emotional states, he says.

Depression treatment is particularly important for those trying to quit smoking. One study found that cognitive therapy significantly improved quit rates for people with a history of depression. Various antidepressants have been effective in small studies, and a large double-blind trial using the drug Zoloft is underway.

Fiore has found that having just one cigarette in the first two weeks of a cessation program predicted about 80 percent of

NICOTINE IN THE NINETIES

Smoking just doesn't have the cachet it once did. Instead of a mark of worldliness and *joie de vivre,* it's become something of a social disease, banned from airplanes, restaurants, and, in some localities, public parks. Except on billboards and in magazine ads, the smoker him- or herself is less likely to be the object of admiration than of pity and contempt.

The change in smoking's status is no doubt in part responsible for the 40 percent decline in its prevalence since 1964. And it would seem logical that those people who are still smoking in the face of such adversity are an increasingly hard-core, heavily addicted bunch, unable to quit.

Alexander Glassman conjectures that as the social environment grows more hostile to smoking, the genetic component of the behavior will become more evident. And as the number of smokers drops, an increasing percentage will have psychiatric problems, particularly depression.

But the change hasn't yet been documented. "Actually, I don't think the data support the idea that today's smokers are very different from years back," says Fiore. "The average number of cigarettes they smoke today isn't dramatically different from 20 years ago—about 22 per day."

One thing that has happened is a change in the sociodemographics of smoking. "More and more, it's a behavior predominantly exercised by disadvantaged members of society: 40 percent of high-school dropouts smoke, compared to 14 percent of college grads. Poor people are more likely to smoke than wealthy. It's getting marginalized," he says.

If nothing else, today's antismoking climate has eliminated much denial about the true nature of the cigarette habit. "Smokers are much more aware of being hooked," says Saul Shiffman. "You can't tell how dependent you are if access is easy. If you can smoke at your desk and at a restaurant, you can delude yourself, as people have for decades: 'I like to smoke but I can take it or leave it.' It's hard to say that when the only place you can smoke is outside when it's hailing and 20 degrees."—C.S.

relapses at six months. Even when the withdrawal symptoms are gone, a single lapse can rekindle the urge as much as ever.

In the critical first weeks without cigarettes, a key to relapse prevention is avoiding, or severely limiting, alcohol, which not only blunts inhibitions, but is often powerfully bound to smoking as a habit. Up to one-half of people who try to quit have their first lapse with alcohol on board.

Watch your coffee intake, too. It can trigger the urge to smoke. And nicotine stimulates a liver enzyme that breaks down caffeine, so when you quit, you'll get more bang for each cup, leading to irritability, anxiety, and insomnia—the withdrawal symptoms that undermine quit efforts.

Try to change your routine to break patterns that strengthen addiction: drive to work a different way; don't linger at the table after a meal. And don't try to quit when you're under stress: vacation time might be a good occasion.

And if you do have a lapse? Don't trivialize it, because then you're more likely to have another, says Shiffman. But, "if you make it a catastrophe, you'll reconfirm fears that you'll never be able to quit," a low self-esteem position that could become a self-fulfilling prophecy. "Think of it as a warning, a mistake you'll have to overcome."

Try to learn from the lapse: examine the situation that led up to it, and plan to deal with it better in the future. "And take it as a sign you need to double your efforts," Shiffman says. "Looking back at a lapse, many people find they'd already begun to slack off; early on, they were avoiding situations where they were tempted to smoke, but later got careless."

Don't be discouraged by ups and downs. "It's normal to have it easy for a while, then all of a sudden you're under stress and for 10 minutes you have an intense craving," says Shiffman. "Consider the gain in frequency and duration: the urge to smoke is now coming back for 10 minutes, every two weeks, rather than all the time."

If lapse turns into relapse and you end up smoking regularly, the best antidote to despair is getting ready to try again. "Smoking is a chronic disease, and quitting is a process. Relapse and remission are part of the process," says Fiore. "As long as you're continuing to make progress toward the ultimate goal of being smoke-free, you should feel good about your achievement."

ALCOHOL and TOBACCO: A Deadly Duo

Kristine Napier

Kristine Napier, M.P.H., R.D., is a Cleveland-based freelance writer. She studied alcohol/tobacco interactions during her graduate work.

Cancer of the upper respiratory and alimentary tracts claimed over 23,000 lives in 1989 and 57,000 additional cases were diagnosed. The majority of individuals who fall prey to this type of cancer are males who abuse both alcohol and tobacco.

THE RISK

The fact that the risk of developing cancer of the esophagus, lip, tongue, mouth, pharynx or larynx, increases dramatically in people who are heavy users of alcohol and tobacco is substantiated by 30 years of collective research. Studies demonstrate that the risk to individuals dually addicted far outweighs the risk to individuals who abuse only one substance. This confirmed link between alcohol and tobacco abuse and an increased risk in upper alimentary and respiratory tract cancer makes this type of disease among the most preventable.

THE CORRELATION BETWEEN SMOKING AND DRINKING

It has been observed that individuals who drink alcohol have a greater tendency to smoke than non-drinkers. One of the first studies to establish and quantify the degree of association between drinking and smoking was reported in 1972. The investigation compared 130 alcoholic men hospitalized for alcohol withdrawal to 100 non-alcoholic psychiatric outpatients. Ninety-four percent of the alcoholic men smoked one or more packs of cigarettes per day, as compared to only 46 percent of the non-alcoholics, who smoked one or more packs per day.

Another study, which compared male and female alcoholics enrolled in an army drug and alcohol rehabilitation program to non-alcoholic army personnel and their relatives, affirmed the smoking-drinking association. The report found that individuals who were alcoholics smoked an average of 49 cigarettes per day, but that the non-alcoholic subjects smoked only 13 cigarettes per day. In addition, the study established a high correlation between the number of cigarettes smoked and the grams of alcohol consumed by alcoholics, as opposed to a very weak association for the non-alcoholic control group.

In a similar report, 58 percent of the non-drinkers were non-smokers, but the individuals who were alcoholics did not abstain from smoking. The finding that smokers who did not drink smoked significantly less than smokers who did drink was further substantiated in additional studies.

WHY DO MANY DRINKERS SMOKE MORE?

Studies released in the late 1950s, correlating heavy coffee consumption with smoking and drinking, suggested that a strong oral drive caused drinkers to smoke more frequently. However, new evidence suggests that a strong oral drive is not the culprit.

In one study, alcoholics who had successfully stopped drinking demonstrated no appreciable increase in smoking. In fact, some even smoked less with alcohol abstinence. If a strong oral drive was responsible for the drinking-smoking association, one would expect an increase in smoking during periods of alcohol abstinence.

An alternative theory claimed that drinkers smoked more due to social pressure. However, a study showing that alcoholics who drank alone smoked just as much as alcoholics who drink in the company of other people

Reprinted with permission from *Priorities* magazine, Spring 1990, pp. 6-7. Published by the American Council on Science and Health, New York, NY.

dispelled this theory. The most plausible explanation is that drinkers smoke more than non-drinkers due to a greater physiological need for nicotine.

Nicotine, the main psychoactive component of tobacco, is a potent chemical. It has a stimulating effect on the nervous system, causing, among other things, increased heart rate and mental stimulation. Once addicted to nicotine, a person may experience tremors or shakiness as blood levels of nicotine decrease to critically low levels. The smoker will crave another cigarette as blood levels reach this threshold to avoid these uncomfortable symptoms. Alcohol apparently causes blood levels of nicotine to fall more rapidly in smokers by activating enzymes in tissues which metabolize drugs. For example, rats pretreated with ethanol cleared nicotine from their blood more rapidly than rats not receiving ethanol. This research, coupled with numerous independent observations, strongly suggests that drinkers must smoke more in order to maintain the blood nicotine levels upon which they have become dependent.

WHY IS THERE MORE CANCER AMONG ALCOHOL AND TOBACCO USERS?

Investigations are under way to find an answer to this question. Laboratory studies have shown that alcohol enhances the metabolism of several tobacco associated carcinogens, including nitrosamines. It is known that tobacco and its smoke contain many classes of chemical carcinogens which must be activated to react with DNA and initiate steps towards carcinogenesis. Important in this activation process are cytochrome P-450 enzymes, which are induced by alcohol in heavy drinkers. Thus, alcohol and smoking are synergistic in increasing cancer risk.

Since alcohol increases the metabolism and hence the need for nicotine, it follows that the success of smoking cessation programs will be improved if drinking habits of patients are controlled. Treatment of incipient alcoholism thus becomes a prerequisite for the ultimate success of behavior modification aimed at the elimination of smoking.

Alcohol in perspective

True or false?

1. An ounce-and-a-half of 80-proof vodka or whiskey contains more alcohol than a 12-ounce can of beer.
2. A woman gets more intoxicated than a man from the same amount of alcohol.
3. Most Americans drink little or no alcohol.
4. Fatalities caused by alcohol-impaired driving are declining.
5. Measured in real dollars, the cost of alcoholic beverages has risen steadily during the last 40 years.

Answers

1. False. They contain the same amount. So does a five-ounce glass of wine.
2. True. The box on page 5 explains why.
3. True. Abstainers account for about 35% of the adult population, and light drinkers another 35%. Light drinkers, in the official definition, are those consuming two drinks a week or less. Moderate drinkers, who average one-half to two drinks a day, account for another 22%. Heavier drinkers—8% of us—consume more than two drinks a day.
4. True. The percentage of road crashes involving alcohol declined from 57% to 49% over the past decade. And the greatest decline was among teens and young adults. This is attributed to new laws setting the minimum drinking age at 21 in all states and to widespread educational efforts.
5. False. It cost less (in inflation-adjusted dollars) to drink in 1992 than it did in 1951. That's not a good thing—see below.

Double messages

Alcohol, a natural product of fermentation, is probably the most widely used of all drugs. It has been a part of human culture since history began and part of American life since Europeans settled on this continent. "The good creature of God," colonial Americans called it—as well as "demon rum." At one time, beer or whiskey may have been safer to drink than well water, but there have always been many other reasons for drinking: the sociability of drinking, the brief but vivid sense of relaxation alcohol can bring, and the wish to celebrate or participate in religious and family rituals where alcohol is served. In some cultures, abstention is the rule. In others, the occasional use of alcohol is regarded as pleasurable and necessary—but such use is carefully controlled and intoxication frowned upon. Tradition and attitude play a powerful role in the use of this drug.

Some people, unfortunately, drink because of depression and/or addiction to alcohol. Apart from such needs, powerful social and economic forces encourage people to drink. For starters, alcoholic beverages are everywhere—from planes and trains to restaurants and county fairs. Also, drink is cheap. The relative cost of alcohol has declined in the last decades. Since 1967 the cost of soft drinks and milk has quadrupled, and the cost of all consumer goods has tripled, but the cost of alcohol has not even doubled. This is because the excise tax on alcohol is not indexed to inflation. Congress has raised the federal tax on beer and wine only once in 40 years (in 1990). The tax on hard liquor has been increased only twice—small raises in 1985 and 1990. Opinion polls have shown that the public is in favor of raising federal excise taxes on alcohol, but the alcohol industry successfully fights increases. Furthermore, about 20% of all alcohol is sold for business entertainment and is thus tax deductible, making it that much less costly to whoever pays the bar bill.

Finally, the alcohol, advertising, and entertainment industries tirelessly promote the idea that it's normal, desirable, smart, sophisticated, and sexy to drink. In print, on television, and at the movies, we see beautiful, healthy people drinking. Beer ads associate the product with sports events, fast cars, camaraderie, and sex. Hollywood's stars have always imbibed plentifully, on and off camera: "Here's looking at you, kid," echoes down the ages. Among modern American male writers, alcoholism has been a badge of the trade: Hemingway, Fitzgerald, and Faulkner were all alcoholics. In *The Thirsty Muse*, literary historian Tom Dardis cites the deadly effect of alcohol on male American writers, many of whom made a credo of heavy drinking.

Considering all these pro-drinking forces, it is amazing that 35% of us over 18 never drink, and another 35% drink lightly and only occasionally. It's equally amazing that our drinking levels have been declining for the past 10 years. But it's estimated that only 8% of us consume more than half of all the alcohol. Still, out-and-out alcoholism is only one factor in the grief caused by drinking, and alcohol problems are not a simple matter of the drunk versus the rest of us.

Alcohol's toll

It's a rare person in our society whose life goes untouched by alcohol. Alcohol causes, or is associated with, over 100,000 deaths every year, often among the young. In 1990, alcohol-related traffic crashes killed more than 22,000 people—almost the same number as homicides. Half the pedestrians killed by cars have elevated blood alcohol levels. At some time in their lives, 40% of all Americans will be involved in an alcohol-related traffic crash. Alcoholism creates unhealthy family dynamics, contributing to domestic violence and child abuse. Fetal alcohol syndrome, caused by drinking during pregnancy, is the leading known cause of mental retardation. After tobacco, alcohol is the leading cause of premature death in America. The total cost of alcohol use in America has been estimated at $86 billion annually, a figure so huge as to lose its meaning. But money is a feeble method for measuring the human suffering.

In a free society, banning alcohol is neither desirable nor acceptable. But government, schools, and other institutions could do more than they do to protect the public health, teach the young about the dangers of alcohol, and treat alcoholics. As individuals and as citizens, we could all contribute to reducing the toll alcohol exacts on American life.

Alcohol and the body: short-term effects

Five ounces of wine, 12 ounces of beer, and 1.5 ounces of 80-proof spirits—all average servings—put the same amount of pure alcohol (about 1/2 to 2/3 ounce) into the bloodstream. But how fast it gets into the blood depends on many things. Some alcohol is absorbed through the stomach lining, enabling it to reach the bloodstream very quickly. If the stomach is empty, absorption is even faster: food slows it down. Aspirin in the stomach can hasten alcohol absorption. Since the alcohol in beer and wine is less concentrated, it tends to be absorbed more slowly than straight whiskey (and presumably you drink beer and wine more slowly than a shot of whiskey). But downing two beers in an hour raises blood alcohol concentration (BAC) more than one drink of whisky sipped for an hour. It's the alcohol that counts. A BAC of 0.10 is defined as legal intoxication in most states (0.08 in California, Maine, Oregon, Utah, and Vermont). It's hard to predict BAC accurately, since so many factors affect it. But a 150-pound man typically reaches a BAC of 0.10 if he has two or three beers in an hour. Any BAC impairs driving ability.

It takes the body about two hours to burn half an ounce of pure alcohol (the amount in about one drink) in the bloodstream. Once the alcohol is there, you can't hurry up the process of metabolizing it. You can't run it off, swim it off, or erase the effects with coffee. Leaner, larger people will be less affected by a given amount of alcohol than smaller ones with more fatty tissue—women, for instance. The effects of a given BAC are also greater in older people than in younger.

Every cell in the body can absorb alcohol from the blood. Of the short-term effects, none is more dramatic than those on the central nervous system. At first the drinker gets a feeling of ease and exhilaration, usually short-lived. But as BAC rises, judgment, memory, and sensory perception are all progressively impaired. Thoughts become jumbled; concentration and insight are dulled. Depression usually sets in. Some people get angry or violent. Alcohol induces drowsiness but at the same time disrupts normal patterns of sleeping and dreaming. It also adversely affects sexual performance.

The most unpleasant physical after-effect of too much alcohol is a hangover: dry mouth, sour stomach, headache, depression, and fatigue. Its cause is over-indulgence—not, as some believe, "mixing" drinks or drinking "cheap booze." No remedy has ever been found for hangovers.

Different for a woman

The alcohol industry has tried for some time to hitch a ride on women's quest for equality. Liquor ads promote the idea that if a woman can work like a man, she can, and indeed should, drink like a man. Nothing could be further from the truth.

Today 55% of women drink alcoholic beverages, and 3% of all women consume more than two drinks a day. But the ads don't tell a woman that she'll get more intoxicated than a man from the same amount of alcohol. Alcohol is distributed through body water, and is more soluble in water than in fat. Since women tend to be smaller than men and have proportionately more fatty tissue and less body water than men, the blood alcohol concentration resulting from a given intake will be higher for a woman than for a man of the same size. Recent research also shows that the stomach enzyme that breaks down alcohol before it reaches the bloodstream is less active in women than in men.

This may explain why excessive drinking seems to have more serious long-term consequences for women. They develop cirrhosis (liver disease) at lower levels of alcohol intake than men, for instance, and alcohol also puts them at increased risk for osteoporosis.

Finally, pregnant women who drink heavily risk having babies with fetal alcohol syndrome—characterized by mental retardation, structural defects of the face and limbs, hyperactivity, and heart defects. Because no level of alcohol consumption during pregnancy is known to be safe, pregnant women (as well as women planning pregnancy or having unprotected intercourse) are advised not to drink and to continue to abstain while breastfeeding. The amount of alcohol that passes into breast milk is smaller than the amount that crosses the placenta during pregnancy, but recent studies suggest that even a small amount can inhibit motor development in an infant. The idea that drinking beer promotes milk supply and benefits the baby is a myth.

The heart effect: worth drinking for?

Much recent research shows that moderate drinkers have a lower risk of developing heart disease. Supposedly, this beneficial effect comes from alcohol's ability to raise HDL cholesterol, the "good" type that protects against atherosclerosis. Some researchers have suggested that only one kind of beverage—for example, red wine—is protective. But it's more likely to be alcohol itself. Still, it's only moderate drinking that's helpful, and some people can't stick to moderation, while others (pregnant women) shouldn't drink at all. Few doctors suggest that nondrinkers begin drinking to protect their hearts.

Heavy drinking: long-term effects

Chronic, excessive use of alcohol can seriously damage nearly every organ and function of the body. When alcohol is burned in the body it produces another, even more toxic substance, acetaldehyde, which contributes to the damage. Alcohol is a stomach irritant. It adversely affects the way the small intestine transports and absorbs nutrients, especially vitamins and minerals. Added to the usually poor diet of heavy drinkers, this often results in severe malnutrition. Furthermore, alcohol can produce pancreatic disorders. It causes fatty deposits to accumulate in the liver. Cirrhosis of the liver, an often fatal illness, may be the ultimate result. Though alcohol is not a food, it does have calories and can contribute to obesity.

The effects of heavy drinking on the cardiovascular system are no less horrific. For many years doctors have observed that hypertension and excessive alcohol use go together, and according to a number of recent studies, heavy drinkers are more likely to have high blood pressure than teetotalers. Heavy alcohol consumption damages healthy heart muscle and puts extra strain on already damaged heart muscle. And it can damage other muscles besides the heart.

Some of the worst effects of alcohol are directly on the brain. The most life-threatening is an acute condition leading to psychosis, confusion, or unconsciousness. Heavy drinkers also tend to be heavy smokers and are also more likely to take and abuse other drugs, such as tranquilizers. Excessive drinking, particularly in combination with tobacco, increases the chance of cancers of the mouth, larynx, and throat. Alcohol appears to play a role in stomach, colorectal, and esophageal cancers, as well as possibly liver cancer.

What causes alcoholism?

Alcoholism is a complex disorder: the official definition, recently devised by a 23-member committee of experts, is "a primary, chronic disease with genetic, psychosocial, and environmental factors influencing its development and manifestations. The disease is often progressive and fatal. It is characterized by impaired control over drinking, preoccupation with the drug alcohol, use of alcohol despite adverse consequences, and distortions in thinking, most notably denial."

Alcohol use, by itself, is not sufficient to cause alcoholism. Medical science cannot yet explain why one person abstains or drinks rarely, while another drinks to excess—or why some heavy drinkers are able to stop drinking, while others continue until they die of cirrhosis. One area currently under intensive investigation is heredity. Are children of heavy drinkers more likely to fall victim to alcohol than others?

The answer is yes, but not just because these children were raised in an adverse environment. Studies have shown that, even when raised in nonalcoholic households, a significant number of children of alcoholic parents become alcoholics. This suggests that the ability to handle alcohol may be in part genetically determined. Not long ago, researchers claimed to have located an alcoholism gene, setting off a bitter controversy and raising the possibility of testing children, job applicants, and even fetuses for latent alcoholism. But if there are alcoholism genes, they remain to be identified, and a test for potential alcoholism is a long way off. Researchers point to differences in blood enzymes among alcoholics and non-users—but do not know whether the difference is responsible for the alcoholism or the result of it. Perhaps the chemistry of the body will prove to be the key to whether a person can drink moderately or not. Though most investigators believe that alcoholism has genetic, as well as environmental, causes, this does not mean that any individual is "doomed" to be an alcoholic. Alcoholic parents don't always produce alcoholic children. And many alcoholics come from families where no one ever drank.

Alcoholism is treatable

One problem in treating alcoholism is that it is hard to recognize. A person who is chronically drunk in public is obviously an alcoholic. But not all alcoholics display their problem by falling down in the street, losing their jobs, causing traffic crashes, or getting arrested. Many drink secretly or only on weekends, only in the evening, or even only once a month. Some may drink from depression, while others are sensation-seekers. They may successfully hold down a job or practice a profession. Yet at some point, whatever their drinking patterns, they have lost their ability to control their use of alcohol.

Many of the serious physical and personal consequences of alcoholism can be halted or reversed if drinking is discontinued soon enough. There are many different approaches to alcoholism: Alcoholics Anonymous and similar 12-step programs, individual or group psychotherapy, hospitalization and detoxification, and other methods. No single system will work for everyone. For some people, a combination of methods can help. Others may do as well with individual counseling. Family therapy may help others. The families of alcoholics also need therapy and other forms of social support. Scientific data about treatment are inconclusive. The crucial factor, most experts agree, is for the drinker to recognize that a problem exists and to seek the kind of treatment he or she needs.

Does Moderate Alcohol Consumption Prolong Life?

Excerpts from the ACSH booklet by Dr. R. Curtis Ellison

R. Curtis Ellison, M.D.

R. Curtis Ellison, M.D., is a Professor of Preventive Medicine and Public Health at Boston University School of Medicine.

Through the ages, conventional wisdom has been that the moderate intake of alcoholic beverages is consistent with a long and healthy life. Modern medicine became particularly interested in the effects of alcohol consumption on mortality in the 1950s and '60s when coronary heart disease became a major cause of death in the United States and in most other industrialized countries. Primarily from epidemiologic studies designed to identify factors associated with high death rates from coronary heart disease, it became apparent that these rates were lower among drinkers of small to moderate amounts of alcohol than among non-drinkers. However, these studies did not often explore effects of alcohol consumption on overall mortality rates. Specifically, it was not known whether increases in death from other diseases that are associated with alcohol abuse, such as cirrhosis of the liver and certain cancers, offset the apparent beneficial effects of low to moderate alcohol intake on mortality from coronary heart disease. This article takes a look at the net effects of drinking alcoholic beverages on the risk of the drinker's death.

DOES ALCOHOL PROTECT AGAINST CORONARY HEART DISEASE?

While searching for the risk factors for coronary heart disease in comparisons among countries as well as among individuals, epidemiologists identified a potential benefit from alcohol consumption on mortality from heart disease. In the past three decades, almost every follow-up epidemiologic study has demonstrated that individuals who drink small to moderate amounts of alcohol have a lower risk than non-drinkers of dying from coronary heart disease. Among drinkers, the categories with the lowest coronary heart disease rates vary across studies, ranging from less than one drink per day to three to five drinks per day. In most studies, individuals who state that they normally consume six or more drinks per day, or who admit to having problems with alcohol abuse, have rates of dying from heart disease higher than both non-drinkers and moderate drinkers.

In general, cirrhosis and alcohol-related cancers are associated with alcohol abuse and not with the consumption of small to moderate amounts of alcohol.

Many of the early studies were criticized for including in the category of non-drinkers both lifetime abstainers and ex-drinkers. Many ex-drinkers may have given up drinking due to alcoholism or other health problems (including cancer and heart disease) and thus would be expected to have a greater risk of early death. Other follow-up studies have demonstrated, however, that even when only lifetime abstainers or healthy abstainers make up the non-drinker category, the risk of coronary heart disease for non-drinkers is still higher than it is for moderate drinkers.

EFFECTS OF ALCOHOL ON OTHER DISEASES

Although there is little doubt that the moderate consumption of alcoholic beverages is associated with a lower risk of coronary heart disease, the risk of death from non-cardiac diseases or other causes depends on how much someone drinks.

Moderate Alcohol Intake There are a number of diseases or conditions that are often attributed to the use of

Reprinted with permission from *Priorities* magazine, Summer 1993, pp. 16-18. Published by the American Council on Science and Health, New York, NY.

alcohol (*e.g.*, cirrhosis of the liver, certain types of cancer, accidents). In general, cirrhosis and alcohol-related cancers are associated with alcohol abuse and not with the consumption of small to moderate amounts of alcohol.

However, even moderate amounts of alcohol may be related to the risk of death from hemorrhagic stroke. On the other hand, the risk of thrombotic stroke, the much more common type of stroke in the U.S. and Europe, is reduced by moderate amounts of alcohol. Therefore, the net effect of moderate alcohol intake in these parts of the world is a lowering of the risk of stroke.

Questions still remain on the apparent relation between moderate alcohol intake and breast cancer. Certain studies indicate that the risk of breast cancer in women may increase with only moderate levels of alcohol intake. However, other studies indicate no such relationship. It will require further research to clearly define what role, if any, alcohol plays in breast cancer.

Excessive Alcohol Intake Alcoholics and other abusers of alcohol generally are at increased risk for a number of diseases and causes of death. Driving while intoxicated causes the most accidental alcohol-related deaths. Rates of suicide are also increased for alcohol abusers. Furthermore, excessive drinkers experience increased rates of oral, pharyngeal, esophageal and stomach cancer. This is presumably due to the direct toxic effect of alcohol, and probably other substances in alcoholic beverages, on the tissues lining the upper gastrointestinal tract. Frequently, rates of such cancers are much higher, or even seen almost exclusively, among drinkers who also smoke cigarettes. Indeed, the combination of heavy drinking and smoking is particularly harmful.

EFFECTS OF ALCOHOL CONSUMPTION ON TOTAL MORTALITY

One approach to determine the net effects of an exposure (such as alcohol consumption) on disease rates is to calculate the rates for all diseases that may be related to the exposure and then attempt to balance the beneficial and harmful effects. When considering death as the outcome, however, we can simply look at total, or all-cause, mortality to judge the net effects of varying levels of alcohol consumption.

The best way to judge the net effects of alcohol consumption on a variety of causes of death is to look at all-cause mortality in follow-up studies, where data on alcohol use are collected prior to the development of disease or death.

The net effects of alcohol consumption on all-cause mortality were recently reported in nine follow-up cohort studies. All of the studies show that the relative risk of dying from any cause is lower for individuals in at least one category of alcohol consumption than for individuals consuming no alcohol. While the changes were not always statistically significant for each category in each study, the general pattern is very clear. Usually, the lowest risk of death is found in the categories reflecting moderate consumption (one to two drinks per day or individuals classified as "moderate drinkers").

In comparison with non-drinkers (even when the category is limited to healthy, lifetime abstainers), the risk of dying of any cause is lower for individuals who consume moderate amounts of alcohol.

Some of the studies included ex-drinkers and lifetime abstainers in the non-drinking category. The greater the proportion of ex-drinkers in the non-drinking category, the higher the death rate is expected to be for that category.

Fortunately, a number of the studies separated the non-drinking category into ex-drinkers and lifetime abstainers. In each of these studies, moderate drinkers had lower death rates than even lifetime abstainers. Results are the same when only healthy abstainers are included in the non-drinking category. Thus, these studies do not support the contention that the inclusion of ex-drinkers or sick individuals in the non-drinking category is the reason that moderate drinkers have lower rates of cardiovascular and other diseases. Overall, the data indicate that, in comparison with non-drinkers (even when the category is limited to healthy, lifetime abstainers), the risk of dying of any cause is lower for individuals who consume moderate amounts of alcohol.

DOES ALCOHOL CONSUMPTION PROLONG LIFE?

In reviewing the results of the studies summarized above, two things become clear. First, individuals who reported that they consumed small to moderate amounts of alcohol had lower death rates than non-drinkers. Thus, on the average, the lives of moderate drinkers were prolonged. The second message from the epidemiologic studies is that those individuals who consumed large amounts of alcohol had higher death rates than non-drinkers (and usually much higher than moderate drinkers). Therefore, on the average, the lives of heavy drinkers were shortened.

How sure can we be that it was the consumption of alcoholic beverages that improved mortality rates in these studies? It is always difficult to prove scientifically that some factor that is associated with an effect causes that effect. It is still possible, though unlikely, that it is not alcohol consumption itself but some lifestyle factor associated with the moderate consumption of alcohol that tends to lead to a prolongation of life.

The decision to drink alcohol must be an individual choice, based not only on average values from epidemiologic studies, but on individual characteristics and the recognition of all of the potential implications of the decision.

However, the accumulating evidence strongly suggests that it is the consumption of alcoholic beverages that results in the lower risk of death among moderate drinkers in epidemiologic studies. The evidence includes the following factors:

- a marked consistency of the findings of lower total mortality among drinkers in both men and women, in different ethnic groups and in different geographic areas of the world;
- a consistency across different age groups;
- a reduction of coronary atherosclerosis following alcohol intake in animal studies;
- a large number of identified mechanisms (increase in HDL-cholesterol, decrease in platelet aggregation, *etc.*) by which alcohol would be expected to reduce the risk of heart disease;
- higher death rates among non-drinkers even when ex-drinkers or individuals with other diseases are excluded.

MANY LIFESTYLE FACTORS AFFECT LONGEVITY

Many factors other than alcohol consumption affect life span. Genetics probably plays the largest role in determining longevity. However, diet, smoking habits, physical activity, obesity, use of seat belts and many other lifestyle factors play a role as well. When thinking of alcohol and life span, it is important to remember that any potential prolongation of life associated with moderate drinking varies markedly according to individual characteristics, especially other health-related habits and medical conditions.

IMPLICATIONS FOR INDIVIDUALS

Many factors should be taken into account when someone is considering whether or not to drink alcoholic beverages. Inappropriate use can lead to addiction, as well as to an increased risk of accidents, violence and a number of severe and even fatal diseases. The societal and personal costs of alcohol abuse are great. Women at increased risk of breast cancer may decide that it is preferable not to drink because of the possibility of a relation between alcohol and this disease. Thus, it is not possible to make blanket recommendations for everyone in the population.

Even physicians find it difficult to know whether it is safe (or advisable) for a given individual to drink. We must rely on the answers to questions such as, "Is there a family history of alcoholism?" "Has that individual ever abused alcohol or other substances?" "Does heart disease or certain cancers tend to run in the family?" "What is the individual's age, sex, body size?" "Is the individual taking medications or ill with a disease?" Such information helps determine how alcohol affects an individual and, to some extent, the risk that the individual will become an abuser of alcohol. We know that, on the average, the consumption of small to moderate amounts of alcohol results in few adverse effects and large beneficial effects in terms of preventing heart disease. However, we can never be sure, *a priori,* that an individual who begins to drink will not become an alcoholic. The decision to drink alcohol must be an individual choice, based not only on average values from epidemiologic studies, but on individual characteristics and the recognition of all of the potential implications of the decision.

Nutritional Health

The "wellness movement" has had a significant impact on the way Americans view their responsibility toward health maintenance. Today it is generally recognized that an individual's lifestyle is the primary determinant of health and longevity. This new attitude regarding lifestyle has fostered tremendous consumer interest in the area of nutrition. The food industry has responded to this new-found interest by introducing new products and promoting old ones on the basis of exaggerated health benefits. The challenge for the consumer is to make wise nutritional choices when confronted and bombarded with seductive and unsubstantiated health claims. Unfortunately, this is not an easy task because much of the nutritional advice we receive is conflicting and controversial. One recent example of this conflicting dietary advice has been the recommendation that all Americans should lower their intake of salt. From the mid-1970s and continuing through most of the 1980s, most nutrition experts encouraged Americans to reduce their salt intake as a way to prevent hypertension. Today, however, there is a difference of opinion as to whether there should be a blanket recommendation for a reduction in dietary salt. On the other hand, "The Salt Shake Out" by Bonnie Liebman asserts that the salt industry, and not sound scientific evidence, is behind the movement to minimize the dangers of dietary salt. She argues that a high dietary salt intake not only increases one's blood pressure, but it also contributes to the development of osteoporosis and stomach cancer. This is a prime example of the type of conflicting information that consumers are inundated with, and it raises the question, "Who should you trust for nutritional advice?"

Examples of conflicting nutritional advice are rampant and are largely due to the fact that nutritional science is in its infancy and, thus, is fraught with contradictions and controversies. Until nutritional science reaches maturity, advice coming from nutrition experts will be tentative at best. Another example that illustrates the controversial nature of nutritional advice is the debate among nutrition experts concerning the recently adopted U.S. Department of Agriculture (USDA) Food Guide Pyramid. The role of the USDA Food Guide Pyramid is to serve as a fundamental dietary guideline for planning nutritionally sound meals. This new dietary guideline breaks all foods into six groups that graphically represent the relative amount that each food group should contribute to one's diet. According to this new dietary guideline, Americans should eat 11 to 20 servings of plant foods a day compared to only 4 to 6 servings of animal foods. Opponents of this new dietary guideline have developed their own food guide, "The Mediterranean Diet Pyramid," which they claim is based solely on sound scientific evidence. According to this dietary guideline, red meat should only be consumed a few times each month. It also recommends that consumers limit their use of poultry and egg products to a couple of times per week. Needless to say, the meat and poultry industries oppose the Mediterranean Diet Pyramid. The article titled "The Mediterranean Diet" compares the USDA Food Guide Pyramid and the Mediterranean Diet Pyramid.

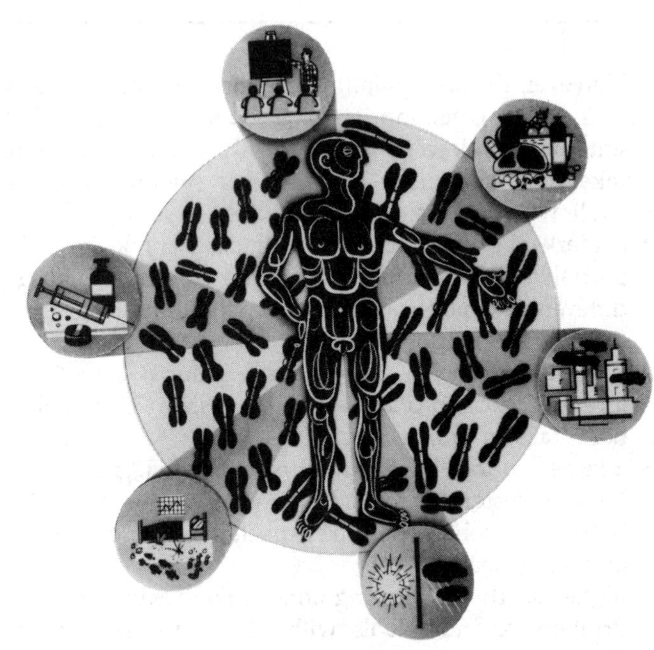

For years the majority of Americans paid little attention to nutrition, other than to eat three meals a day and, perhaps, take a vitamin supplement. While this dietary style was generally adequate for the prevention of major nutritional deficiencies, medical evidence began to accumulate linking the American diet to a variety of chronic illnesses. The most ominous finding was the link between dietary fat and coronary heart disease. The exact nature of this connection has been the focus of numerous studies, and, as a result, the role that dietary fats play in the process of atherosclerosis has been well documented. Recommendations based on these studies strongly suggest that Americans should reduce their intake of saturated fats and substitute monounsaturated or polyunsaturated fats whenever possible. This appears to be particularly true for individuals under stress. The article "The New Thinking about Fats" discusses why the type of fat we eat may be as important as the amount when it comes to preventing heart disease.

Unit 5

The National Research Council (NRC) currently recommends that Americans trim back their dietary fat intake so that it constitutes no more than 30 percent of one's total caloric intake. The NRC also recommends that saturated fats should be limited to less than 10 percent. While these dietary recommendations may be prudent, compliance with them can be challenging. One of the major obstacles blocking compliance is the fact that many consumers have misconceptions regarding the NRC's dietary recommendations. The most common misconception is that any food that derives more than 30 percent of its calories from fat should be eliminated from one's diet. The NRC's dietary recommendation is not concerned with the percentage of fat calories found in specific foods, but instead emphasizes the importance of keeping one's total daily diet at or below the 30 percent fat ratio. "How's Your Diet?" is a nutrition quiz designed to assist in assessing one's dietary consumption of total fat, saturated fat, cholesterol, sodium, sugar, fiber, and vitamins A and C.

As a result of all the bad press that dietary fats have gotten, millions of Americans are making a concerted effort to cut the fat content of their diets. The food category in which consumers have had the least success in reducing their fat consumption has been in the area of snack foods. "Snack Attack" by Patricia Long examines the fat content of various snack foods and suggests that the problem with snacking is not the eating between meals, but rather the food choices that are made at such times.

While fats have increasingly come under scrutiny as a source of health problems, carbohydrates have been given high ratings for health. Nutritionists generally agree that Americans should eat more carbohydrates, particularly the complex type, as they are a good source of vitamins, minerals, and fiber. While complex carbohydrates generally receive high marks for their nutritional value, highly refined forms, such as sugar, do not fare nearly as well. Over the last 20 years, dietary sugar (sucrose) has been linked to the etiology of obesity, heart disease, diabetes, dental caries, and periodontal disease. As a result, millions of Americans have made the switch to artificial sweeteners. Does this switch represent a positive change? Health authorities now generally agree that while sugar is a source of empty calories, the only demonstrable health hazard it poses appears to be dental. If you have made the switch to artificial sweeteners for health reasons other than diabetes or dental problems, then perhaps it is time to reconsider sugar.

Over the past few years, dietary fiber has become a hot issue in dietary circles. Several studies reported that individuals eating high-fiber diets demonstrated a lower incidence of colon cancer and lower blood cholesterol levels. In response to these findings, several noted health authorities have encouraged Americans to increase their consumption of dietary fiber.

The use of dietary supplements is another highly controversial topic in the area of nutrition. Today approximately 33 percent of Americans take a vitamin supplement regularly. For some, this consists of a simple multiple vitamin; others, however, rely on megadosing. Most nutritional experts agree that eating a varied and balanced diet is the single best way to meet all your nutritional needs, but not everyone eats a balanced diet. For those who do not, supplements may be necessary. At the present time, there is no definitive evidence to demonstrate that vitamins can actually bolster ones health, but a group of vitamins known as the antioxidants has generated considerable interest in this regard. In "Taking Vitamins: Can They Prevent Disease?" *Consumer Reports* examines the use of the antioxidant vitamins and presents recent research findings regarding their potential for disease prevention.

Another nutritional concern that has received considerable attention in the last few years is the problem of osteoporosis, particularly in women. Currently, most authorities agree that many Americans do not get sufficient amounts of dietary calcium. There is, however, considerable debate on how this deficit is best corrected.

Of all the topical areas in health, nutrition is certainly one of the most interesting, if for no other reason than the mere rate at which dietary recommendations change. Despite all the controversy and conflict, the one message that seems to remain constant is the importance of balance and moderation in everything we eat.

Looking Ahead: Challenge Questions

Given the controversies that abound in the area of nutrition, what guidelines should an individual use to make dietary decisions?

If you were asked to advise someone on how he or she might reduce the fat content of their diet, what advice would you give?

Given what we now know about the link between salt and hypertension, do you think it is a good idea for the National Research Council to continue its widespread advocacy of dietary salt restrictions? Defend your answer.

What restrictions, if any, should be placed on the use of nutritional supplements?

What dietary changes could you make to improve your diet? What is keeping you from making those changes?

How's Your Diet?

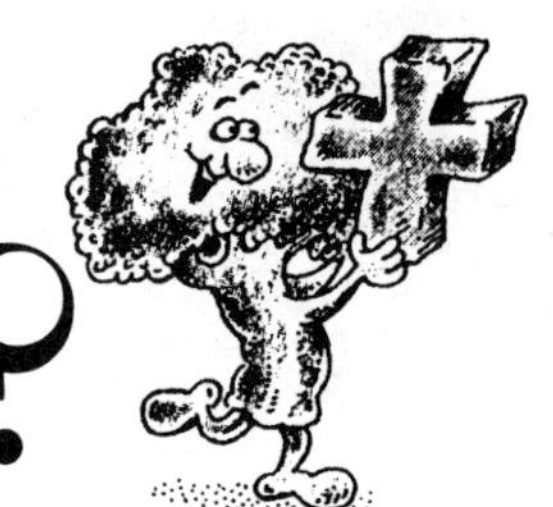

The 40 questions below will help you focus on the key features of your diet. The (+) or (–) numbers under each set of answers instantly pat you on the back for good habits or alert you to problems you may not even realize you have.

The Grand Total rates your overall diet, on a scale from "Great" to "Arrgh!"

The quiz focuses on fat, saturated fat, cholesterol, sodium, sugar, fiber, and vitamins A and C. It doesn't attempt to cover everything in your diet. Also, it doesn't try to measure precisely how much of these key nutrients you eat. (For that, we recommend the DINE nutrition software. [Contact CSPI at (202) 332-9110.])

What the quiz will do is give you a rough sketch of your current eating habits and, implicitly, suggest what you can do to improve them.

And don't despair over a less-than-perfect score. We didn't get a +117 either.

INSTRUCTIONS

■ Under each answer is a number with a + or – sign in front of it. Circle the number that is directly beneath the answer you choose. That's your score for the question. (If you use a pencil, you can erase your answers and give the quiz to someone else.)

■ Circle only one number for each question, unless the instructions tell you to "average two or more scores if necessary."

■ *How to average.* In answering question 18, for example, if you drink club soda (+3) and coffee (–1) on a typical day, add the two scores (which gives you +2) and then divide by 2. That gives you a score of +1 for the question. If averaging gives you a fraction, round it to the nearest whole number.

■ If a question doesn't apply to you, skip it.

■ Pay attention to serving sizes. For example, a serving of vegetables is ½ cup. If you usually eat one cup of vegetables at a time, count it as two servings.

■ Add up all your + scores and your – scores.

■ Subtract your – scores from your + scores. That's your GRAND TOTAL.

QUIZ

1. How many times per week do you eat unprocessed red meat (steak, roast beef, lamb or pork chops, burgers, etc.)?

(a) 0 +3 (b) 1 or less +2 (c) 2-3 0 (d) 4-5 –1 (e) 6 or more –3

2. How many times per week do you eat processed meats (hot dogs, bacon, sausage, bologna, luncheon meats, etc.)? ***(OMIT products that contain one gram of fat or less per serving.)***

(a) 0 +3 (b) less than 1 +2 (c) 1 0 (d) 2-3 –1 (e) 4 or more –3

3. What kind of ground meat or poultry do you usually eat?

(a) regular or lean ground beef –3 (b) extra lean ground beef –2

(c) ground round –1 (d) ground turkey +1 (e) Healthy Choice +3

(f) don't eat ground meat +3

4. Do you trim the visible fat when you cook or eat red meat?

(a) yes +1 (b) no –3 (c) don't eat red meat 0

5. After cooking, how large is the serving of red meat you usually eat? ***(To convert from raw to cooked, reduce by 25 percent. For example, 4 oz. of raw meat shrinks to 3 oz. after cooking. There are 16 oz. in a pound.)***

(a) 8 oz. or more –3 (b) 6-7 oz. –2 (c) 4-5 oz. –1 (d) 3 oz. or less 0

(e) don't eat red meat +3

6. What type of bread, rolls, bagels, etc., do you usually eat?

(a) 100% whole wheat +3 (b) whole wheat as 1st or 2nd ingredient +2

(c) rye, pumpernickel, or oatmeal +1 (d) white, French, or Italian –1

7. How many times per week do you eat deep-fried foods (fish, chicken, vegetables, potatoes, etc.)?

(a) 0 +3 (b) 1-2 0 (c) 3-4 –1 (d) 5 or more –3

8. How many servings of non-fried vegetables do you usually eat per day? ***(One serving = 1/2 cup. INCLUDE potatoes.)***

(a) 0 –3 (b) 1 0 (c) 2 +1 (d) 3 +2 (e) 4 or more +3

9. How many servings of cruciferous vegetables do you usually eat per week? ***(ONLY count kale, broccoli, cauliflower, cabbage, Brussels sprouts, greens, bok choy, kohlrabi, turnip, and rutabaga. One serving = 1/2 cup.)***

(a) 0 –3 (b) 1-3 +1 (c) 4-6 +2 (d) 7 or more +3

10. How many servings of vitamin-A-rich fruits or vegetables do you usually eat per week? ***(ONLY count cantaloupe, apricots, or cooked carrots, pumpkin, sweet potatoes, spinach, winter squash, or greens. One serving = 1/2 cup.)***

(a) 0 –3 (b) 1-3 +1 (c) 4-6 +2 (d) 7 or more +3

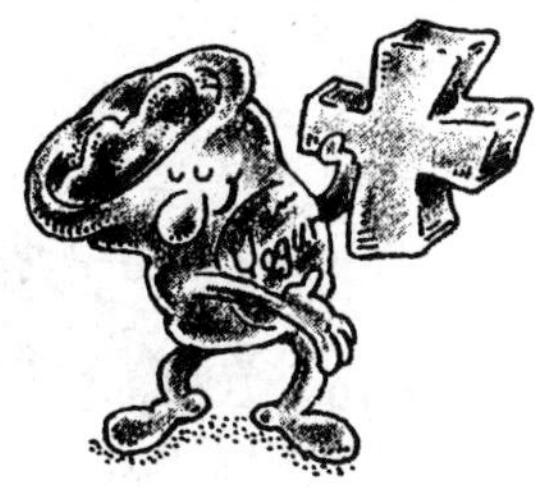

11. How many times per week do you eat at a fast-food restaurant? ***(INCLUDE burgers, fried fish or chicken, croissant or biscuit sandwiches, topped potatoes, and other main dishes. OMIT plain baked potatoes, broiled skinned chicken, or low-fat salads.)***

(a) 0 (b) less than 1 (c) 1 (d) 2 (e) 3 (f) 4 or more
+3 +1 0 −1 −2 −3

12. How many servings of grains do you eat per day? ***(One serving = 1 slice of bread, 1 large pancake, 1 cup cold cereal, or ½ cup cooked cereal, rice, pasta, bulgur, wheat berries, kasha, or millet. OMIT heavily-sweetened cold cereals.)***

(a) 0 (b) 1-3 (c) 4-5 (d) 6-8 (e) 9 or more
−3 0 +1 +2 +3

13. How many times per week do you eat fish or shellfish? ***(OMIT deep-fried items, tuna packed in oil, and mayonnaise-laden tuna salad– a little mayo is okay.)***

(a) 0 (b) 1 (c) 2 (d) 3 or more (e) 0 (vegetarians)
0 +1 +2 +3 +3

14. How many times per week do you eat cheese? ***(INCLUDE pizza, cheeseburgers, veal or eggplant parmigiana, cream cheese, etc. OMIT low-fat or fat-free cheeses.)***

(a) 0 (b) 1 (c) 2-3 (d) 4 or more
+3 +1 −1 −3

15. How many servings of fresh fruit do you eat per day?

(a) 0 (b) 1 (c) 2 (d) 3 (e) 4 or more
−3 0 +1 +2 +3

16. Do you remove the skin before eating poultry?

(a) yes (b) no (c) don't eat poultry
+3 −3 0

17. What do you usually put on your bread or toast? ***(AVERAGE two or more scores if necessary.)***

(a) butter or cream cheese −3 (b) margarine −2 (c) peanut butter −1
(d) diet margarine −1 (e) jam or honey 0 (f) 100% fruit butter +1
(g) nothing +3

18. Which of these beverages do you drink on a typical day? ***(AVERAGE two or more scores if necessary.)***

(a) water or club soda +3 (b) fruit juice +1 (c) diet soda −1
(d) coffee or tea −1 (e) soda, fruit "drink," or fruit "ade" −3

19. Which flavorings do you most frequently add to your foods? ***(AVERAGE two or more scores if necessary.)***

(a) garlic or lemon juice +3 (b) herbs or spices +3 (c) olive oil −1
(d) salt or soy sauce −1 (e) margarine −2 (f) butter −3 (g) nothing +3

20. What do you eat most frequently as a snack? ***(AVERAGE two or more scores if necessary.)***

(a) fruits or vegetables +3 (b) yogurt +2 (c) crackers +1
(d) nuts −1 (e) cookies or fried chips −2 (f) granola bar −2
(g) candy bar or pastry −3 (h) nothing 0

21. What is your most typical breakfast? ***(SUBTRACT an extra 3 points if you also eat bacon or sausage.)***

(a) croissant, danish, or doughnut −3 (b) whole eggs −3
(c) pancakes or waffles −2 (d) cereal or toast +3
(e) low-fat yogurt or cottage cheese +3 (f) don't eat breakfast 0

22. What do you usually eat for dessert?

(a) pie, pastry, or cake −3 (b) ice cream −3
(c) fat-free cookies or cakes −1 (d) frozen yogurt or ice milk 0
(e) non-fat ice cream or sorbet +1 (f) fruit +3 (g) don't eat dessert +3

23. How many times per week do you eat beans, split peas, or lentils?

(a) 0 (b) 1 (c) 2 (d) 3 (e) 4 or more
−3 0 +1 +2 +3

24. What kind of milk do you drink?

(a) whole −3 (b) 2% fat −1 (c) 1% low-fat +2
(d) ½% or skim +3 (e) don't drink milk 0

25. Which items do you choose at a salad bar? ***(ADD two or more scores if necessary.)***

(a) nothing, lemon, or vinegar +3 (b) fat-free dressing +2
(c) low- or reduced-calorie dressing +1 (d) regular dressing −1
(e) croutons or bacon bits −1
(f) cole slaw, pasta salad, or potato salad −1

26. What sandwich fillings do you eat most frequently? ***(AVERAGE two or more scores if necessary.)***

(a) regular luncheon meat −3 (b) cheese −2 (c) roast beef −1
(d) peanut butter 0 (e) low-fat luncheon meat +1
(f) tuna or chicken salad +1 (g) fresh turkey breast or bean spread +3
(h) don't eat sandwiches 0

27. What do you usually spread on your sandwiches? ***(AVERAGE two or more scores if necessary.)***

(a) mayonnaise −2 (b) light mayonnaise −1
(c) catsup, mustard, or fat-free mayonnaise +1
(d) nothing +2

28. How many egg yolks do you eat per week? ***(ADD 1 yolk for every slice of quiche you eat.)***

(a) 2 or less (b) 3-4 (c) 5-6 (d) 7 or more
+3 0 −1 −3

29. How many times per week do you eat canned or dried soups? ***(OMIT low-sodium, low-fat soups.)***

(a) 0 +3 (b) 1-2 0 (c) 3-4 −2 (d) 5 or more −3

30. How many servings of a rich source of calcium do you eat per day? ***(One serving = 2/3 cup milk or yogurt, 1 oz. cheese, 1 1/2 oz. sardines, 3 1/2 oz. canned salmon (with bones), 5 oz. tofu made with calcium sulfate, 1 cup greens or broccoli, or 200 mg of a calcium supplement.)***

(a) 0 −3 (b) 1 +1 (c) 2 +2 (d) 3 or more +3

31. What do you usually order on your pizza? ***(Vegetable toppings include green pepper, mushrooms, onions, and other vegetables. SUBTRACT 1 point from your score if you order extra cheese.)***

(a) no cheese with vegetables +3 (b) cheese with vegetables +1
(c) cheese 0 (d) cheese with meat toppings −3
(e) don't eat pizza +2

32. What kind of cookies do you usually eat?

(a) don't eat cookies +3 (b) fat-free cookies +2
(c) graham crackers or ginger snaps +1 (d) oatmeal −1
(e) sandwich cookies (like Oreos) −2
(f) chocolate coated, chocolate chip, or peanut butter −3

33. What kind of frozen dessert do you usually eat? ***(SUBTRACT 1 point from your score for each topping you use—whipped cream, hot fudge, nuts, etc.)***

(a) gourmet ice cream −3 (b) regular ice cream −2
(c) frozen yogurt, ice milk 0 (d) sorbet, sherbet, or ices +1
(e) non-fat frozen yogurt or fat-free ice cream +1
(f) don't eat frozen desserts +3

34. What kind of cake or pastry do you usually eat?

(a) cheesecake, pie, or any microwave cake −3
(b) cake with frosting −2 (c) cake without frosting −1
(d) unfrosted muffin, banana bread, or carrot cake 0
(e) angelfood or fat-free cake +1 (f) don't eat cakes or pastries +3

35. How many times per week does your dinner contain grains, vegetables, or beans, but little or no animal protein (meat, poultry, fish, eggs, milk, or cheese)?

(a) 0 −1 (b) 1-2 +1 (c) 3-4 +2 (d) 5 or more +3

36. Which of the following "salty" snacks do you typically eat? ***(AVERAGE two or more scores if necessary.)***

(a) potato chips, corn chips, or pre-popped popcorn −3
(b) tortilla chips, reduced-fat potato chips, or microwave popcorn −2
(c) salted pretzels −1 (d) light microwave popcorn 0
(e) unsalted pretzels +1 (f) fat-free tortilla or potato chips +2
(g) homemade air-popped popcorn +3 (h) don't eat salty snacks +3

37. What do you usually use to sauté vegetables or other foods? ***(Vegetable oil includes safflower, corn, canola, sunflower, and soybean.)***

(a) butter or lard −3 (b) margarine −2 (c) vegetable oil −1
(d) olive oil +1 (e) broth +2 (f) water or cooking spray +3

38. What kind of cereal do you usually eat?

(a) whole grain (like oatmeal or Shredded Wheat) +3
(b) low-fiber (like Cream of Wheat or Corn Flakes) 0
(c) sugary low-fiber (like Frosted Flakes) −1 (d) regular granola −2

39. With what do you make tuna salad, pasta salad, chicken salad, etc?

(a) mayonnaise −2 (b) light mayonnaise −1 (c) non-fat mayonnaise 0
(d) low-fat yogurt +2 (e) non-fat yogurt +3

40. What do you typically put on your pasta? ***(ADD one point if you also add sautéed vegetables. AVERAGE two or more scores if necessary.)***

(a) tomato sauce, with or without a little parmesan +3
(b) white clam sauce 0 (c) meat sauce or meat balls −2
(d) Alfredo, pesto, or other creamy or oily sauce −3

YOUR GRAND TOTAL

+59 to +117	GREAT!	You're a nutrition superstar. Give yourself a big (non-butter) pat on the back.
0 to +58	GOOD	You're doing just fine. Pin your Quiz to the nearest wall.
−1 to −58	FAIR	Hang in there. Tape CSPI's Nutrition Scoreboard poster to your refrigerator for a little friendly help.
−59 to −116	ARRGH!	Stop lining the cat box with *Nutrition Action Healthletter*. Empty your refrigerator and cupboard. It's time to start over.

3

The Mediterranean Diet

Medical advances often come from basic science laboratories, where researchers study the molecules and proteins involved in a disease. But some of the most important knowledge about the causes of heart disease has resulted from *epidemiological* studies, in which researchers study large populations of people to identify "risk factors" for diseases. Such research often requires years of careful data collection and analysis. Over the past four or five decades, this painstaking approach has already shown that heart attacks are more common in people who smoke or have high blood pressure, a high cholesterol level, or diabetes.

During this same time period, epidemiologists also noted remarkably low rates of heart attack and of some other diseases in the countries around the Mediterranean Sea. For example, in 1959 the coronary heart disease death rate for American men between the ages of 55 and 59 was nearly eight times that of Greek men of the same age — 748 per 100,000 versus 95 per 100,000. Rates of other chronic diseases such as breast and colon cancer were also very low in this region, and life expectancy was about four years longer than in the U.S. and northern Europe.

The lower heart-attack rate in the Mediterranean countries could not be explained by the known risk factors for heart disease. So researchers began to evaluate other differences between the peoples of these countries and the rest of the Western world. Over time, attention has increasingly focused on the traditional Mediterranean diet.

Ironically, the "Mediterranean diet" is not as common in that region as it once was, because diets throughout much of the world have become steadily "Americanized," with the addition of processed and fast foods made with saturated and partially hydrogenated fats. But during the 1960s, the daily fare for most people around the Mediterranean included very little meat and only moderate amounts of dairy products; olive oil was the principal fat. Can this Mediterranean diet help reduce the risk of heart disease? If so, what elements of the cuisine might be most effective? And what are the similarities and differences between such a diet and the one recommended by the U.S. Department of Agriculture (USDA)?

Occasional treats

The core of the traditional Mediterranean cuisine was an abundance of fruits and vegetables as well as large quantities of bread, pasta, couscous, rice, and other grains. Legumes (such as peas, beans, and lentils) and nuts were also eaten frequently. However, meats were used mainly as condiments, accents to meals, or occasional treats for holidays. Red meat was consumed only a few times per month, or somewhat more often in very small portions. The Mediterraneans ate modest quantities of other foods from animal sources, including dairy products (especially cheese and yogurt), fish and poultry; and they drank wine in moderation, primarily at meals. Sweets played a small role in the diet, and fruit was the main form of dessert. Vigorous physical labor was a way of life in this agrarian society.

From *Harvard Heart Letter,* November 1993, pp. 1-5.

The most conspicuous feature of the Mediterranean diet of the 1960s was olive oil. Olive trees abound in the region, and consequently olive oil accounted for most of the fat in the Mediterranean cuisine, ranging from 28% of total calories in southern Italy to 40% in Crete. Like other fats, olive oil is rich in calories, but it is a monounsaturated fat — a chemical form that is markedly different from the saturated fats found in meats.

Olive oil and other "monos" like canola and peanut oils seem to have beneficial effects on both low-density-lipoprotein (LDL) and high-density-lipoprotein (HDL) cholesterol. LDL cholesterol contributes to the buildup of fatty deposits in the arteries, thereby raising the risk of heart disease, while HDL helps to remove such deposits. A diet low in fat and high in complex carbohydrates tends to reduce LDL *and* HDL cholesterol. However, a diet rich in olive oil can lower the "bad" LDL cholesterol and *raise* the "good" HDL cholesterol — cutting heart-attack risk in two ways at once.

Mounting support

Several studies have demonstrated olive oil's positive effects on blood-fat levels. In a study from the Netherlands, 48 healthy male and female volunteers between the ages of 18 and 59 years old were divided into two similar groups and given special diets for five weeks. One group received a low-fat diet that was high in unrefined carbohydrates, including bread, legumes, vegetables, fruits, and jam; the second group ate a diet rich in olive oil, including a special bread made with olive oil. Total cholesterol fell to the same extent in both groups. But the "good" HDL fell an average of 7.3 mg/dl on the high carbohydrate diet, whereas it actually rose 1.1 mg/dl on the olive-oil-rich diet.

Another recent study showed that the substitution of olive oil for saturated fat appeared to be at least as healthy as the diet recommended by the American Heart Association (AHA). Researchers from Columbia University tested the effect of various fats on the cholesterol levels of 36 healthy male medical and dental students. One-third of the participants ate an average American diet, in which 38% of the calories come from fat (18% saturated, 10% monounsaturated, and 10% polyunsaturated). Another third ate the AHA/USDA-recommended diet, with 30% of the calories from fat (10% each from saturated, monounsaturated, and polyunsaturated). The final group followed a Mono diet, which was the AHA diet with an extra 8% of monounsaturated fat replacing equivalent calories from complex carbohydrates.

Total cholesterol fell by 1% in those on the average American diet, by 8% on the AHA diet, and by 10% on the Mono diet. Furthermore, the participants who ate the Mono diet tended to have higher levels of the "good" HDL cholesterol than did those on the AHA diet. The Mono diet also resulted in significantly better ratios of total cholesterol to HDL cholesterol than did the average American and AHA diets — indicating a lower heart-attack risk.

People with diabetes may reap additional benefits from monounsaturates. Researchers at the Center for Human Nutrition in Dallas compared two diets with the same number of calories — one rich in carbohydrates and the other in monounsaturates — in a group of patients with diabetes. The Mono diet resulted in decreased insulin requirements, lower blood sugar, and a better lipid profile than did the carbohydrate diet.

What about polyunsaturates?

Is olive oil any better than vegetable oils that are high in polyunsaturated fats, such as corn and soybean oils? These vegetable oils are as effective as olive oil in reducing total cholesterol while maintaining high levels of the "good" HDL, but the long-term effects of diets rich in polyunsaturates are not known, since there have been no studies of large population groups that have consumed high levels of these fats for a lifetime.

Some polyunsaturated fats are needed as precursors for the production of prostaglandins, which are essential for regulating clotting and other bodily functions. Since olive oil actually contains polyunsaturated fatty acids, a diet rich in olive oil should be sufficient for the body's needs.

A new pyramid

To convert the Mediterranean diet of the 1960s to a recommended diet for Americans in the 1990s, researchers have proposed a Mediterranean food pyramid (*see illustration*) that includes a generous daily intake of fruits and vegetables. This aspect of the recommendations is in harmony with both the U.S. National Cancer Institute and the USDA guidelines, which urge a minimum of two or more servings of fruit and three or more servings of vegetables every day.

The Mediterranean and USDA approaches diverge in other areas, however. The Mediterranean pyramid recommends only small quantities of dairy products, whereas the USDA guide suggests quite a bit more — two to three servings a day. The USDA rationale for higher dairy-product consumption is based on the belief that calcium may help prevent osteoporosis. Both guides suggest low-fat or skimmed-milk dairy products as a way to reduce the intake of saturated fats.

Plenty of breads, grains, and cereals are recommended by both pyramids; but the Mediterranean diet emphasizes whole-grain foods, while the USDA guide makes little distinction between them and refined products. The effects of dietary fiber from whole grains on cholesterol are controversial. In one study, people who ate two ounces (dry weight) of oat bran every day had a 16% drop in LDL cholesterol. In another study, however, when oat brain was substituted for other carbohydrates, the change in cholesterol was much smaller. Thus, the jury is still out on whether whole-grain foods are substantially better at lowering lipids than are other grain products. It is important to remember, however, that whole grains are rich in several micronutrients, many of which are lost when the grains are processed into refined products.

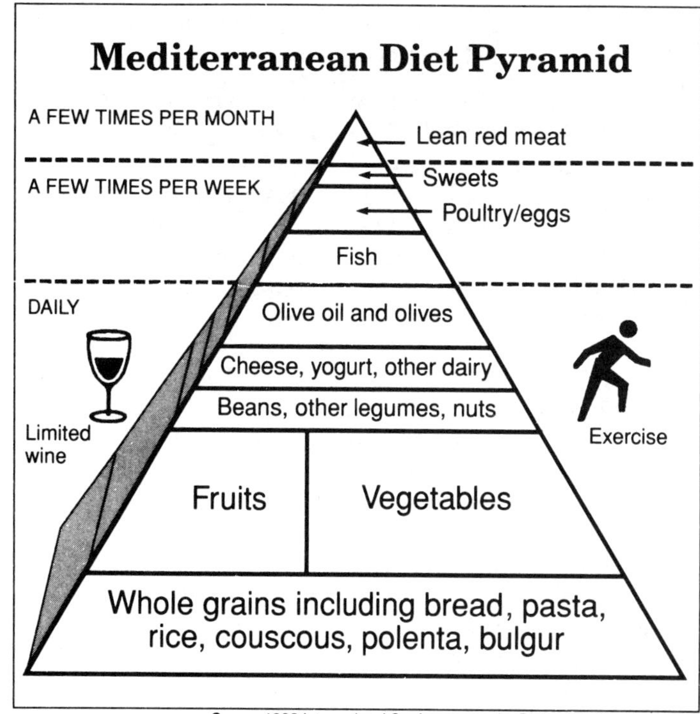

Source:1993 International Conference on the Diets of the Mediterranean
Preliminary concept; subject to modification.

Following the Mediterranean tradition, the new pyramid suggests the option of one glass of wine a day for women and up to two glasses for men, with the caveat that drinking should be avoided whenever consumption would put the individual or others at risk. Many studies have suggested that moderate consumption of alcohol raises HDL levels, lowers the risk of heart disease, and reduces overall mortality. For women, however, the decision of whether to drink or not is complicated, since substantial evidence indicates that even one or two drinks per day increases the risk of breast cancer.

Given current knowledge about the health benefits of physical activity and the role it played in the lives of the Mediterraneans, the proposed guide recommends daily exercise. Many studies have linked a physically active lifestyle to a lower heart-disease risk. Even moderate exercise, if done regularly, can improve an unfavorable cholesterol profile by lowering both the "bad" LDL cholesterol and triglycerides and raising the "good" HDL cholesterol.

Only on Sunday

In the proposed Mediterranean food guide, "lean red meat" is represented by a tiny triangle sitting at the top of the pyramid, with the admonition to eat it no more than a few times per month. In Crete in the 1960s, one pound of red meat was divided among six to eight people at one meal, and the meat was far leaner than the beef in the U.S. today. In fact, in Crete the per capita consumption of red meat *and* poultry together averaged only 1.2 ounces per day.

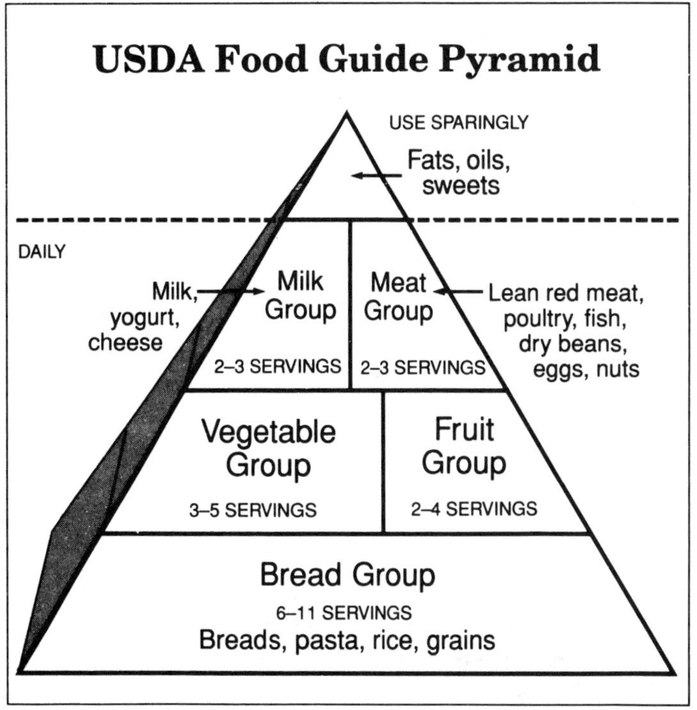

Source: U.S. Department of Agriculture

On the Table

Proponents of a Mediterranean menu contend that dieting need not be an unpleasant experience. At a conference on this cuisine held early this year, nutritionists and other health professionals were served traditional Mediterranean meals. Here is one of the lunches: Barley croutons soaked in grated tomato and herbs; warm bean stew with fennel and tomato; bulgur salad with beets, onions, and potatoes; simmered wild greens with olive oil and lemon dressing; olive oil biscuits with cumin and sesame; fresh orange wedges; graviera cheese laced with honey; and wine.

A Mediterranean diet does not have to be all or nothing, however. It is one excellent way to eat in a healthy manner and provides additional options for people trying to reduce harmful fats and cholesterol in their diet. But many of the healthful components in the Mediterranean diet can be found in other cuisines. People could "mix and match" — healthy Mexican food one day (perhaps chicken enchilada with salsa and black bean soup), Greek the next (tabouli, lentil soup, and a Greek salad), Thai the next (chicken satay with peanut butter sauce and stir-fried vegetables), and Japanese another (miso soup with rice and vegetables tempura).

The USDA Food Guide Pyramid is not so restrictive about red meat. It combines meat, chicken, fish, and legumes in the "Meat Group" category and recommends two to three 3-ounce servings a day. Some nutritionists believe that this "lumping together" allows the false impression that current nutrition research condones up to 9 ounces of red meat per day (63 ounces per week, or 3.9 pounds). Many studies suggest that a high intake of red meat is associated with increased risks of coronary heart disease, colon cancer, and possibly other cancers.

The Mediterranean food guide recommends that fish be eaten a few times a week. Many salt-water fish are rich in omega-3 fatty acids, and some nutritionists speculate that these fatty acids may have helped protect the Mediterranean people against heart disease. One modern investigation — of 852 middle-aged Dutch men — found that those who ate the equivalent of two fish meals a week reduced their heart-disease risk over a 20-year period, but subsequent studies have yielded conflicting results. The Mediterranean food guide also suggests that small portions of poultry and eggs be eaten no more than a few times per week.

Unanswered questions

Unanswered questions persist regarding the Mediterranean diet: Some skeptics question the safety of a diet in which 25–40% of calories come from fat, and others wonder whether olive oil was the key ingredient that lowered chronic-disease rates and extended life expectancy in the Mediterranean. Perhaps the plant-based diet, or the inhabitants' vigorous physical activity (necessary for tending crops and livestock), or some other element of their lifestyle accounted for the low rate of heart disease in that region of the world. Most likely, a combination of influences was responsible.

In the meantime, epidemiologists and other medical scientists are continuing to conduct studies about how the Mediterranean diet and lifestyle

Some Examples of Carbohydrates and Fats

Complex or unrefined carbohydrates: Grains (brown rice, oats, wheat, barley, corn), legumes (chick peas, black-eyed peas, lentils, lima, kidney, pinto, soy, and black beans), vegetables, and whole fruits.

Refined or simple carbohydrates: White table sugar, brown sugar, corn syrup, molasses, honey, fruit sugars, white flour, white bread, candy, alcohol, and some processed foods and commercially baked goods.

Fiber: Undigestible parts of carbohydrates from plants. Found in the skins, stems, or seeds of fruits, vegetables, whole grains, breads, and cereals.

Monounsaturated fats: Olive, peanut, sesame, and canola oils and most nuts and seeds.

Polyunsaturated fats: Soybean, corn, cottonseed, safflower, and sunflower oils.

Saturated fats: Red meat, poultry skin, lard, butter, hard cheeses, some vegetable oils (palm, coconut, and cocoa butter), and partially hydrogenated oils.

Partially hydrogenated fats: Oils hardened by the addition of hydrogen and used in margarines, vegetable shortening, and many commercially baked goods.

achieved such healthy results. Nutritionists agree on certain points: Saturated-fat intake and meat consumption must be reduced in the American diet, and a major shift toward foods from plant sources is necessary for optimal health. It is also clear that many components of the Mediterranean diet — olive oil, fruits, vegetables, legumes, whole wheat, and nuts — are sources of antioxidants, which appear to help prevent LDL, the "bad" cholesterol, from forming fat deposits on the walls of the blood vessels (see *Harvard Heart Letter*, March 1993).

Diets rich in monounsaturated fats appear to be at least as healthy as very low-fat diets — and may be an even better way to improve the lipid profile. However, if people simply add olive oil to an existing diet that already includes large amounts of saturated and partially hydrogenated fats, then they may negate the beneficial effects of olive oil. In addition, since all fats, including olive oil, have 9 calories per gram — more than twice the 4 calories contained in a gram of carbohydrate or protein — it is important that monounsaturates be substituted for other calories; if the Mediterranean diet results in significant weight gain, the value of the diet will be undermined. Finally, any diet should be accompanied by regular aerobic exercise — such as brisk walking, biking, or swimming — and by a program to reduce other risk factors, including high blood pressure, smoking, and obesity.

The new thinking about fats

As most people see it, fat is the nutritional villain, clogging the arteries and settling around the waist. Americans have one of the fattiest diets in the world: about 37% of our calories now come from fats, up from 32% at the start of the century. The largest portion of our fats comes from animal sources—especially meat and whole-milk dairy products—and is thus highly saturated and accompanied by cholesterol. Thanks to recent research, we now know that the fat scenario is more complicated than it once seemed. Are hydrogenated vegetable oils (found in margarines, for example) necessarily better for us than animal fats (such as butter)? Should we adopt a "Mediterranean diet" that is rich in olive oil? Here are answers to these and other questions.

What are fats? Why are they high in calories?

Technically called lipids, the fats in foods are mostly triglycerides, which consist of three fatty acids attached to a glycerol molecule. Fats are the most concentrated source of food energy, supplying nine calories per gram; carbohydrates and proteins have four calories per gram. High-fat foods are thus always high-calorie foods. And a high-fat diet may increase the chance of obesity, which in turn increases the risk of cardiovascular disease, diabetes, and other disorders.

What's the difference between saturated and unsaturated fats?

All fats are combinations of saturated and unsaturated fatty acids, which is why fats are described with terms such as "highly saturated." Fatty acids vary in length and in degree of saturation (that is, how many hydrogen atoms they carry), both of which help determine whether a fat is solid or liquid (oil) at room temperature.

Saturated fatty acids carry all the hydrogen atoms they can hold. Highly saturated fats come chiefly from animal sources and include butter, milk fat, and the fat in meats; two vegetable oils—coconut and palm kernel oils—are also highly saturated.

Unsaturated fatty acids do not have all the hydrogen atoms they can carry. If a pair of hydrogen atoms is missing, these fatty acids are called **monounsaturated** (olive, peanut, and canola oils are largely monounsaturated). If two pairs or more of hydrogen atoms are missing, the fatty acids are called **polyunsaturated** (corn, safflower, and sesame oils are primarily polyunsaturated). Plants and fish are the important sources of unsaturated fats. These fats generally are liquid at room temperature.

Should I avoid all fat?

That would be very difficult—and undesirable. You need to consume some fat to stay healthy. For instance, it supplies "essential" fatty acids—so named because the body can't make them and must get them from foods—which are crucial for proper growth and development. Essential fatty acids are the raw materials for several hormonelike compounds, including prostaglandins, that help control vital bodily functions. However, you don't need to consume any *saturated* fatty acids; your body makes all it needs. Fat also aids in the absorption of the fat-soluble vitamins (A, D, E, and K) and helps maintain healthy skin and hair.

Are all saturated fats bad?

Highly saturated fats raise overall cholesterol levels in the blood, especially LDL ("bad") cholesterol. Yet even this seemingly clear-cut fact has been complicated by recent research that has examined the interactions of various fatty acids in the body. At least one saturated fatty acid, stearic acid (a major component of the fat in beef, pork, and the cocoa butter in chocolate), appears to have a neutral effect on blood cholesterol. However, this has little or no practical implication, since no one eats isolated stearic acid, except in laboratory studies. In any case, what may be true of stearic acid alone isn't true of sirloin steaks, burgers, pork chops, and other foods rich in stearic acid. These foods still have two strikes against them—they contain other saturated fatty acids (notably palmitic acid) that clearly raise cholesterol in the blood, and most are high in cholesterol.

Is cholesterol a fat?

No, though it is also classified as a lipid. Cholesterol is a vital part of all cell membranes and nerve fibers and serves as a building block for hormones. It is the cholesterol that circulates in the blood that is so often discussed and measured. That's because this cholesterol can accumulate in the walls of blood vessels, leading to atherosclerosis and possibly heart attack or stroke.

Comparing oils (one tablespoon)

All vegetable oils contain 120 calories and 13.5 grams of fat per tablespoon (butter and margarine have 100 calories and 11.5 grams per tablespoon; lard 115 calories and 13 grams of fat). Look for an oil that is low in saturated fatty acids and, preferably, high in monounsatured fatty acids.

TYPE	UNSATURATED		SATURATED
	MONO (g)	POLY (g)	(g)
BEST			
Almond	10	2	1
Canola (rapeseed)	8	4	1
Olive	10	1	2
Peanut	6	5	2
GOOD			
Corn	3	8	2
Cottonseed	2	7	4
Safflower	2	10	1
Sesame	5	6	2
Soybean	3	8	2
Sunflower	3	9	1
Walnut	3	9	1
WORST			
Coconut	1	—	12
Palm	5	1	7
Palm kernel	2	—	11
Butter	3	1	7
Margarine, stick	5	4	2
Lard	6	2	5

Cholesterol is found only in foods from animal sources, such as meats, eggs, and dairy products, which are usually also rich in saturated fats. If it were simply a matter of the cholesterol from food going directly into our bloodstream, we would only have to worry about how much cholesterol we eat. But the liver usually synthesizes most of the cholesterol in the body—a process only partly regulated by the amount of cholesterol eaten. Surprisingly, the amount and type of fat you eat generally affects blood cholesterol levels much more than the cholesterol in the foods you eat. Thus limiting your cholesterol intake but not your consumption of saturated fats can result in high blood cholesterol.

What's wrong with safflower oil and other polyunsaturates?

Highly polyunsaturated vegetable oils—such as safflower, sunflower, and soybean—used to be considered the most healthful oils because they dramatically lower overall cholesterol levels, especially LDL. But in recent years nutritionists have focused on the possible negative effects of these oils. First of all, large amounts of highly polyunsaturated fats also lower HDL ("good") cholesterol, and scientists now believe that a *low* HDL level is an independent risk factor for heart disease (monounsaturates may not lower HDL as much). In addition, studies on animals have found that large amounts of highly polyunsaturated vegetable oils increase the risk of several types of cancer—but that's not necessarily true for humans. (For more on fat and cancer, see page 126.)

What are those hydrogenated fats in margarine?

Manufacturers hydrogenate—that is, add hydrogen atoms to—soybean, corn, and other liquid oils to make them more solid and stable. This gives margarines and some puddings a creamy consistency, for instance, and prolongs the shelf life of crackers, cookies, potato chips, and other foods that contain the semi-solid oils. Because they are less likely to turn rancid, hydrogenated oils are also often used to cook french fries in restaurants. Usually oils are only partially hydrogenated; totally hydrogenated oils are suitable for few foods. Depending on the degree of hydrogenation, these artificially saturated vegetable fats may be no better for you than comparably saturated animal fats.

Most important, hydrogenation transforms many of an oil's unsaturated fatty acids, making them more saturated and changing their structure in other subtle ways—they are thus called *trans* fatty acids. Scientists have been concerned that these trans fats may increase the risk of coronary artery disease and perhaps other health problems. While a diet high in regular unsaturated fat lowers total blood cholesterol, a diet high in trans fats lowers it much less—or may even raise it—by increasing LDL cholesterol. In addition, trans fats lower HDL cholesterol, the type that carries cholesterol out of the arteries. This may help explain why a study from Harvard published in March in *Lancet* found that women who ate lots of foods high in trans fatty acids (especially margarine) had a 50% higher risk of coronary artery disease than women who ate these fats rarely. Another study, reported in the *American Journal of Cardiology* in April, found that people with coronary artery disease have significantly elevated levels of trans fatty acids in their blood.

A few years back, the National Academy of Sciences concluded that there was little or no cause for concern about trans fats because they make up only a small amount of our fat intake. Critics claim, however, that in recent years Americans have been consuming two to three times as much trans fat as was previously estimated—especially since food makers, pressured to reduce the use of highly saturated tropical oils (such as palm and coconut), have generally replaced them with hydrogenated oils. The fact is, no one really knows how much trans fat we eat. For one thing, food manufacturers often change the types of oils they use and the degree of hydrogenation of the oils. In addition, nutrition labels don't specify how much trans fats are in foods.

So should I avoid margarine and go back to butter?

Butter, lard, and coconut oil contain more saturated fat than margarine, so they probably raise blood cholesterol more than margarine. Butter and lard also contain cholesterol, while margarine doesn't. Still, if your diet is otherwise low in fat, you needn't worry about occasionally eating small amounts of butter, margarine, or any high-fat food.

If, however, you eat lots of margarine and many processed foods that contain hydrogenated oils, try to cut back. In general, the more solid the vegetable oil, the more hydrogenated, and therefore the more trans fatty acids it has—that's why tub and liquid "squeeze" margarines are preferable to stick margarine. "Diet" margarines are even better, since they are very soft and contain more water and only half the fat of other margarines. When possible, use liquid vegetable oil (except coconut or palm oil) in cooking rather than butter or margarine. You can even use a little olive oil on your bread instead of either spread.

Is olive oil the way to go, then?

Olive oil, as well as other highly monounsaturated oils such as canola and nut oils, may not only help lower overall blood cholesterol level and artery-damaging LDL cholesterol, but also maintain the level of heart-healthy HDL cholesterol. Monounsaturated fats may also result in less oxidation of LDL (this chemical process appears to trigger a chain of events that causes plaque to build up in artery walls and that subsequently leads to a heart attack). Though the evidence is weaker, some studies have also suggested that olive oil can help lower blood pressure and control blood sugar levels. Highly monounsaturated oils are especially good for cooking: when overheated, they develop fewer "free radicals"—chemical agents that may be dangerous to human cells—than polyunsaturated oils do.

The recent surge in popularity of olive oil can probably be traced to the Seven Countries Study begun in 1958, which found that Mediterranean peoples, such as the Italians and Greeks, whose chief dietary fat is olive oil, have relatively low cholesterol levels and low rates of coronary artery disease, despite a fat intake as high as ours. It is important to remember, however, that the "Mediterranean diet" typically contains much more fruit and vegetables and less meat than ours, and these Europeans are generally more active than we are.

Still, no responsible scientists recommend that Americans simply swallow olive or canola oil by the tablespoon. Like other oils, they are 100% fat and contain 120 calories per tablespoon, and thus may cause you to gain weight. The important part of the equation is to use olive oil to *replace* animal fats and highly polyunsaturated oils.

What's special about the fat in nuts?

Like olive oil, most nuts are high in monounsaturated fat, and several recent studies have suggested that nuts may offer beneficial effects. For instance, a study published in the *Journal of the American College of Nutrition* in 1992 found that people on a low-fat diet lowered their total and LDL cholesterol levels significantly when they started eating 3.5 ounces of almonds a day (the percentage of calories derived from fat in their diet rose from 28% to 37%). Another study, using walnuts instead of almonds and published in the *New England Journal of Medicine,* found similar results (the percentage of fat calories stayed the same—30%). And a study of Seventh Day Adventists suggested that those who ate nuts most often had the lowest risk of heart attack (see *Wellness Letter,* February 1993). These results are promising, but it is still too early to recommend a daily handful of nuts—which are very high in calories—as a way to ward off heart attacks.

How strong is the evidence that fat causes cancer?

The strongest evidence concerns the link between a high fat intake and colon cancer. For other kinds of cancer, fat's role remains controversial (the *Wellness Letter* discussed the debate about breast cancer and fat in March 1993). Nonetheless, a low-fat diet makes sense if you're concerned about cancer, particularly since it helps guard against becoming overweight or obese, which in itself may be a risk factor for certain cancers, as well as for diabetes and heart disease.

Many scientists have noted that, with a few exceptions, countries with a high national fat intake also have the highest cancer rates. Some studies have found that a diet high in fat—saturated or unsaturated—increases the risk of cancer of the colon and breast, and possibly of the ovary, uterus, and prostate. Most recently, a study presented to the American Cancer Society found that among nonsmoking women, the risk of an uncommon form of lung cancer increases dramatically along with saturated-fat intake.

The mechanism for the link between a high-fat diet and cancer has not been determined, but there are theories. A diet high in fat affects the secretion of some sex hormones, which might cause cancer in the reproductive organs. Moreover, high-fat diets increase the amount of bile acids in the colon, which may be converted there by bacteria into carcinogenic by-products.

What about the polyunsaturated fat in fish?

Fish contains a type of long-chain polyunsaturated fatty acids commonly called omega-3s, which make the blood's platelets less likely to form a clot, thus reducing the chances of an artery blockage and heart attack. Get your omega-3s from fish, not from supplements, since many questions remain about the safety, effectiveness, and proper dosage of fish oil in liquid or capsule form.

The bottom line

Eat less fat, period. Virtually all health organizations and government agencies recommend that Americans reduce their fat intake so that less than 30% of all calories consumed each day come from fats. That translates to less than 66 grams of fat in a 2,000-calorie daily diet. Some health professionals advocate that total fat consumption should drop to 25% or even 20%.

Eat less saturated fat. Less than 10% of your calories should come from saturated fat, such as that in cheese, butter, and meat.

Limit your polyunsaturated fats. Less than 10% of your calories should come from polyunsaturated fat, such as that in safflower oil, soybean oil, and sunflower oil. Especially limit your intake of hydrogenated vegetable oils, found in so many processed foods. For instance, instead of stick margarine, which contains lots of hydrogenated fat, choose a tub margarine, which doesn't. The softer the spread, usually the less hydrogenated.

Eat monounsaturated fats in place of other fats. Olive and canola oils are the best choices among vegetable oils because they are highest in monounsaturated fat and among the lowest in saturated fat: use them instead of butter or margarine, when possible. You can also choose a peanut butter sandwich *instead of* a hamburger. Since avocados are another source of monounsaturates, opt for guacamole instead of cheese dip. But, of course, even better choices would be fish instead of the fatty hamburger, and salsa instead of the cheese dip, since the goal is to cut down on all fats.

TAKING VITAMINS

CAN THEY PREVENT DISEASE?

Should you take vitamin pills—or simply eat well?

If economics had not already claimed the title, nutrition might well be considered the dismal science. The ups and downs of nutrition advice have come to seem as capricious as the fluctuations of the stock market. In recent years, Americans have been told that margarine might be as bad for them as butter; that iron supplements, long promoted as a cure for "tired blood," might contribute to heart disease; and that repeated dieting could be more hazardous than staying overweight. But none of those flip-flops was as confusing and disturbing as the Great Vitamin Scare of 1994.

By last April, when the scare occurred, many scientists were beginning to believe that vitamin supplements could be a highly effective, relatively inexpensive, and virtually risk-free form of preventive medicine. In particular, they were excited by a trio of "antioxidants": vitamin C, vitamin E, and beta-carotene, a substance that is partly converted to vitamin A in the body. These nutrients are believed to help protect the body's cells from free radicals, destructive molecules that are thought to cause wide-ranging damage. Free radicals may damage a cell's DNA in ways that eventually lead to cancer; may interact with cholesterol in the bloodstream in a way that leads it to clog the arteries; may help cause cataracts, rheumatoid arthritis, and other ills; and may underlie much of the aging process. Free radicals arise from normal metabolic processes, as well as from toxic substances such as air pollution and cigarette smoke.

Anything that fights free radicals would be a boon to health, and the antioxidants have looked like a top contender. Test-tube experiments, animal research, and studies of large populations—comparing people who get higher and lower levels of antioxidants in their diets or from supplements—have all shown benefits from vitamin C, vitamin E, and beta-carotene. After more than a decade of cautious interpretation, some nutrition experts were ready, by last year, to declare that the evidence for antioxidants was compelling. Several even admitted that they had started taking vitamin pills themselves.

But a major piece of the puzzle was still missing. Scientists were waiting for the results of controlled clinical studies: studies where large groups of people were chosen at random to receive either nutritional supplements or placebos, then followed for a number of years. In April, a team of researchers announced that one of the first such studies had been completed—and it was a bombshell.

The study, done with support from the National Cancer Institute (NCI), had tested the effect of beta-carotene supplements on more than 29,000 male smokers in Finland. Most researchers were expecting beta-carotene to lower the risk of lung cancer. More than a dozen population studies had already shown that people who ate foods rich in beta-carotene, and people who had high blood levels of the nutrient, had a relatively low lung-cancer risk. So scientists were dumbfounded to learn that after about six years, the incidence of lung cancer was 18 percent *higher* in the Finnish men who took beta-carotene than in those who didn't.

The study had bad news about vitamin E, too. While some of the men had taken beta-carotene, others took vitamin E. (Some got both nutrients, and some got placebos.) The men who took vitamin E had a lower risk of prostate cancer, but an increased death rate from hemorrhagic, or bleeding-related, strokes. The apparent effects of vitamin E were minimal after the proper statistical adjustments were made, but were a cause for concern nevertheless.

The reactions were quick. The NCI urged researchers studying beta-carotene to inform people in their studies of the possible risk. A leading nutrition advocacy group that had advised people to take supplements the year before now warned the public to "shelve the beta-carotene." Some scientists dismissed the study as seriously flawed, while others said it reinforced the need to proceed with caution.

The Finnish study could turn out to be a watershed. A report in July, showing that antioxidants don't prevent a precursor of colon cancer, added weight to the view that they are not helpful. But the Finnish results also could be a statistical fluke. Either way, the study makes it more important than ever for consumers to understand the science of supplementation.

Can vitamins hurt?

Several months after the Finnish study, Dr. Philip Taylor, chief of NCI's cancer prevention studies branch, took a philosophical view of the unexpected results. The study, he said, simply reflects "the beauty and the frustration" of science. "Just about the time we think it all fits, someone steps in our sandpile and everything goes in every direction."

As the sand has started to settle, scientists are trying to figure out just what the Finnish study means. One confounding factor is that the study involved a group of men at extremely high risk: middle-aged men who had smoked a pack a day for 36 years, on average. It's hardly surprising that nutritional supplements did nothing to prevent lung cancer in men whose lungs were probably severely damaged to begin with. Supplements could have quite different effects on healthy people.

GOOD SOURCES OF BETA-CAROTENE

The following foods all have at least 1 milligram of beta-carotene per serving, a significant amount. While there is no official U.S. RDA for beta-carotene, 3 milligrams is equivalent to 5000 IU, the U.S. RDA for vitamin A. All nutrient levels are approximate, and will vary.

Food	Serving size	Beta-carotene
FRUITS		
Apricots, dried	10 halves	6.2 mg.
Cantaloupe	½	4.8
Apricots, fresh	2	2.5
Grapefruit, pink or red	½	1.6
Mango	½	1.4
Watermelon	1 slice	1.1
VEGETABLES [1]		
Sweet potato	1 medium	10.0
Chicory, raw	1 cup	6.2
Carrot, raw	1 medium	5.7
Spinach	½ cup	4.9
Turnip greens	½ cup	3.9
Pumpkin	½ cup	3.7
Collard greens	½ cup	3.4
Swiss chard	½ cup	3.2
Kale	½ cup	3.0
Winter squash	½ cup	2.9
Spinach, raw	1 cup	2.3
Spaghetti squash	½ cup	1.9
Mustard greens	½ cup	1.9
Beet greens	½ cup	1.8
Dandelion greens	½ cup	1.4
Bell peppers, sweet red, raw	½ cup	1.1
Romaine lettuce, raw	1 cup	1.1
Broccoli	½ cup	1.0
JUICES AND SOUPS		
Carrot juice	1 cup	24.2
Gazpacho	1 cup	11.7
Tomato juice	1 cup	2.2
Vegetable soup	1 cup	1.9
Manhattan clam chowder	1 cup	1.9
Vegetable and beef stew	1 cup	1.7
Split-pea soup	1 cup	1.4

[1] Cooked, unless otherwise specified.

Source: United States Department of Agriculture/National Cancer Institute

No one can yet explain why beta-carotene actually appeared harmful in this study. In the other ongoing controlled clinical trials in which people are taking beta-carotene supplements, subjects are monitored periodically for signs of harm, and no ill effects have been reported.

People have also taken vitamin E safely for long periods and at much higher levels than the modest amount used in the Finnish study. There is some evidence that taking extra vitamin E may interfere with blood clotting in people with certain medical problems, including those who take anticoagulant drugs—and that problem could theoretically increase the risk of hemorrhagic stroke. These anticlotting effects have been observed only at doses 16 times as high as the level the Finns used. Nevertheless, people who take these drugs, or who take aspirin regularly to prevent heart disease, should probably consult a doctor before adding vitamin E to their regimen. (No one has ever shown that taking vitamin E alone can put healthy people at such a risk.)

With no compelling evidence of harm, other clinical trials of antioxidants are continuing unchanged. "I consider [the Finnish study] a little yellow flag that says there may be some effects of long-term use that no one suspected," says Harvard researcher Julie Buring, who heads the Women's Health Study, one of several major studies underway. "But one study doesn't prove anything, especially against a body of evidence to the contrary."

The bulk of the evidence still suggests that antioxidants are safe, at least in the moderate doses now being used in most studies. Vitamin C can cause diarrhea and other problems, but only at doses above 1000 milligrams a day—and most scientists doubt that beta-carotene and vitamin E supplements will prove to be harmful. Whether they will be helpful, however, is another question.

The trials of research

Although controlled clinical trials provide the clearest evidence of a vitamin's effects, they are costly, cumbersome, and time-consuming. As an alternative, researchers have turned largely to "observational" studies: studies in which they examine the health and habits of hundreds or thousands of people, and try to see how different factors correlate with their rates of illness or death. One type of study compares people with a certain disease to healthy people, to see whether there are noteworthy differences in the diets of the two groups. Another approach is to follow a large group of healthy people over several years and compare the diets of those who later become sick with the diets of those who don't. This kind of research can be useful and illuminating—but since the comparison groups have not been randomized, all the possible variables can never be accounted for.

In all the research that has been done on diet, antioxidants, and disease, the strongest and most consistent pattern has been the benefit of eating a variety of fruits and vegetables. According to one comprehensive review, people who ate a lot of produce had a significantly lower-than-average risk of cancer in 128 of 156 studies. In most of the studies, people who ate the fewest fruits and vegetables had at least twice the cancer risk of people who ate the most.

No matter how strong the association, however, such studies can't *prove* that specific antioxidants in fruits and vegetables prevent cancer. There are too many other factors to consider. For instance, people who eat diets rich in fruits and vegetables may have a healthy lifestyle overall. The studies are also limited by uncertainties about the nutritional composition of even familiar foods, and a poor understanding of how well the body absorbs certain nutrients.

While fruits and vegetables are rich in the antioxidant vitamins and beta-carotene, they also contain hundreds of other compounds, many of which are just beginning to show promise against disease. Fruits and vegetables contain more than 500 compounds related to beta-carotene, many of which actually appear to be more potent cancer-fighters in test-tube and animal experiments. Scientists also recently discovered that a compound in broccoli called sulforaphane—unrelated to any known vitamin—can block the growth of tumors in experiments with rats.

Since food chemistry is so complex, some researchers have tried to gauge the effects of individual vitamins by measuring their levels in the blood—reasoning that blood levels of vitamin C, say, will directly reflect the amount a person eats. But that, too, has its problems. The vitamin level in a person's blood at any given time reflects only what they ate on that particular day, and not necessarily what they eat from week to week. Moreover, measurements of blood levels don't account for the way the body uses vitamins—still a mysterious area.

Although observational studies of vitamins are not definitive, and the results of controlled clinical trials are still largely lacking, some patterns have already emerged. In those cases, the data are consistent enough to give researchers hope that they have found evidence of a real benefit. And several patterns suggest that the payoff could be great: Antioxidants may help prevent the nation's two biggest killers.

Cancer and heart disease

As research on the effects of eating fruits and vegetables has shown, it's still very difficult to figure out precisely which antioxidants may help prevent which kinds of cancer. It may turn out that no single antioxidant is as powerful as a combination.

Nevertheless, a number of studies have analyzed food content or measured blood levels and found that specific antioxidants seem to reduce the risk of specific cancers. In many studies, beta-carotene has shown a protective effect against lung cancer. A diet rich in vitamin C seems to reduce the risk of cancers of the mouth, esophagus, stomach, and pancreas in several studies, although some other studies have failed to find this effect. There is less evidence that vitamin E guards against cancer, but there are some hints. One large study showed that people who had taken vitamin E supplements regularly were half as likely as a comparable group to develop mouth and throat cancers.

One major clinical trial has also suggested that antioxidants can prevent cancer, though the meaning of the results is still being debated. The study, published last September, followed nearly 30,000 middle-aged men and women in Linxian, China, a rural area where rates of stomach and esophageal cancer are among the world's highest.

After five years, the NCI-sponsored study found that those who took beta-carotene, vitamin E, and selenium—a mineral with antioxidant-related activity—had significantly lower death rates from cancer and from all causes combined. But the supplements may have made the subjects healthier, in part, simply by correcting their nutritional deficiencies.

Another clinical trial, reported in July, found that beta-carotene and vitamins C and E had no benefit against a condition that sometimes leads to colon cancer. But the 751 subjects were tracked for just four years, which might not be long enough to see an effect, says Harvard's Julie Buring.

There is a good biochemical reason to expect that antioxidants could help heart disease. Theoretically, they should be able to prevent a chemical change that takes place in LDL-cholesterol—the "bad," potentially harmful form of cholesterol—that would otherwise lead the cholesterol to accumulate and clog the arteries. Vitamins C and E seem to have this preventive effect in test-tube studies, and a small study of monkeys has shown a cardiovascular benefit from vitamin E.

So far, research on people has been promising as well. Two ongoing observational studies at Harvard—the Nurses Health Study and the Health Professionals Follow-Up Study, with more than 80,000 women and 40,000 men, respectively—found that people who took at least 100 international units (IU) of vitamin E for two years or more were about 40 percent less likely to develop heart disease than those with the lowest intakes.

The same two studies also found a modest protective effect for beta-carotene, as did a study of 1,300 elderly people followed for about five years. The Physicians' Health Study, a randomized clinical trial at Harvard, is now testing the effect of giving beta-carotene supplements to about 22,000 healthy male physicians. An early analysis of 333 doctors who had a history of angina or heart surgery showed that those who took beta-carotene were 50 percent less likely to suffer a heart attack or stroke. Those results are very preliminary, however, and the study will not be completed until next year.

For vitamin C, the results are mixed. In 1992, investigators at the University of California at Los Angeles School of Public Health reported that people who took in high levels of the vitamin were less likely to die of cardiovascular disease. The study followed more than 11,000 people for 14 years. But other large-scale studies have failed to find the same connection.

How much do you need?

For all the promising leads, the value of antioxidants in preventing disease is still unproven. But the research has already had one profound effect. It has called into question the traditional notion that a well-balanced American diet provides all the vitamins anyone needs for optimal health.

Inspired by the rising tide of interest in antioxidants and other nutrients, the Food and Nutrition Board of the National Research Council last year held the first of several meetings to consider expanding the focus of the nation's Recommended Dietary Allowances (RDAs), from which the Government derives the U.S. RDAs. (RDA levels vary by age and gender; U.S. RDAs are set at a level high

GOOD SOURCES OF VITAMIN C

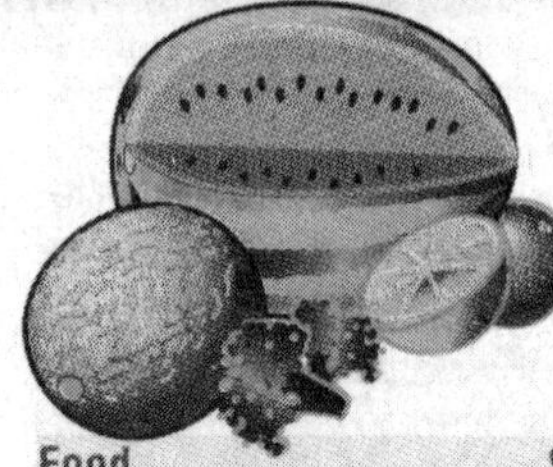

The following foods all have at least 20 milligrams of vitamin C per serving, a third of the U.S. RDA. All nutrient levels are approximate, and will vary.

Food	Serving size	Vitamin C
FRUITS		
Papaya	½	94 mg.
Orange, California navel	1	80
Cantaloupe	⅓	75
Kiwi	1	75
Orange, Florida	1	68
Currants, black	¼ cup	51
Grapefruit, pink or red	½	47
Watermelon	1 slice	46
Strawberries	½ cup	41
Grapefruit, white	½	39
Mango	½	29
Starfruit (carambola)	1	27
VEGETABLES [1]		
Bell peppers, sweet red, raw	½ cup	95
Chili peppers, hot red or green, raw	¼ cup	91
Broccoli	½ cup	58
Brussels sprouts	½ cup	48
Bell peppers, sweet green, raw	½ cup	45
Kohlrabi	½ cup	45
Snow peas (edible pod)	½ cup	38
Sweet potato, baked	1 medium	28
Cauliflower	½ cup	28
Kale	½ cup	27
Potato, baked with skin	1 large	26
Cabbage, red	½ cup	26
Tomato, raw	1 medium	24
Cabbage, bok choy	½ cup	22
Turnip greens	½ cup	20
JUICES		
Orange juice	6 fl. oz.	93
Grapefruit juice	6 fl. oz.	70
Cranberry juice cocktail	6 fl. oz.	67
Tomato juice	6 fl. oz.	34

[1] Cooked, unless otherwise specified.

Source: ESHA Research, Salem, Ore.

enough to cover most of the population.) Until now, the dietary allowances have been defined as the amounts of vitamins and minerals needed to prevent outright deficiency diseases, such as scurvy and rickets. The new approach could include the recommendation to take certain nutrients in greater amounts to reduce the risk of chronic disease.

There are two issues here. The first is that many Americans do not even meet the current U.S. RDAs, as Government studies have shown. Both people in poverty and well-to-do dieters may take in too few calories to get the U.S. RDAs from food alone. Many elderly people are short on essential nutrients, either because their appetite is dwindling or because medical conditions or treatments interfere with their ability to absorb nutrients from food.

What are vitamins, anyway? Vitamins are complex molecules that are essential to a number of bodily functions, from energy metabolism to maintenance of the nerves, blood, and bone. The body can break vitamins down, but can't produce them: You have to get vitamins from outside sources in order to live.

Millions of people with subtle deficiencies might benefit from taking a daily multivitamin/mineral supplement. In one study, for example, elderly men and women clearly benefited from taking a daily multiple supplement: Their immune systems were strengthened and they suffered fewer infections.

The second issue, however, is that even people who get recommended levels of vitamins and minerals may not be getting enough for optimal health. For example, the U.S. Public Health Service now advises women of childbearing age to get higher-than-RDA levels of the B-vitamin folic acid to prevent birth defects.

Most controlled clinical trials of antioxidants are using levels much higher than the U.S. RDAs. Some studies use 100 to 400 IU of vitamin E a day, while the U.S. RDA is 30 IU; others use 500 to 1000 milligrams of vitamin C, which has a U.S. RDA of 60 milligrams. While there is no RDA for beta-carotene, 3 milligrams (5000 IU) will provide the U.S. RDA for vitamin A—and researchers are using three to five times that much.

What to do now?

There will be no clear scientific consensus on antioxidants until more studies are completed. Within the next five years, several controlled clinical trials will yield new information about the effects of taking those supplements. Most scientists counsel patience until those results are in, and don't recommend that the public start taking supplements at this time.

Some nutrition experts say that waiting won't help. "This idea that clinical trials will give definitive answers is really holding out false hope," says nutrition scientist Jeffrey Blumberg, chief of the antioxidant research laboratory at Tufts University in Boston. Many trials are conducted in high-risk groups to shorten the length of time needed to see results, but the results may not apply to healthy individuals, he notes. And because each clinical trial can test only a few nutrients at one or two doses, questions will always remain.

Dr. Blumberg believes that the totality of the evidence, despite its inconsistencies, supports taking antioxidants now. "Americans are dying prematurely of heart disease and cancer," he argues. "Are we so uncertain that we want to discourage supplements? Generations can pass before the answers are complete."

But other observers remain wary of acting on incomplete evidence. Epidemiologist Tim Byers, chief of the chronic disease prevention branch at the Centers for Disease Control and Prevention, agrees that having "every last answer" isn't necessary to make personal or policy decisions about supplements. "But we're still not close enough to make those decisions," he says. "If we believe fruits and vegetables are protective because of antioxidant activity, does it work to just pull out one antioxidant and take it in high doses? I think the answer may be no."

To James Olson, professor of biochemistry at Iowa State University in Ames, the difficulty of reaching absolute conclusions may mean consumers have to make an informed guess. "There will always be uncertainties about any single nutrient," he observes. "Whether to take a leap of faith is more an issue of philosophy than it is of science."

Recommendations

If you want to try to improve your health by increasing your vitamin intake, there is one strategy that no scientist would dispute: Eat more fruits and vegetables. Those foods contain hundreds of substances that have the potential to improve health —not just the handful of compounds that have been isolated and packaged in pills. Moreover, a diet loaded with produce tends to be high in fiber and low in fat.

If you choose carefully—and eat five to nine servings of fruits and vegetables a day, as Government guidelines now recommend—you can take in the relatively high levels of antioxidants that various studies have found to be protective. It's fairly easy to get 250 to 500 milligrams of vitamin C, which is abundant in oranges, cantaloupe, and peppers, among other foods. And selecting good sources of beta-carotene, such as sweet potatoes, apricots, and carrots, can add up to 10 to 15 milligrams (or 17,000 to 25,000 IU) a day. The tables on pages 562 and 563 show particularly good sources of those vitamins.

Vitamin E poses more of a problem. With the exception of fortified cereals, the main dietary sources of vitamin E are polyunsaturated vegetable oils. You can get the U.S. RDA for this vitamin fairly easily in a few tablespoons of sunflower oil, safflower oil, or mayonnaise. But to take in 100 to 400 IU, the amount used in many studies, would require either eating a heavy dose of fatty foods or taking supplements.

Some people will choose to take one or more antioxidant supplements. Others may choose to take a multivitamin/mineral supplement—to get a combination of antioxidants, to get overall "nutritional insurance," or both.

If you decide to take supplements, you should know that the vitamin industry has not been effectively regulated by either the U.S. Food and Drug Administration or the U.S. Pharmacopeia, an independent group that sets standards for drugs. There are no guarantees that these pills contain what they're supposed to, or even that they break down enough to dissolve and be absorbed by the body. And the prices of pills vary widely, with no indication of whether price relates to quality. . . .

The Salt Shakeout

Bonnie Liebman

"I don't worry about how much salt I eat because my blood pressure is low," says 27-year-old Karen Brown of Washington, D.C.

What a relief. What a mistake.

Myths about salt are almost as common as salt shakers. That's partly because of the astute public relations professionals at the industry's Salt Institute, and partly because some scientists disagree—so what else is new?—about the dangers of salt.

Yet after exhaustively reviewing all the evidence, every major health authority, from the U.S. Surgeon General to the National Academy of Sciences, has urged Americans to cut back on salt—or sodium, to be precise.

And it's not just your blood pressure that's at stake.

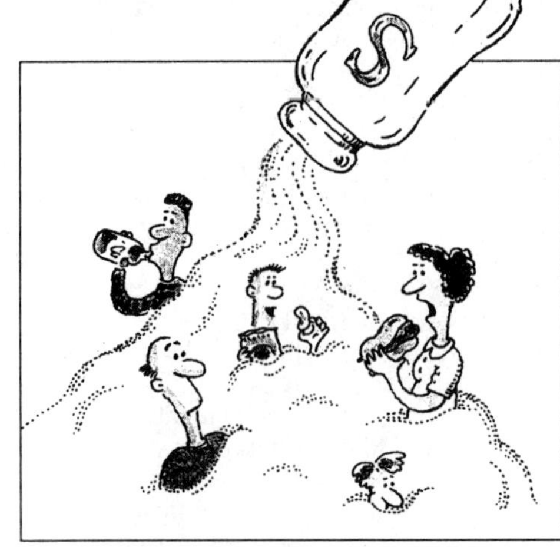

"Hypertension Research Challenges Role of Salt," declared the headline in *The New York Times* in December of 1991. Does that mean you don't have to worry about sodium?

Call that Myth Number One.

"The recommendations that today's high salt intake be reduced are based not on any one study," says Jeremiah Stamler, a renowned cardiovascular disease expert at Northwestern University Medical School in Chicago. "They're based on hundreds of studies, over many decades, using every method of medical research."[1]

Fretting over salt needn't raise your blood pressure. Just don't fall for the "I don't have to worry about salt" trap. That—and half a dozen other myths—could get you into trouble.

Myth. *If you don't have high blood pressure, you don't have to worry about salt.*

Sorry. Fifty million Americans have high blood pressure, which means at least 140 over 90. But just because your pressure isn't *high* doesn't mean it's *optimal*—that is, below 120 over 80.

"The risk of dying of heart disease or stroke doesn't start to rise at 140 over 90, but at a systolic pressure of 120 or a diastolic pressure of 80," says Rose Stamler, a researcher at the Northwestern University Medical School and Jeremiah Stamler's wife. "And sodium has an effect on blood pressure across all levels."

Even though the risk is greater for people with the highest blood pressures, she adds, "so many of us are between 120 and 139 systolic and 80 and 89 diastolic that we contribute more than a third of the preventable deaths caused by above-optimal pressure."

Add those "in-between" people to the 50 million or so with "high" pressure, and we're talking about 80 percent of Americans aged 35 or above with blood pressures that increase their risk of both heart disease and stroke. We're talking about an epidemic.

Myth. *If your blood pressure is low, it'll stay low.*

Even if your pressure is optimal now, if you live in an industrialized country, it's likely to rise as you get older.

In the INTERSALT study that Rose Stamler helped organize, systolic blood pressure rose an average of 15 points between the ages of 25 and 55.

HOW HIGH IS HIGH?

High blood pressure
140/90 or higher

Blood pressure that increases risk of disease
120–139/80–89

Optimal blood pressure
below 120/80

140	90
130	85
120	80

"That's not small stuff," she says. "If lifetime salt intake were lower by about one teaspoon a day—that's 2,300 mg of sodium—blood pressure would still rise with age, but the increase would be six, not 15 points. That would mean a 16 percent drop in coronary heart disease deaths, and 23 percent fewer stroke deaths at age 55."

And if those numbers don't impress you, consider this: "Cutting back on salt may have a small impact on your blood pressure," says Jeffrey Cutler, a hypertension expert at the National Heart, Lung and Blood Institute in Washington. "But that can have a strong impact on whether you'll cross a threshold and your doctor will treat you with medication."

Myth. *Most people's blood pressures aren't sensitive to salt.*

That's based largely on widely publicized—thank you, Salt Institute—but flawed studies.

"These are really poor studies," says Rose Stamler. "Most were small—a half dozen or a dozen people. Most were short-term, which has nothing to do with a lifetime of exposure. And most were not repeated in the same people to see how their responses vary from time to time."

That's because most of the studies were designed not to estimate the number of people who are salt-sensitive, but to understand *how* salt might raise blood pressure, says Cutler. "I think they've been misused."

"You and I may react differently to the same salt intake," says Rose Stamler, "just as when I eat a lot of fat and cholesterol, my serum cholesterol won't go as high as my husband's.

"As with anything in biology, there's a variation in response. But most of us are sensitive to one degree or another."

Myth. *High blood pressure is the only danger posed by salt.*

You can add these to the list:

■ **Osteoporosis.** It causes 1.5 million fractures a year and affects 20 million Americans, mostly older women. And most people don't know that much of their bone mass has vanished until what's left of a hip or leg breaks.

Shop Around

Cutting down on salt should be the food industry's job, since it's responsible for the salt surplus in our diets. You can encourage salt cutting by buying lower-salt brands. And avoid high-sodium foods—those with at least 480 mg of sodium. That's 20 percent of the "Daily Value" that's on new food labels.

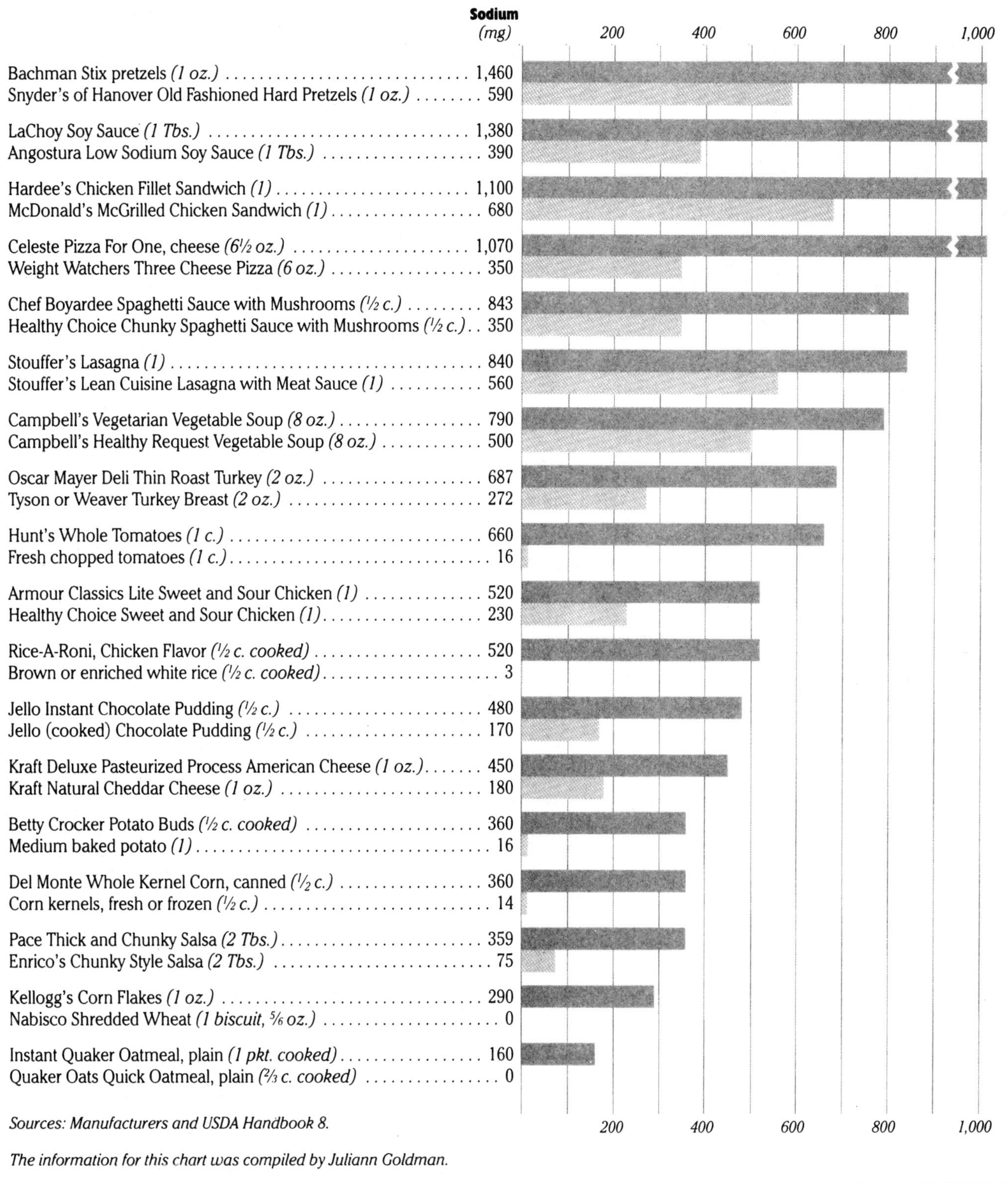

Food	Sodium (mg)
Bachman Stix pretzels *(1 oz.)*	1,460
Snyder's of Hanover Old Fashioned Hard Pretzels *(1 oz.)*	590
LaChoy Soy Sauce *(1 Tbs.)*	1,380
Angostura Low Sodium Soy Sauce *(1 Tbs.)*	390
Hardee's Chicken Fillet Sandwich *(1)*	1,100
McDonald's McGrilled Chicken Sandwich *(1)*	680
Celeste Pizza For One, cheese *(6½ oz.)*	1,070
Weight Watchers Three Cheese Pizza *(6 oz.)*	350
Chef Boyardee Spaghetti Sauce with Mushrooms *(½ c.)*	843
Healthy Choice Chunky Spaghetti Sauce with Mushrooms *(½ c.)*	350
Stouffer's Lasagna *(1)*	840
Stouffer's Lean Cuisine Lasagna with Meat Sauce *(1)*	560
Campbell's Vegetarian Vegetable Soup *(8 oz.)*	790
Campbell's Healthy Request Vegetable Soup *(8 oz.)*	500
Oscar Mayer Deli Thin Roast Turkey *(2 oz.)*	687
Tyson or Weaver Turkey Breast *(2 oz.)*	272
Hunt's Whole Tomatoes *(1 c.)*	660
Fresh chopped tomatoes *(1 c.)*	16
Armour Classics Lite Sweet and Sour Chicken *(1)*	520
Healthy Choice Sweet and Sour Chicken *(1)*	230
Rice-A-Roni, Chicken Flavor *(½ c. cooked)*	520
Brown or enriched white rice *(½ c. cooked)*	3
Jello Instant Chocolate Pudding *(½ c.)*	480
Jello (cooked) Chocolate Pudding *(½ c.)*	170
Kraft Deluxe Pasteurized Process American Cheese *(1 oz.)*	450
Kraft Natural Cheddar Cheese *(1 oz.)*	180
Betty Crocker Potato Buds *(½ c. cooked)*	360
Medium baked potato *(1)*	16
Del Monte Whole Kernel Corn, canned *(½ c.)*	360
Corn kernels, fresh or frozen *(½ c.)*	14
Pace Thick and Chunky Salsa *(2 Tbs.)*	359
Enrico's Chunky Style Salsa *(2 Tbs.)*	75
Kellogg's Corn Flakes *(1 oz.)*	290
Nabisco Shredded Wheat *(1 biscuit, ⅚ oz.)*	0
Instant Quaker Oatmeal, plain *(1 pkt. cooked)*	160
Quaker Oats Quick Oatmeal, plain *(⅔ c. cooked)*	0

Sources: Manufacturers and USDA Handbook 8.

The information for this chart was compiled by Juliann Goldman.

"Spinal crush fractures and [hip] fractures are already a major scourge of the elderly and an important cause of discomfort, deformity, loss of independence, and mortality," explains osteoporosis expert Ailsa Goulding of the University of Otago Medical School in Dunedin, New Zealand, in the *New Zealand Medical Journal.*[2] As the population ages, she adds, the ranks of the bone-poor will swell.

Most people rightly think of too little calcium as a cause of osteoporosis, but too much sodium is another culprit. The reason is simple: The more sodium you excrete, the more calcium you lose. No one knows if the sodium pulls calcium out of your bones or compels your kidneys to excrete it.[3]

"On average, urinary calcium increases by about [23 mg] for every teaspoon of salt consumed," explains Goulding. "An uncompensated calcium loss of 23 mg per day is large enough to dissolve one percent of the skeleton annually—that is, ten percent in a decade!"

That's okay if you consume enough calcium to compensate for the loss, but most people don't. Reducing sodium intakes to about 1,600 mg a day would lower the calcium we excrete by about a third, notes Goulding. Excess sodium is as important a calcium-waster as excess protein.

And it's not just older folks who should be concerned. The best strategy for avoiding osteoporosis is to build up your bone mass before the age of 35. Says Goulding: "If you wish to grow a strong skeleton when you are young and conserve bone mass as you get older, it is sensible to spare the salt."

■ **Stomach cancer.** Worldwide, it's still one of the most common malignancies. But in the U.S., death rates from stomach cancer have plunged by more than 75 percent since the 1930s.

The risk is still excessive among African-Americans, Latino-Americans, Native-Americans, and immigrants from high-risk areas like Asia. Yet no one can afford to ignore stomach cancer, because when it strikes, it's a killer.

Of the 25,000 Americans who are diagnosed each year, only 13 percent survive another five years. This is one cancer you want to avoid...and avoiding excess salt may help.

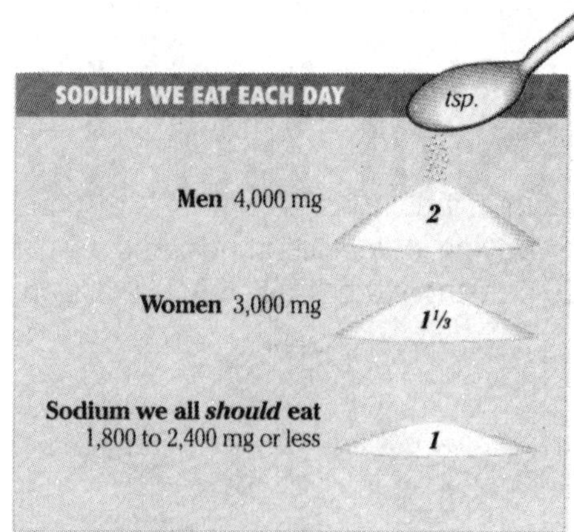

Not that it's the only cause. "In the case of stomach cancer, three factors appear to be dominant: infection [with a bacterium called *Helicobacter pylori*], excessive salt intake, and a diet low in fresh fruits and vegetables," explains Pelayo Correa in *The New England Journal of Medicine*.[4] Correa is a stomach cancer expert at the Louisiana State University Medical Center in New Orleans.

Excess salt irritates the stomach lining, causing cells to reproduce more often. That alone could increase the risk of cancer. And in animal experiments, salt also makes cancer-causing chemicals more potent. That would explain why researchers have found a greater salt intake among Japanese, Chinese, Italians, and Americans who have stomach cancer.[5]

It might also help explain why U.S. rates have fallen so swiftly since the 1930s. Before then, we used salt instead of refrigerators to preserve many foods (though we also ate fewer fresh fruits and vegetables).

But we're still not home free. In a recent study in Buffalo, New York, stomach cancer patients were more likely to have consumed roughly 3,000 mg or more of sodium a day.[6] That's what the average American woman eats. The average man eats 4,000 mg.

Myth. *The easiest way to cut the salt is to throw out your shaker.*

That helps. But only 15 percent of the sodium the average American consumes comes from the shaker. Another ten percent occurs naturally in foods. By far, the most comes from processed foods.

And it's not even salty-tasting foods like potato chips and french fries that do the most damage. At McDonald's, a large order of fries has less sodium than a serving of any sandwich, biscuit, danish, hotcakes, cookies, salad dressing, or apple pie.

Want to really avoid salt? Watch out for *most* brands of frozen dinners or pizza, processed meat (like hot dogs or bacon), processed (American-style) cheese, canned or dried soup, salad dressing, canned meats, beans, or vegetables, tomato sauce, restaurant and fast food, and . . . whew!

At least some companies are now helping. A decade ago, manufacturers said people wouldn't eat frozen dinners and canned soups if the sodium were much below 1,000 mg. Then along came Healthy Choice, and suddenly it became possible to slice that number by at least a half.

As for that shaker, why not fill it with herbs or use a squeeze of fresh lemon juice instead?

Myth. *The only way to treat high blood pressure is with drugs.*

The National Heart, Lung and Blood Institute urges physicians to "vigorously encourage their [high blood pressure] patients to adopt...lifestyle modifications."[7]

That means not just cutting sodium, but losing weight (especially around the waist); limiting alcohol to no more than two drinks a day; doing regular aerobic exercise; and getting adequate amounts—that is, the Recommended Dietary Allowance (RDA)—of potassium, calcium, and magnesium (though the evidence is not conclusive that the minerals will help).

[1] *British Medical Journal 302*: 811-824, 1991.
[2] *New Zealand Medical Journal 103*: 120, 1990.
[3] *Journal of Nutrition 123*: 1615, 1993.
[4] *New England Journal of Medicine 325*: 1170, 1991.
[5] *Journal of the National Cancer Institute Monographs 12*: 75, 1992.
[6] *Nutrition and Cancer 13*: 19, 1990.
[7] *Archives of Internal Medicine 153*: 154, 1993.

Snack Attack

Patricia Long

Patricia Long is a contributing editor.

SITTING IN BAR 234, a windowless, fluorescent-lit room, it's difficult to tell day from night, lunchtime from dinnertime. But the place fairly well shouts snack. The walls are lined with 22 mechanical dispensers that disgorge everything from Care Free gum to Famous Amos cookies, from pickles to Lay's potato chips, from Ultra Slim-Fast to the latest vending triumph, French fries cooked with hot air.

A uniformed U.S. Army major walks in the door and heads toward a machine. He presses his face up against the glass and plunks in a few quarters. I sidle up.

"Fritos, eh?"

"Excuse me?"

"Fritos. Kinda high in fat and salt, aren't they?"

Maybe I shouldn't be so confrontational with a guy trained in combat techniques. But orders are orders, and mine are to explore the workaday snacking habits that cost Americans $13.4 billion a year. Find out why we shove $2.5 billion of that into vending machines, yet of our 60 favorite selections, only three of them aren't extremely heavy in sugar or fat—Snak-Ens party mix, Snyder's hard pretzels, and Fig Newtons (and they're numbers 12, 42, and 43 in the ranking). I'm after the answer to perhaps America's most intriguing dietary question: Is there some way for even the stuff in vending machines to improve our national diet, rather than ruin it?

Bar 234 is named for its location on the second floor at the junction of corridors three and four in the world's largest office building: the Pentagon, situated outside Washington, D.C. The Pentagon is a perfect test environment, because offices—along with schools and factories—are where the nation's snacking culture truly thrives. While a visitor could easily get lost in the nearly 18 miles of corridors and among the 23,000 employees, there's little hazard of starving. At almost every turn sits a vending machine. Les Barnett, the Pentagon's snack vendor, figures that between the machines in the halls, in Bar 234, and in one other snack bar, every week he sells about 5,000 candy bars, 2,900 packages of cookies, crackers, and nuts, and 7,000 bags of chips, pretzels, and pastries.

One of those bags of chips is now being torn open by the major, a polite man.

"I tend to snack if I'm edgy," he says. "I feel guilty only when I get on the scale in the morning and weigh too much. Then I skip my snack that day." He hesitates, figuring how to upgrade his image from a Fritos-only type. "Once in a while I get a granola bar."

I haven't the heart to point out that regular granola bars aren't much better than Fritos. They're loaded with sugar and get between 38 and 55 percent of their calories from fat. But otherwise the major has the right idea. When his weight rises, he cuts back on snacking for a while. That's one good thing about being in the military: Twice yearly mandatory weight checks keep most personnel from letting themselves go to pot.

An army lieutenant colonel whom I corner at the burrito machine confirms this. "Because we're military," he says, "we're theoretically healthier than the rest of the drone population." He pauses as the smell of buttered popcorn—more than half its calories from fat—wafts over us. He shakes his head. "Someone convinced someone in this building that popcorn consumed in industrial-size bags will not make you pudgy."

Here's a man, I think, who's not deceived by marketing, who understands that while plain air-popped popcorn boasts less than 10 percent of calories from fat, the microwave kind we're smelling is in the same fat league as fried chicken. I ask him what he snacks on.

"Diet Coke and doughnuts."

He notes my surprise. "Put it this way," he says, backpedaling. "Working in this building is like attending one continuous meeting. I don't get regular meal breaks, so I just have to lay my hands on whatever's not moving."

No matter how you figure it, combining a diet soda with a greasy doughnut is living by a weird credo: "Sugar is bad, fat isn't." True, sugar offers little more than calories, but it's not the demon fat is. Too much fat is linked to cancer, obesity, and heart disease. That's why we're advised to hold fat to under 30 percent of calories.

That's also why one look at the way we snack will tell you we're in big trouble.

AMERICANS ARE VERY concerned about nutrition. Just ask them. Fifty-eight percent of those surveyed by the Food Marketing Institute believe fat in food is a "serious health hazard." But how many are doing anything about it? According to one food industry survey, some 86 percent of adults admit to eating between meals. As for what they're eating—well, the overall top-selling snack food in America is potato chips. From vending machines it's the Snickers bar.

"Everybody says, 'Boy, we'd really like to see some healthier snacks in vending machines,'" says Tim Sanford, executive editor of the trade magazine *Vending Times*. "And that's exactly what they mean. They don't want to buy them, they just want to see them."

Consider what happened to Ruth Ward-Gross, vice president of Vendmark Inc. in Eagan, Minnesota. To celebrate "nutrition week" in a local health center, she replaced all the vending snacks with healthier ones such as raisins and trail mix, leaving only one exception—a slot

The Vending Machine Top 30

SOME WE GREW UP ON; others only recently hit the popularity chart. Either way, these classic snack foods aren't going to disappear from machines anytime soon, despite the fact that (or maybe *because*) most are heavy in fat and sugar. Still, say nutritionists, it's okay to eat them every once in a while, if you follow the advice on these pages.

In the meantime, see how your tastes match up with those of America's other snackers, and then take a look at the real price of your favorite vending machine pick.

	% of calories from fat	calories
1. **Snickers bar** *(2.07 oz)*	42	280
2. **M&M's peanut candies** *(1.74 oz)*	47	250
3. **Reese's peanut butter cups** *(1.6 oz)*	54	250
4. **M&M's plain chocolate candies** *(1.69 oz)*	39	230
5. **Butterfinger bar** *(2.1 oz)*	39	280
6. **Baby Ruth bar** *(2.1 oz)*	43	290
7. **Pay Day bar** *(1.85 oz)*	43	250
8. **3 Musketeers bar** *(2.13 oz)*	28	260
9. **Hershey's almond bar** *(1.45 oz)*	55	230
10. **Cheetos** *(1 oz)*	54	150
11. **Twix caramel cookie bar** *(2 oz)*	45	140
12. **Snak-Ens snack mix** *(1 oz)*	17	133
13. **Milky Way bar** *(2.15 oz)*	32	280
14. **Famous Amos Chocolate Chip cookies** *(1 oz or 3 cookies)*	36	150
15. **Act II Microwave Popcorn** *(3 cups popped)*	51	140
16. **Fritos corn chips** *(1 oz)*	60	150
17. **Almond Joy bar** *(1.76 oz)*	50	250
18. **Nestlé Crunch bar** *(1.55 oz)*	47	230
19. **Oreo cookies** *(1 oz or 3 cookies)*	36	150
20. **Lay's potato chips** *(1 oz)*	60	150
21. **Planters peanuts** *(1 oz)*	74	170
22. **Doritos Nacho Cheese tortilla chips** *(1 oz)*	45	140
23. **Kit Kat bar** *(1.4 oz)*	47	220
24. **Mr. Goodbar** *(1.65 oz)*	55	260
25. **Planters cheese peanut butter sandwiches** *(1.4 oz or 6 sandwiches)*	45	200
26. **Nature Valley Oats 'N Honey granola bar** *(.83 oz)*	36	120
27. **Milky Way Dark bar** *(1.76 oz)*	33	220
28. **Cheez-It crackers** *(.5 oz or 12 crackers)*	51	70
29. **Starburst Original Fruit Chews** *(2.07 oz)*	19	240
30. **M&M's peanut butter candies** *(1.63 oz)*	45	240

Excludes gum. Based on vendors' dollar purchases for the year ending June 1992. Ranking source: DEBS, Ann Arbor, Michigan. Vended samples vary in size.

full of Snickers. Within two days she got a call for more Snickers. "That's the reality," she says.

And we're ashamed about it. Fully one in three snackers confess to feelings of guilt, according to a 1990 survey. Of those, nearly half say they feel worse about snacking than they do about lying about their weight or age or letting the answering machine take a call when they're home. A third think it's worse than breaking a date, taking a phony sick day, or cheating on taxes.

"I'll see someone in front of a machine," says Barnett, the Pentagon's vendor, "and I'll ask if something's wrong. 'No, I'm just looking,' they'll say. They'll stand there, and you can almost hear them thinking, *I really should get something healthy, but I really want such-and-such. I had a late lunch, I'm having an early dinner, I'm too fat.* It just goes on and on."

But, really, is all this guilt warranted?

Not in theory. Studies on both animals and humans show that snacks—if complementary to regular meals—can help you feel more alert, lose weight, and lower your levels of "bad" cholesterol.

For one thing, standard mealtimes aren't always in synch with the body's rhythms. "After lunchtime your circadian performance rhythms are on a downswing," says Bonnie Spring, a psychologist at The Chicago Medical School. "Fatigue will peak around one to three in the afternoon." Reports Robin Kanarek, a psychologist at Tufts University in Medford, Massachusetts, "Somebody looking at a computer screen—at letters or numbers or whatever—does worse after lunch than before." British researcher Andrew Smith describes the feeling archly: "Lethargic, feeble, clumsy, and muzzy."

Kanarek's research confirms that a snack can reverse the letdown. In two experiments, she asked 18 men to either skip or eat a moderate lunch. Hours later some got no snack (actually, a diet soda), while others got a snack (in one, a chocolate bar, in the other, a yogurt). Then the men took tests measuring memory, math reasoning, reading speed, and attention span. It didn't matter much whether the men had lunched or not. Those eating calories at snacktime scored higher than those who didn't.

If we could manage it, eating tiny meals all day long—a meal pattern researchers refer to, not surprisingly, as nibbling—would actually cut more than our muzziness. For instance, our weight and our heart disease rates. Lab animals fed two large daily meals—known as gorging

No-Guilt Everyday Snacks

NUTRITIONISTS WHO understand human nature agree that a once-every-week-or-so splurge on your snack of illicit choice (*Oh, Lorna!*) can actually help you manage your cravings and diet. But how are you supposed to satisfy your desires the *other* days?

These 21 snacks are low in fat or high in nutritional value (some are both), not too caloric, and tasty to many. (In other words, tofu didn't make the list.)

ANYTIME

Low in fat and filled with vitamins, minerals, or fiber

	% of calories from fat	calories
Nonfat yogurt with fruit *(8 oz)*	0	100
Baby carrots *(3 oz)*	4	40
Fresh fruit *(pear)*	6	98
Bagel *(1)*	6	152
Raisin bran *(1.4-oz box)*	6	111
Fig bar *(1)*	15	60
Graham crackers *(.5 oz or 2 crackers)*	15	60
Instant oatmeal *(1-oz package)*	18	100

ONCE A DAY

Low to moderate in fat

	% of calories from fat	calories
Hard candy *(1 piece)*	0	22
Nonfat pudding *(4 oz)*	0	100
Rice cakes *(2)*	8	70
Pretzel twists *(10)*	8	229
Air-popped popcorn *(1 cup)*	9	31
Animal crackers *(.5 oz or 5 crackers)*	26	70
Gingersnaps *(.5 oz or 3 cookies)*	30	60
Saltines *(5)*	30	60
Whole wheat crackers *(.5 oz or 3 crackers)*	30	60

WHEN YOU'RE ACTIVE

Fatty, but high in vitamins and minerals

	% of calories from fat	calories
Trail mix *(1 oz)*	57	131
Roasted pumpkin seeds *(1 oz)*	73	148
Roasted peanuts *(1 oz)*	76	163
Sunflower seeds *(1 oz)*	82	176

All of the above items have no cholesterol or only moderate amounts; people on low-salt diets should always check labels for sodium content.

—experience large surges in insulin. Some studies show that because insulin converts glucose into body fat, big-meal eaters have more weight problems than the critters who eat the same amount, but spread out over the day.

Weight-conscious people especially should eat something every four or six hours, say diet experts. Anything less, and the body thinks it's starving so slows down its metabolism (not exactly what a weight-watcher wants). It also grows famished; the liver stores only about 340 calories' worth of fuel to maintain steady blood sugar levels. In other words, the I-didn't-eat-anything-all-day diet is bound to fail, explains Evelyn Tribole, a Beverly Hills, California, dietitian and author of *Eating on the Run*. "If you have a light meal at lunch and no snack, then work out and don't eat dinner until seven o'clock, you are too hungry to exercise any self-control."

Such big meals lead to higher levels of cholesterol. In one study, David Jenkins, a nutrition researcher at the University of Toronto, fed two groups of men identical food. One group polished it off as three meals, the other as 17 snacks. Sure enough, snackers experienced drops in "bad" cholesterol levels, lowering their risk of heart disease. Researchers believe the insulin surges that follow big meals prompt the liver to generate more of the cholesterol that helps cause heart disease.

But before you start nibbling, look at what happens when lab animals are given *unlimited* access to either wholesome Purina rat chow or an assortment of tasty chocolate cookies, peanut butter, and marshmallows. They turn up their little noses at the boring chow, gorge on the snacks, and grow very, very fat.

You don't need a research study to know humans do the same thing. Big lunch at noon, candy at two, potato chips at four, and so on into the evening. "The downside to nibbling in real life is that most people don't have any self-control," says Jenkins. "They gain weight."

SO WHAT'S A snack lover to do? Here's what the experts advise:

THINK OF SNACKS AS MINI-MEALS

The way nutritionists see it, we'd be healthier if we skipped candy, chips, cookies, and other typical snack foods altogether or ate them only occasionally. Instead, we'd snack on "meal-type" foods, such as fruit salad, instant oatmeal,

New and Improved

STROLL THE SNACK aisle of any grocery store these days and you might think you've blundered into the health-food section. Cookies are sweetened with fruit juice, while tortilla chips sport ingredients like beets, carrots, and flax seed.

If you eat any of the four C's—cookies, cakes, chips, chocolate bars—it can't hurt to see if you like the lighter alternatives. Though some still have loads of sugar or salt, all of the newcomers are a *lot* lower in fat.

CHIPS

Some chip makers now bake instead of fry. But a "baked-not-fried" claim isn't the same as "fat free." For taste, some companies spike their dough with shortening; others spray fat on after baking.

	% of calories from fat	calories
OLD-TECH		
Regular tortilla chips	47	142
Regular potato chips	62	158
NEW-TECH		
Guiltless Gourmet Baked Tortilla Chips	11	110
Childers Oven Toasted Potato Chips	0	98
Mr. Phipps Tater Crisps	30	120

COOKIES AND CAKES

Commercial bakers are replacing fat with fruit pectin or vegetable gums—xanthan gum, for example, or cellulose gel—which help keep the products moist.

	% of calories from fat	calories
OLD-TECH		
Regular blueberry muffin	34	210
Regular oatmeal raisin cookie	41	44
Regular granola bar	38	134
NEW-TECH		
Entenmann's Fat Free Blueberry Muffin	0	150
R.W. Frookie Oatmeal Raisin Fat Free Cookie	0	45
Health Valley Fat Free Granola Bar	0	140

CHOCOLATE BARS

Bars are now being made with two new ingredients. Caprenin, a manufactured fat, provides about half the calories per gram of most fats. Polydextrose, a lower-calorie bulking agent, replaces some of the candies' carbohydrates.

	% of calories from fat	calories
OLD-TECH		
Milky Way *(2.15 oz)*	32	280
Hershey's *(1.55 oz)*	54	240
NEW-TECH		
Milky Way II *(2.05 oz)*	24	190
Hershey's Reduced Calorie and Fat *(1.37 oz; in test marketing)*	30	150

strawberry yogurt, snack-size cans of tuna, and bagels.

At the very least, we should avoid having our snacks make matters worse. Deep inside the Pentagon I meet an air force senior airman whose regular meals are high in fat and cholesterol. For breakfast, he says, he eats ham and cheese omelettes, bacon, toast, juice, and vitamins; for lunch, pizza; and for dinner, fried chicken, mixed vegetables, and rice.

In between? He consumes two Cokes and two bags of Fritos.

While this man looks fit enough, there's no telling what's happening to his arteries. And it wouldn't take a visit to a health food store every afternoon for snacks to become his healthiest meals. Pretzels, gingersnaps, animal crackers, popcorn (unbuttered, that is), bread sticks, and hard candy are *far* less fatty than what he eats all day. Fresh fruit would be even better. Instead of the soda, he could drink fruit juice (not fruit punch or fruit ade, which are mostly sugar water). Instead of the Fritos, he could eat fig bars, graham crackers, or oatmeal raisin cookies, which all have fiber.

COMPENSATE FOR SNACKS IN YOUR WORKOUT OR NEXT MEAL

"If I want a candy bar," says a senior master sergeant in the air force, "I'll flip it over, look at the grams of fat, and figure out how many miles I have to run to work it off." By that measure, after eating a 250-calorie Reese's peanut butter cup he would run 2.5 miles. (In general, you burn about 100 calories for every mile you walk or run.) His other choice? At dinner he could skip the caloric equivalent of a Reese's: an order of French fries or a cup of ice cream.

Here's one way to handle this internal bargaining: Pretend you're carrying around a grocery bag filled with all your day's food—the perfect number of calories (for the average man and woman, 2,200 and 1,600 respectively). You can eat whenever and however much you want until the bag is empty, but that's all you get. If you use up your allotment with high-calorie candy bars and potato chips, you won't need a very big sack. Fill it with lower-calorie fruits, vegetables, whole grain cereals and crackers, and you'll get to eat a lot more before your hand scrapes bottom.

AVOID MINDLESS SPEED-EATING

Perhaps the sole advantage of vending machines is that they force you to consciously get out of your chair, walk to a machine, and pay money for a single item (provided you don't stock up on *several* candy bars).

Less measured eating styles invite disaster. An air force captain cheerfully pulls out the second drawer of his desk to reveal a stash of Brach's mints and Gummy Bears. He tells me he eats them throughout the day for an "energy high." I tell him he's a candidate for "eating amnesia," what happens when your hand goes to your mouth repeatedly without your brain kicking in.

It's a particular problem with itty-bitty snacks. On the Ritz Bits label, for example, a serving is listed as 22 pieces totaling 70 calories. Three calories per bit seems like nothing, and some out of control snackers will keep munching until the box is empty. That's almost as much food as the average woman needs in a day.

Eating too fast is another problem, because it takes 20 minutes from the start of eating before your body can tell your mind that it's had enough. "It's not like putting your hand on a hot stove, and you instantly know it's hot," says Captain Ellen Stoute, an army dietitian at Walter Reed Army Medical Center in Washington, D.C. "If our bodies worked that way, no one would overeat."

INDULGE YOUR DESIRES—NOW AND THEN

"When I go to a vending machine, I'm usually thinking candy bar," says a woman air force technical sergeant who is a confessed lover of Mars bars. "Sometimes I can even feel my craving."

It's a feeling deep inside all of us. A newborn given a sweetened solution in place of an unsweetened one, say taste researchers, drinks more eagerly—and also looks more contented. So it can be with adults, says Evelyn Tribole. "Don't necessarily swear off all your favorite foods, because deprivation can lead to an overeating backlash. Instead, sit down and savor them."

Sounds reasonable to me. Back in Bar 234, despite the lack of windows, I can tell from my stomach that the day's getting on. I face the machines. Yogurt? (It's got calcium for bones.) Pretzels? (They're low in fat.) Orange juice? (I could use the vitamin C.) The choices seem tortuous.

Then again, maybe not. Smiling, I drop in the coins, remember the part about indulging every once in a while, and press the button . . . for a Reese's.

Exercise and Weight Control

The fitness movement that this country is experiencing began in the early 1970s in response to medical reports that linked Americans' sedentary lifestyle to the rising incidence of cardiovascular disease and obesity. The early advocates of this movement took up jogging and racquet sports as a way to trim off excess pounds and reduce their risk of coronary heart disease. As the movement grew, so did the diversity of the exercise programs being offered. Many people found that jogging was painful and boring, and the popularity of racquet sports diminished in the face of rising costs and competition for facilities. These factors, coupled with a broadening interest in physical fitness, prompted the exploration and development of numerous fitness programs. What type of exercise program is best? The answer varies depending on your fitness goals. One thing is clear, however, if you do not enjoy your fitness program, you will not stick with it. Given the diversity of fitness programs, chances are good that you can find one that is right for you. The article "Which Exercise Is Best for You?" discusses some of the most common fitness goals and provides a comparative analysis of 18 common fitness activities related to these goals.

We have all heard numerous claims as to the health benefits associated with exercise. We may be less clear on exactly how much exercise is necessary to achieve these benefits. For the last 20 years, fitness experts have promoted an exercise regime based on the "no pain, no gain concept." The basic guidelines of this approach to fitness were as follows: frequency—five days a week; duration—20 to 30 minutes of continuous exercise; intensity—40 to 60 percent of one's maximal heart rate. These guidelines, while scientifically valid, were based on studies investigating the impact of exercise on the athletic performance of college-age males. Following these guidelines will, indeed, yield a physically fit individual, but they have proved to be too demanding for most people to incorporate into their lives. Recently, a new set of guidelines dubbed "Exercise Lite" has been issued by the U.S. Centers for Disease Control and Prevention in conjunction with the American College of Sports Medicine. These guidelines still call for 30 minutes of exercise five days of the week, but this is where any similarity to the old guidelines ends. No mention is made of target heart rates, and the 30 minutes can be spread over the course of a day, rather than in consecutive minutes. The primary focus of this approach to exercise is improving one's health, not athletic performance. While "Exercise Lite" may not be enough to prepare one for athletic competition, it will strengthen your heart and bones, and, possibly, add years to your life.

Everyone knows that exercise is good for you, but most people are not aware of the specific health benefits directly attributable to exercise. Unfortunately, many of these benefits can take weeks or even months before they become apparent. Because of this delay, it is very important that individuals choose an exercise program that they will stick with. While the health benefits associated with low levels of activity are not as great as with higher levels of activity, research now indicates low to moderate levels of exercise seem to yield the greatest return for the time and energy invested in exercise. In "The 10 Most Common Sports Injuries," Mark Fuerst discusses 10 common sports injuries and presents some helpful advice on preventing such injuries. "Revive Sore Muscles" by Michael Castleman discusses why your muscles hurt 24 to 48 hours after exercising. He makes suggestions as to how pain can be minimized.

Even though exercise is widely recognized as an effective means for shedding unwanted pounds of body fat, it still rates a distant second to dieting for weight control. The obsession that Americans have about their weight is evidenced by statistics indicating that 90 percent of Americans think they should lose weight. This preoccupation with body weight is primarily due to social factors such as appearance and group acceptance, rather than concerns regarding health. Many of these individuals are either on a diet or have tried to diet at some point in their lives. This obsession is not limited to obese individuals, but it is shared by many with normal, and even low, body weight. Young women of normal body weight who feel they are fat are of particular concern because some of them become so obsessed with their body weight that they turn to starvation as a way to control it. This approach to weight control may result in a medical condition known as anorexia nervosa. Still others with distorted body images resort to vomiting and purging their systems with laxatives in an attempt to control their weight. This condition is known as bulimia. Both anorexia and bulimia are serious eating disorders that may have deadly consequences. Judith Rodin, in "Body Mania," discusses the issue of body image and suggests that how we look has become a significant component of our self-worth. She contends that we have become preoccupied with a quest for the perfect body, and in doing so we have lost much of the joy and pleasures of life.

In 1993 the National Institutes of Health examined several of the leading diet programs in the United States and concluded that most of them were ineffective as long-term weight-management programs. The problem with most of the diets that are promoted as quick ways to lose weight is that they are not designed to be used as a long-term method of weight control; instead, they are geared toward rapid weight loss. Programs such as these should generally be avoided for the following reasons: they promote a rapid weight loss (usually water); they tend to be nutritionally unbalanced; unless they include an exercise component, most of the weight lost will be muscle mass and not fat; they provide no long-term approach to maintaining a weight loss; and repeatedly going on and off diets (the yo-yo effect) not only makes it more difficult to lose weight in the future, but it places one at higher risk for developing coronary heart disease.

Being overweight not only causes health problems, it also carries with it a social stigma. Overweight people are often thought of as weak-willed individuals with little or no self-respect. The notion that weight control problems are the result of personality defects is being challenged by new research findings. Evidence is mounting that suggests physiological and hereditary factors may play as great a role in obesity as do behavioral and environmental factors.

It should be apparent by now that the issue of weight control is both an attitudinal issue as well as a lifestyle issue. Fortunately, a new, more rational approach to the problem of weight control is emerging. This approach is based on the premise that you can be perfectly healthy and look good without being pencil-thin. The primary focus of this approach to weight management is the attainment of your body's "natural ideal weight" and not some idealized, fanciful notion of what you would like to weigh. Proponents of the natural ideal weight concept believe that each of us carry a genetic blueprint for our ideal size and shape, and that we will achieve it through eating a healthful diet and getting a reasonable amount of exercise. "The Best Shape of Your Life" by Anne Alexander discusses why caloric restrictive diets do not work for most people. She explains how a combination of eating smart in conjunction with regular exercise will result in the attainment of your natural ideal weight.

Health researchers changed the focus of the medical community in the late 1980s with the publication of studies indicating that from a longevity perspective, people who maintained or slightly increased their weight between the ages of 47 and 74 lived longer than those that demonstrated a significant weight change either up or down. Medical experts are not certain why a slight weight gain as one ages appears to confer health, but they suspect that those who demonstrated significant changes die sooner due to physiological changes brought on by the yo-yo effect. The U.S. government responded to these findings in 1990 by publishing a new set of dietary guidelines. These guidelines include a new height-weight table that is much more lenient in terms of ideal weight ranges, and it clearly suggests that putting on a few extra pounds as one grows older may be desirable. "Losing Weight: What Works, What Doesn't" takes a comprehensive look at the issues concerning weight control and provides the reader with current research findings regarding these issues.

As America strives to contain the high cost of health care, the role that preventative health practices play in the solution will continue to grow. To this end we must all strive to become more physically active so that we may not only increase our resistance to various disease processes, but enhance our capacity to enjoy all that life has to offer.

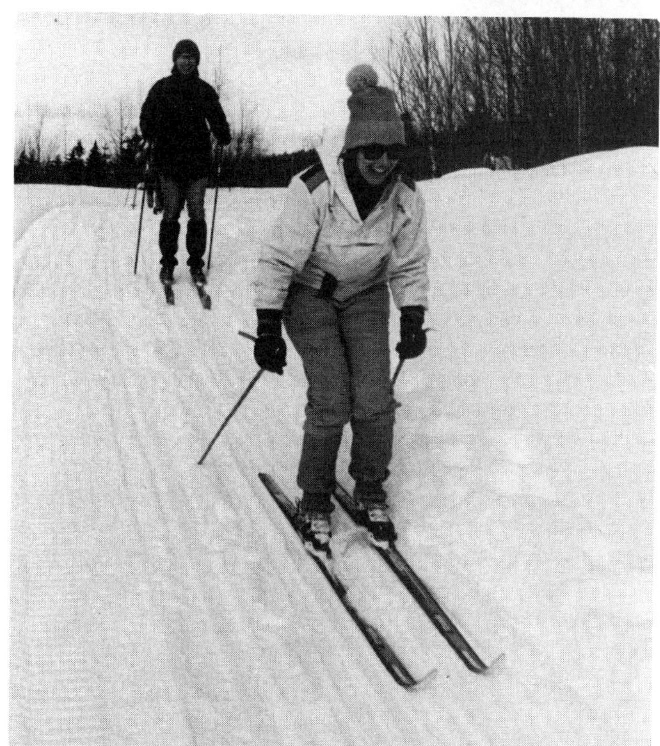

Looking Ahead: Challenge Questions

Explain why the concepts of balance and moderation are crucial to any discussion regarding physical fitness or weight control.

How important is regular exercise to optimal health?

Why should exercise be included in weight-control programs?

What advice would you give someone regarding the prevention of sports injuries?

Are Americans too weight-conscious?

How does American society encourage or contribute to weight control problems? What changes would you suggest?

How do you feel about people who are overweight? Has weight control been a problem for you? If so, what have you done about it?

Do you exercise on a regular basis? Do you think you should?

Revive Sore Muscles

Overdo it one day, and you can barely walk the next. Here's how to get achy legs moving again.

Michael Castleman

MICHAEL CASTLEMAN is a San Francisco-based medical writer and the author of seven books, most recently An Aspirin A Day *(Hyperion, 1993).*

EXHILARATED! That's how you feel when you catch the first glimpse of the pounding Pacific after hiking the Bear Valley Trail at Point Reyes National Seashore in California. The hike feels just right—4 miles with a rise and fall of 400 feet. Out on the water, surfers brave the cold swells. And somewhere in nearby Drake's Bay lies the buried wreck of the San Augustin, a Spanish treasure galleon lost in a storm in 1595 with a cargo estimated to be worth millions. You'd almost trade the ship's booty to keep this feeling forever.

You stop and picnic and dream of napping on the walk back. But your friend has another idea: returning via 1,407-foot Mount Wittenberg.

You hesitate. You're in decent shape, but the hike along the shorter, flatter trail seems challenging enough.

"C'mon," he says. "You can do it."

"Oh, what the hell," you say and bound up the trail. Eventually, you finish feeling none the worse for wear.

But the next morning, your legs feel as old and wrecked as the San Augustin. You've got a bad case of delayed-onset muscle soreness, or DOMS. Now what?

Why it hurts. Unlike sprains, tendinitis, or torn muscles or ligaments that cause sudden, sharp, often excruciating pain during exercise, DOMS pain appears 24 to 48 hours after exercise and causes less severe, dull aching.

Exercise physiologists used to attribute DOMS to lactic acid, a byproduct of muscle metabolism that was thought to accumulate in muscles during exertion and cause soreness afterward as it dissipated. Today we know differently. "Lactic acid has nothing to do with soreness," says exercise physiologist Scott Hasson, an associate professor of physical therapy at Texas Women's University in Houston. "It dissipates within minutes of completing exercise."

Another theory held that exercise drained blood from the muscles, causing an oxygen deficit (ischemia) and muscle spasms experienced as soreness. But according to Bryant Stamford, director of the Health Promotion Center at the University of Louisville School of Medicine in Kentucky, that's not right: Some forms of exercise cause no ischemia but can leave muscles quite sore the day after a workout.

So what causes DOMS? "Microtrauma to muscle fibers," Hasson says. "Any physical activity injures some muscle cells. But when activity level exceeds conditioning level, enough microscopic muscle damage occurs to cause inflammation. A day or two later, the inflammation causes soreness."

Take two what? Within the last few years, studies by Hasson have shed new light on treating DOMS. If inflammation is the cause of DOMS, he reasons, anti-inflammatory medication should help relieve "the moaning after."

In recent experiments, Hasson gave one group of volunteers a standard dose of the anti-inflammatory pain reliever ibuprofen (Advil, Nuprin, Motrin) before a strenuous high-stepping workout. Another group took the drug after the workout. A third group took a placebo. Compared with the placebo takers, both ibuprofen groups showed 50% to 60% less muscle inflammation and reported significantly less soreness.

Then Hasson used acetaminophen (Tylenol) instead of ibuprofen. Acetaminophen relieves pain but not inflammation. This study confirmed that inflammation from microtrauma is the cause of DOMS, and anti-inflammatories are the drug treatment choice.

Aspirin is the world's most popular anti-inflammatory. "Aspirin ought to work as well as ibuprofen," Hasson says, since aspirin is chemically similar to ibuprofen. Aspirin is available not only in the familiar white pills, but as Aspercreme, an ointment that delivers the drug through the skin. "I recommend Aspercreme after exercise to prevent soreness," says physical therapist Alyse Friedman at the University of Maryland Hospital in Baltimore.

Active recovery. When DOMS strikes, most people head for the couch. Not a good idea. "Immobilizing sore muscles limits blood flow to the injured cells," says Mike McCormick, a certified athletic trainer and director of sports medicine at DePaul University in Chicago. "You want to maintain good blood flow to bring oxygen and nutrients to repair the damage."

There are two ways to keep the blood flowing: exercise and massage. "I recommend gentle exercise," McCormick says. "Nothing strenuous, but don't just lay around. Do some stretches or take short walks. In addition to promoting circulation, light exercise helps take your mind off the achiness."

Suki Munsell, director of the Dynamic Walking Institute in Corte Madera, Calif., recommends massage for sore calves and thighs.

The Latest in PAIN

If you haven't heard about ALEVE yet, just wait. Procter & Gamble will be introducing it to the world this summer. Since ALEVE is the first non-prescription pain reliever containing a new analgesic ingredient to hit drugstores in a decade, expect fanfare. Here's a preview:

ALEVE contains naproxen, an anti-inflammatory that has been in the prescription drugs Naprosyn (an arthritis drug) and Anaprox (for menstrual cramps and muscle aches) for 20 years. Now in non-prescription strength, naproxen is going over the counter. The result, according to the doctors and pharmacists that studied ALEVE, is a pain reliever that they rank with ibuprofen, aspirin, and acetominophen for alleviating the symptoms of minor aches and pains.

So what's the big deal about ALEVE? It works for 8 to 12 hours, more than twice as long as the other three. For some people, this could mean a good night's sleep. Since ALEVE spends more time in the body, however, there may be an increased risk of side effects. People with kidney, liver, or stomach problems and those who drink alcohol should consult their physician before reaching for ALEVE.

For strains and sprains, the standard prescription is R.I.C.E.—rest, ice, compression, and elevation. Though rest is no help for DOMS, ice is. The moment professional athletes hit the bench, a trainer wraps their overworked arms or legs in ice packs. "Ice is an anti-inflammatory," McCormick explains.

If you know you've overdone it, apply ice immediately afterward to help minimize soreness the day after. If DOMS develops, an ice pack can help treat the inflammation.

Heat's value in treating DOMS is a matter of some debate. Munsell says a hot bath after exercise can help prevent soreness; Hasson insists that while heat may help injured joints, it's no balm for sore muscles. "Surface-applied heat doesn't penetrate deep enough to increase blood flow," he says. Nonetheless, Hasson recognizes that heat feels good. And if the temperature is high enough, a hot shower might help alleviate soreness temporarily through a counter-irritant effect.

Good irritations. Counter-irritants, like those in Ben-Gay, ICY HOT Balm, Deep-Down Pain Relief Rub, and even homemade salves containing cayenne pepper, represent an ironic twist on muscle pain relief.

Physicians have recognized the effectiveness of counter-irritants for centuries. Ancient Roman soldiers suffering from the cold flailed themselves with stinging nettles because the plant's bite relieved their discomfort. Later, nettles were used to treat arthritis, gout, and other painful ailments. But until the 1960s, no one knew why counter-irritants worked, except for the belief that the surface irritation distracted from deeper pain.

There's more to counter-irritants than distraction. Modern research has shown that they actually trick the brain into ignoring soreness. Pain signals reach the brain along two kinds of nerve fibers—C fibers, which are not covered by a fatty material called myelin, and myelinated fibers that have the fatty covering. C fibers transmit dull, aching, DOMS-type pain. Myelinated fibers transmit sharper pain. "The brain can only process so many pain signals at a time," Hasson explains. "When C fibers and myelinated fibers fire simulataneously, the myelinated fibers override the C fibers, and the person perceives only the sharper pain and sensations of heat, cold, and pressure, not the dull ache. Counter-irritants activate myelinated fibers. Your muscles are still sore, but as long as the myelinated fibers keep firing, you don't perceive it."

Water, water. Most walkers know they should carry a water bottle on extended hikes. Muscle tissue is about 70% water, and without regular hydration, muscle performance suffers. Once DOMS sets in, microtraumatized muscle cells depend on blood to supply the oxygen and nutrients necessary to repair them. Blood is 85% water, and even minor dehydration can impair its ability to heal sore muscles.

Make a point of drinking at least six to eight cups of water a day. And if you know you've overdone a workout, don't compound the problem by drinking alcohol afterward, since alcohol causes dehydration and can inhibit muscle repair.

Pain gain. "Muscle soreness is no fun," says McCormick, "but it's not all bad. It's part of conditioning. When the body repairs injured muscle fibers, they increase in size and strength. The key is to challenge your muscles a little so they grow, but not so much that you suffer DOMS."

How? "Recognize your abilities and never do too much too soon too fast or too often," McCormick advises. "Don't increase the frequency, intensity, or duration of your walks by more than 10% a week, and be especially careful if you're a weekend walker who doesn't get much exercise during the week."

In addition, Munsell suggests warming up before walking and stretching before and after: "Start with a leisurely 5- to 10-minute walk to get the blood flowing to the muscles, and then stretch for about 10 minutes to loosen the tendons and ligaments. Stretching again after walking also helps."

Finally, soreness prevention involves setting an alarm inside your head attuned to the phrase, "Oh, what the hell." Whenever you find yourself saying that, the next thought should be, "No, better not."

the 10 most common sports injuries

. . . and how to prevent and treat them

Mark L. Fuerst

Mark L. Fuerst is a coauthor of The Sports Injury Handbook.

Most weekend warriors are hell-bent on getting the maximum benefit out of their all-too-brief exercise time. That's why so many of us wind up injured, like the tennis player who spends three minutes hitting before his usual Sunday game, then can't figure out why he pulls a hamstring the first time he rushes the net. Fortunately, most of the minor strains, sprains and pulls that come from running one too many miles or even hoisting a heavy bag of groceries aren't difficult to treat.

Learning how to prevent injury in the first place is even more important. The key? Always start your workout slowly, whether you're a new exerciser or a gym rat. Just a few minutes of brisk walking or light jogging warms up muscles so that they're loose, flexible and less vulnerable to strain. (The goal is to raise your body temperature about two degrees—enough to break a sweat—*before* you begin pushing yourself.) Likewise, cooling down gradually after a workout with a five- to 10-minute walk prevents lactic acid, responsible for most postexercise soreness, from building up in muscles. Finally, stretching your major muscle groups *after* you've cooled down, but while your muscles are still warm, increases flexibility and decreases the risk of painful pulls and spasms.

No matter how careful you are, certain activities are likelier than others to land you on your back. In-line skating injuries, for instance, have doubled in the past year. Running causes its share of trouble too. Dr. James Garrick, director of the Center for Sports Medicine at St. Francis Hospital in San Francisco, sees more injured runners in his clinic than any other recreational athletes. "Running jars the body from the feet all the way up to the back," he says.

Here's a look at the injuries you're most likely to face, and what to do about them. (For a nationwide listing of sports medicine specialists, call the American Running & Fitness Association's referral service at 800-776-2732.)

1. Muscle Pull

A muscle pull occurs when a sudden force stretches the muscle fibers beyond their capacity. Besides warming up and stretching, there's not much you can do to prevent this common injury, though it's relatively easy to treat. Immediately icing the injured area for 20 minutes as often as possible will relax the muscle and relieve the spasm until the swelling subsides, usually within a day or two.

As muscles heal, they shorten, which can make them more prone to pulls the next time around. So you'll need to gently stretch the area as soon as you can tolerate it. It may take up to a week for a pulled calf muscle to regain its normal range of motion and up to a month for a pulled hamstring.

2. Neck Stiffness

When you wake up in the morning and can turn your head only one way, a pulled muscle or muscle spasm is probably to blame. Neck pain is common in tennis players who look up to serve or hit a lot of overheads and in cyclists who ride racing bikes, where the back is bent over and the neck tilted up.

Ice works for neck pain too: Apply it during the first 48 hours after the injury for 20 minutes at a time, then gently stretch the area by dropping your chin to your chest and moving it in a semicircle from shoulder to shoulder five times. (Take care not to drop your head back.) Or sit in a chair and grasp the seat with the hand on the same side as the pain. Then lean your trunk and head toward the opposite side, holding the stretch for 20 seconds.

If the pain is especially severe, you may need prescription medication—muscle relaxants or anti-inflammatories such as ibuprofen—as well as physical therapy. And if the pain radiates down your arm to your hand, see a doctor: You may have a pinched or stretched nerve.

3. Shoulder Impingement

Due to its loose-fitting ball-and-socket design, the shoulder is notoriously unstable. The shoulder bones are held together by a group of muscles known as the rotator cuff (specifically, the supraspinatus, infraspinatus, subscapularis and teres minor). When these muscles are weak, the humerus bone can slide around in the joint, trapping the surrounding tendons and causing shoulder impingement—and pain.

Activities that call for lifting the arms overhead can cause or aggravate the

From *American Health*, October 1994, pp. 66-70.

condition. Tennis players may suffer when they hit an overhead or serve; golfers are most vulnerable during the backswing and follow-through.

Strengthening a roughed-up rotator cuff with exercise will help hold the shoulder in place and prevent it from slipping in and out of its socket. (For specific shoulder strengtheners, plus exercises for other oft-injured spots, see "A Workout to Prevent Injury.") If exercise doesn't help, however, or if you also feel numbness or tingling in your hand, see a doctor.

4. Lower-Back Strain

Twist awkwardly or lift a heavy weight, and you may trigger a sudden back spasm, which can make standing, sitting or walking sheer agony. "If the pain is in your mid or lower back, you've probably strained a muscle," says Dr. Robert Cantu, director of sports medicine at Emerson Hospital in Concord, N.H. If it radiates down into the buttocks and leg and continues for more than a day or two, see an orthopedist or a neurosurgeon; you may have sciatica or a spinal disk problem. (If you can't urinate or you lose control of your bladder, get to an emergency room. Both are signs that something may be pressing on spinal nerve roots, and this can cause neurological damage.)

Fortunately, most back injuries heal themselves in a few weeks, with or without treatment. Weak or tense muscles are often the culprit: They're more prone to strain when they're overloaded. Standard doses of aspirin or ibuprofen can ease the pain. So can a few days of bed rest, but don't stay in bed much longer or you risk weakening the muscles further. You also may want to have someone ice your back for 20 minutes at a time for the first few days after you've strained it.

If the symptoms don't quiet down in about 10 days, you may need physical therapy. Your doctor can also give you back, abdomen and hamstring strengtheners to do at home to prevent future problems.

5. Tennis Elbow

Something of a misnomer, tennis elbow, or lateral epicondylitis, is actually an inflammation of the muscles in the forearm and the tendon that attaches these muscles to the elbow. It afflicts golfers (as well as tennis players) and other athletes, especially those who have bad form. "Tennis lessons will ultimately do more good than pain medication," says St. Francis Hospital's Garrick. That's because hitting the ball late on the backhand side or turning your wrist during a serve puts extra stress on the muscles and tendon. "The key," he continues, "is getting your body behind the ball." Golfers with elbow problems should also consider lessons to smooth out their swings.

Exercise (doing reverse wrist curls with a one-pound dumbbell or squeezing a soft rubber ball) can increase forearm strength and flexibility. And ice applied for 20 minutes at a time at least half an hour after your match (when body temperature has returned to normal) can also ease discomfort. If pain persists, your doctor may prescribe drugs such as cortisone to make it easier to strengthen the elbow without too much discomfort.

6. Runner's Knee

You may never jog, much less run, but you can still develop runner's knee, or chondromalacia patella. The telltale symptom—pain around the back of the kneecap or knee—can strike anyone who's relatively active.

Runner's knee is caused by a misalignment of the kneecap, which normally moves up and down in a fixed groove as the knee bends and straightens. When the kneecap is askew, however, it can rub against the surrounding cartilage, wearing it out and resulting in pain and swelling.

Strengthening the quadriceps muscles in front of the thigh can realign the knee and prevent future injury. Start with simple isometric exercises, contracting and relaxing the quadriceps. Then try limited leg extensions. A neoprene sleeve (essentially a soft brace available at most sporting goods stores for under $50), can also hold the kneecap in place. Allan Levy, the team physician for the New York Giants and coauthor of *The Sports Injury Handbook* (John Wiley & Sons, 1993), recommends taking two aspirin four times a day until the knee improves, since studies have shown that aspirin can stimulate cartilage regeneration.

Changing the way your foot strikes the ground can also head off knee trouble, particularly for people who pronate, or roll their foot and ankle inward with each step. Pronation causes the kneecap to rotate inward as well, so that it slides at an angle instead of straight up and down. An arch support (available in drug or sporting goods stores for $10 to $30) helps prevent excessive pronation. If it doesn't work, you may need a custom orthotic. (Contact the American Academy of Podiatric Medicine at 800-438-3355 for a list of podiatrists in your area who prescribe orthotics.) If there's no improvement after a few weeks of strengthening exercises, or if your knee feels swollen, tight or like something is caught in it, have your doctor check for more serious damage.

7. Shinsplints

The bane of casual exercisers, shinsplints can also flare up in more serious athletes, such as runners who switch to lighter shoes or intensify their training. Shinsplint pain, which radiates from deep within the front of the mid shin, is caused by overuse or running and jumping on a hard surface. Repeated jarring (say, the kind inflicted by a high-impact aerobics class) can pull muscle fibers from the shinbone (the tibia in the front of the leg), causing pain and bleeding around the lining of the bone. Some preventive measures: Wear well-cushioned athletic shoes, warm up slowly and exercise on soft surfaces (e.g., run on a track instead of the street and do aerobics on a wood floor rather than a cement one).

An arch support will prevent excessive tugging on the muscle fibers. The soreness should ease within a few days and disappear completely in a few weeks. (If the irritated area is no bigger than the size of a 50¢ piece, or if your shin pain suddenly worsens, see a doctor—you may have a stress fracture.)

8. Ankle Sprain

If you roll off the outside of your foot during a run or walk and overstretch the ligaments in the outer part of the

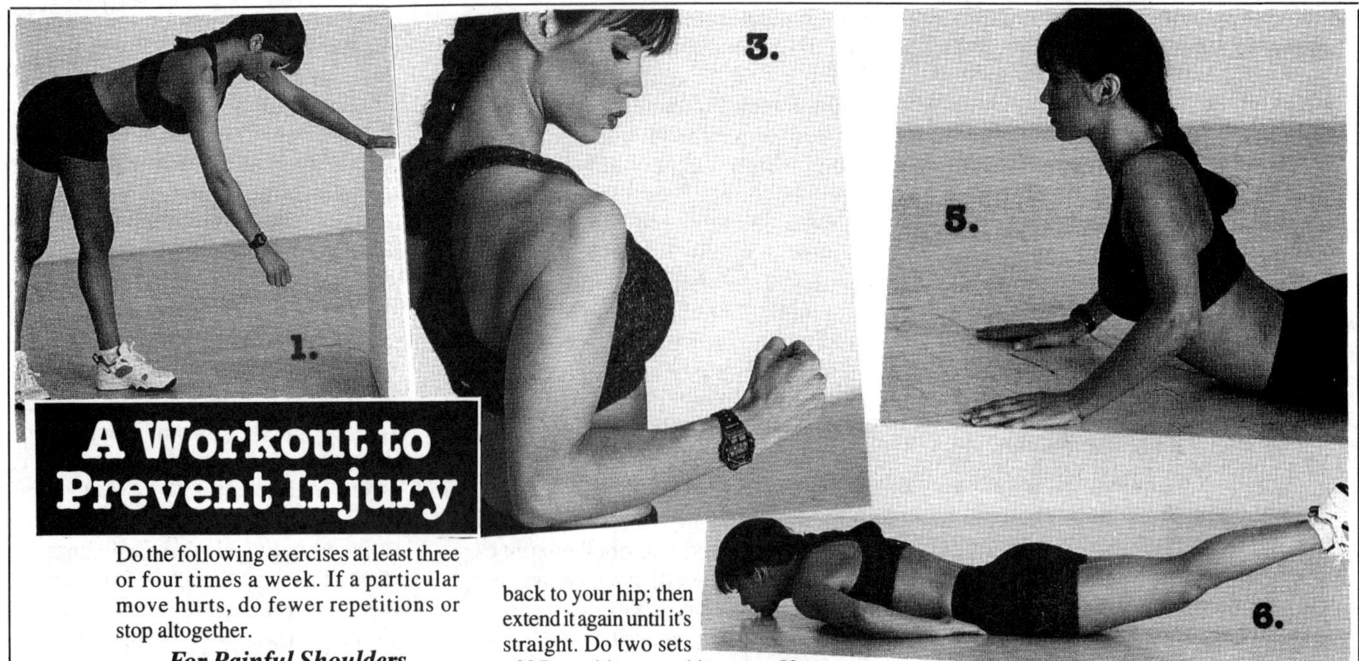

A Workout to Prevent Injury

Do the following exercises at least three or four times a week. If a particular move hurts, do fewer repetitions or stop altogether.

For Painful Shoulders

1. Bent-Over Circle (works the rotator cuff): Bend at the waist until your upper body is parallel to the ground and place your left hand on a chair or a bench for support. Let your right arm hang down and make 25 large clockwise circles, then reverse. Switch arms and repeat. Work up to two sets of 50 repetitions per arm.

2. Lateral Raise (not pictured; works the deltoid muscles): Stand erect with your hands at your sides and your palms facing in. Raise your injured arm to the side until it's parallel to the floor (but no higher). Lower. Do two sets of 25 repetitions, working up to 50 repetitions per set. Repeat with the other arm.

8.

3. Two-Person Saw (works the trapezius and rhomboid muscles): Stand erect and extend your right arm in front of you. Make a fist, thumb up, and pull your arm back to your hip; then extend it again until it's straight. Do two sets of 25 repetitions, working up to 50 repetitions per set. Repeat with the other arm.

4. Shoulder Roll (not pictured; works the rotator cuff): Stand erect and roll your shoulders backward in a circle. Do two sets of 25 repetitions, working up to 50 repetitions per set.

For a Sore Back

5. Chest Raise (works the erector spinae muscles in the lower back): Lie on your stomach with your hands by your shoulders and your palms and chin on the floor. Raise your chest up to eight inches off the ground and hold for 10 seconds. (Don't do this move if you're in pain.) Work up to 10 repetitions.

6. Leg Raise (works the latissimus dorsi and erector spinae muscles): Lie on your stomach with your hands under your pelvis and your chin on the floor. Keeping your legs straight and together, raise them from the thighs up to eight inches off the floor. Hold for 10 seconds, working up to 10 repetitions.

7. Abdominal Crunch (not pictured): Lie on your back with your knees bent, your feet flat and your arms across your chest. Press your lower back against the floor and slowly curl up until your shoulders are six to eight inches off the ground. Hold for 10 seconds and lower. Start with five repetitions, working up to two sets of 25.

For Pulled Hamstrings

8. Hurdler Stretch (works the hamstring and the latissimus dorsi muscles): Stand erect and place your right foot on a chair in front of you. Keeping your back straight, bend at the hips and try to touch your forehead to your knee. Hold for 10 seconds. Start with three repetitions, working up to 12.

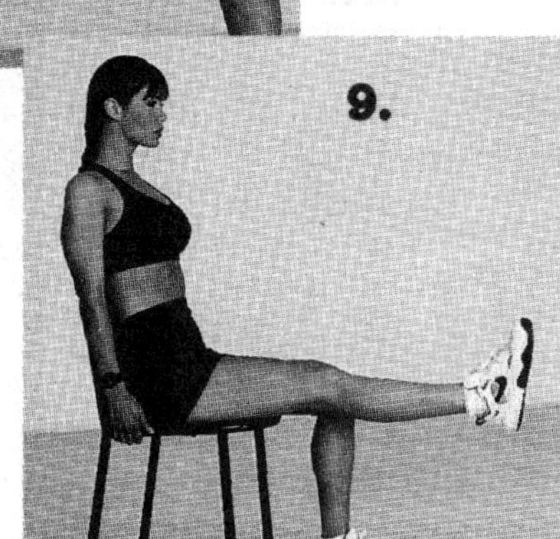

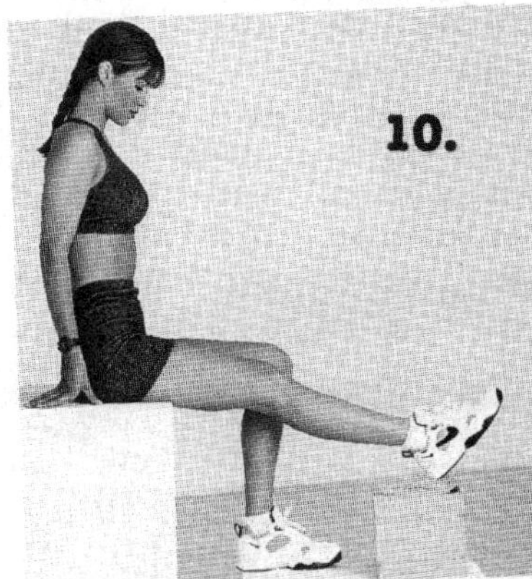

For Tender Knees

9. Isometric Quadriceps Strengthener: Sit in a chair and extend your right leg in front of you, your toes pointed toward the ceiling. Tighten the quadriceps muscle in front of your thigh and hold for five seconds. Relax, then tighten two more times. Repeat with the other leg. Work up to seven sets, interspersed throughout the day.

10. Limited Leg Extension (works the quadriceps): Sit on the edge of a table with your feet dangling. Extend the injured leg straight in front of you, noting the height of your heel from the floor. Then get up, take a stool and pile books on it to a height of six to eight inches below your heel when your leg is fully extended. Sit down and extend your right leg. Slowly lower it until your heel touches the pile of books. (Your knee shouldn't bend more than 30°.) Return to the starting position. Do five sets of 10 repetitions; as you get stronger, add a one- to two-pound ankle weight. Repeat with the other leg. —M.L.F.

ankle, you've suffered a mild ankle sprain. When the ligaments actually tear partway, the sprain is moderate, and when most or all of the fibers tear, the sprain is severe. If you're able to put any weight on your ankle immediately after the injury, it's probably not broken. "If you can't, or if you also feel pain on the inside of your ankle, have it x-rayed," Levy advises.

For any sprain, you'll want to limit internal bleeding and swelling by using the RICE method of treatment, which stands for Rest, Ice, Compression and Elevation. Rest your ankle immediately, even if the discomfort eases after a few minutes. Otherwise, you may later find yourself with a swollen, discolored ankle too sore to stand on. Stay off your feet until the swelling subsides and you can walk easily, usually within 24 hours (you may need crutches for a day or two). Ice your ankle for 20 minutes at a time during the first 48 hours, or until the swelling disappears. Between icings, compress the ankle by wrapping it with an elastic bandage, which also lessens swelling and bruising. For the best results, wrap a sock or a disposable diaper in a horseshoe shape around the anklebone underneath the bandage to fill in the hollows and increase compression. To reduce fluid buildup, elevate the ankle above your heart and rest it on pillows when you sleep.

Once the aching has stopped, you need exercise to restore ankle mobility. Sit in a chair, cross your injured leg over the other and trace the capital letters of the alphabet from A to Z with your big toe (the motion should come from your ankle). Increase the size of the letters as your flexibility improves. To regain your balance, practice standing on one foot at a time with your arms out to the sides, first with your eyes open, then closed. Then walk 15 paces, placing the heel of one foot directly in front of the toe of the other.

An air cast, available in sports medicine clinics and rehabilitation facilities for about $40 to $50, can help you get around as your ankle heals. An orthotic with a built-up area or a lateral flange over the side of the heel also lends extra ankle support. If you're constantly suffering sprains, however, you may need surgery to repair the ligaments.

9. Achilles Tendinitis

Avid basketball or volleyball players are subject to inflammation of the Achilles tendon—the largest in the body—caused by excessive pounding and jumping. More serious is a full or partial tendon tear, which feels "as if you've been shot in the leg," says Emerson Hospital's Cantu, and may call for surgery. Another signal to see your doctor: if the injured tendon looks narrower than the healthy one, or you feel intense pain when you stand on your toes.

Otherwise, rest, ice (20 minutes, several times a day) and aspirin or ibuprofen will relieve swelling and pain. Stretching the injured tendon helps too. Stand on your toes for 10 seconds, then lower. When you can do three repetitions easily, try raising up on one foot at a time.

Once the tendon has healed, which will probably take about two weeks, strengthen it by standing with your forefeet on a raised surface, such as the bottom step of a staircase. Drop your heels below the level of the surface until you feel a stretch in the back of your calves and hold for 10 seconds. Repeat until your calf is fatigued. A commercial arch support or an orthotic can counteract pronation, which may be causing the condition.

10. Arch Pain

If you feel a dull ache along the length of your arch, it's a good bet that you've got plantar fasciitis, an inflammation of the shock-absorbing, fibrous connective tissue that covers the sole. It's common among runners, people with high, rigid arches or anyone who has been sedentary and suddenly plunges into an exercise program. Poorly fitting shoes or a weight gain of 10 to 20 pounds can exacerbate the condition.

The injury occurs when the plantar fascia is overstretched or partially torn, and the pain is at its worst when you put your weight on your foot or push off during a power walk or a run. You're also likely to wince when you get up in the morning or after you've been sitting for a long time. That's because the muscle fibers start to heal when there's no weight on the foot, but they're pulled apart again as soon as you stand. Daily icing can provide relief: Fill a paper cup with water, freeze it, then apply the ice to the heel and arch, stroking in a circular motion for 10 minutes several times a day. (Peel away the paper as the ice melts.)

Stretching also helps keep the area supple. Sit on the edge of a table and let your legs dangle straight down. Loop a towel under the ball of your injured foot, grasping each end. Keeping your knee bent, slowly pull up on the towel to flex your forefoot for 10 seconds; repeat four or five times, working up to 10 repetitions. Also, put a heel pad in your slippers (and street shoes) and wear them as soon as you get out of bed, since just a few barefoot steps is all it takes to stretch the plantar fascia and start the problem all over again.

WHICH EXERCISE IS BEST FOR YOU?

The wrong exercises can make you sweat in vain. Here's how to choose the right ones.

Most health-conscious people know the many benefits of exercise—that exercise reduces the risk of disease, increases stamina, builds strength, burns calories, and relieves stress. But they may not know which exercise best suits their particular goals.

An inappropriate exercise can wreck a budding exercise habit. An overweight person who plunges into a vigorous running program, for example, may end up sore—and sorely disappointed—when the exercise proves too hard on overburdened joints and fails to burn off more than a pound or two after a month of panting and sweating.

This report will help you identify the most effective workouts that can enable you to achieve each of the five most important goals of exercise.

1. Preventing disease

Any regular exercise that requires sustained movement, such as walking or bicycling, reduces the risk of several life-threatening diseases, including coronary heart disease, hypertension, diabetes, and possibly cancer. The harder you work out, the greater the reduction in risk. But the sharpest risk reduction occurs when previously inactive people start doing even a little exercise, not when moderately active people start exercising strenuously.

To get that modest, disease-preventing dose of exercise, you don't need to climb into exercise clothes or sweat through formal workouts. Gardening, dancing, even shopping expeditions are all moderately good exercise. You could even squeeze exercise into your daily routine—for example, by walking short distances instead of taking the car, bus, or elevator, or by attacking household chores vigorously. (For more ways to take the boredom and inconvenience out of exercise, see CRH, 7/93).

It's not clear whether strength training helps prevent all the diseases that aerobics do. But strength training may be the best exercise for cutting the risk of osteoporosis, the brittle-bone disease. Strengthening workouts exert much more pressure on the bones, particularly the spine, than nonweight-bearing exercises such as swimming or cycling, or even moderately weight-bearing exercises like walking or jogging. That pressure stimulates the flow of bone-hardening calcium into the skeleton. Indeed, one study, not yet published, found that weight lifters have 15 percent denser spinal bones than either runners or people who don't exercise. While runners had denser thigh bones than inactive people, the weight lifters' thigh bones were even denser than the runners', by an additional 11 percent.

2. Boosting aerobic fitness

Aerobic (or cardiovascular) fitness is the ability of the heart and the lungs to supply the muscles with enough oxygen, so you don't get winded or fatigued when you run for a bus, climb stairs, or walk more than a few blocks. To improve aerobic fitness, you need to work out more often—at least three times per week—than you would to reduce your risk of disease. You also need to exercise more intensely, enough to push your heart rate to between 60 and 90 percent of its maximum rate—a rate calculated by subtracting your age from 220. (Before regularly exercising close to your maximum heart rate, get an O.K. from your doctor.)

Jogging typically pushes the heart rate into that aerobic benefit zone, but it's too demanding for many people, and it puts considerable stress on the knees, shins, and feet. Listed below are some good, low-impact alternatives:

■ **Brisk walking, with arms swinging.** To increase the aerobic benefit, carry 1- to 3-pound hand or wrist weights or walk on hilly terrain rather than on flat roads.

■ **Low-impact aerobic dance.** You can boost the aerobic intensity by increasing the arm movements you make at or above shoulder level. Arm movements make the heart pump blood against the force of gravity.

■ **Swimming.** Note that overweight people may have to work harder to get a good aerobic workout in a swimming pool, since their extra body fat lets them float more easily.

■ **Step aerobics.** This exercise involves stepping on and off a low bench while moving your arms, usually in time to music. (For more information, see CRH, 10/92; or get an instructional video, available at many libraries and video stores.)

■ **Stair-stepping or cross-country-skiing machines.** Using a machine with movable bars that you pump with your hands increases the aerobic benefit of stair stepping. (Stationary cycling machines with movable bars can also provide a good aerobic workout without making you pedal uncomfortably fast.)

People who just want to maintain their current level of fitness can get by with somewhat less exercise than it would take to improve their stamina—say, two workouts per week instead of three or four, 20 minutes per session instead of 30, or 60 percent of the maximum heart rate instead of 70 to 90.

3. Building strength

After age 30 or so, people often begin to lose muscle. When they get older, they may start having trouble with everyday tasks such as opening windows or carrying grocery bags. Worse yet, they may eventually be unable to climb stairs or even walk normally, maintain their balance, or get up out of a chair.

Strength training—mainly weight lifting—can help prevent or reverse that deterioration, even among people in their 80s or 90s. (Weight lifting may even improve aerobic fitness in older people, particularly if they move rapidly from one maneuver to the next, an approach known as circuit training.)

The most effective way to build strength—the ability to lift a heavy suitcase, for example—is to pick a weight you can lift only about six to eight times. (**Warning:** People with high blood pressure should avoid such "power lifting.") To increase endurance—the ability to carry that suitcase for several blocks—pick a lighter weight that you can lift 15 to 20 times. Performing 8 to 12 repetitions of an intermediate weight builds both strength and endurance.

For fastest results, repeat each set of repetitions two or three times, three or four days per week. If you just want to maintain your current strength, you can get by with one set performed twice a week; even a single session per week will slow muscle loss substantially.

Weight machines, barbells, dumbbells, or any heavy object around the house, such as a plastic jug filled with water, can be used to provided resistance for strength training. However, older people, particularly if they're frail, may want to avoid barbells, since they're harder to control and more likely to fall on you.

After age 30, people often start to lose muscle.

Strengthening the upper body. For people who don't have much time for exercise, here's a streamlined strength-training regimen, involving just four exercises, that works the major upper-body muscles:

■ **Push-ups.** Lie face down with your palms on the floor beside your shoulders. Without arching your back, push up with your arms to raise your body from your toes. If that's too difficult, push up from your knees or do the exercise in a standing position, leaning forward with your hands against a wall. Stop just before your elbows lock. To make the push-ups harder, elevate your knees or feet.

■ **Biceps curl.** Hold a weight at your side in one hand, palm facing forward. Keeping your elbow stationary, raise the weight to your shoulder, then lower it again.

■ **Upright row.** Hold the weights in front of your thighs, with your palms facing your legs. Raise the weights to your armpits without rotating your wrists, them lower the weights.

■ **Partial sit-ups.** Lie on your back, with your arms at your sides. Bring your knees partway up, keeping your feet flat on the floor. Raise your head and shoulders until your shoulder blades come up off the floor, then return to the starting position. To increase the difficulty, lock your hands behind your head, lift your upper body farther off the ground, or do the sit-ups on an incline, with your buttocks higher than your head.

Strengthening the legs. Aerobic exercise that vigorously works the legs will prevent young and middle-aged people from losing muscle in their lower body. But most older people, as well as younger ones who don't exercise their legs, could benefit from lower-body strength training. Here's a simple, effective exercise for improving leg strength:

■ **Partial squats.** Stand with your back to a wall, with your feet about six inches from the wall and spread slightly beyond shoulder width. Keeping your back against the wall and your feet flat on the floor, slowly crouch down until your thighs are almost parallel to the floor, then return to the starting position.

To increase the difficulty, hold a weight in your hands or strapped to your waist. **Warning:** People with knee or back problems should not do partial squats. Taken together, these two exercises are a good alternative:

- **Leg extension.** Sit in a chair, with your feet on the floor and weights strapped to your ankles. Keeping your thigh stationary, raise one foot by straightening your knee, then bring the foot back down to the floor.
- **Hamstring curl.** Stand erect, holding the back of a chair and wearing ankle weights. Lift your foot behind you as high as possible by bending your knee, then lower your foot to the floor.

People who want to increase their strength dramatically will need to do more than just those four to six basic exercises. The book "Get in Shape, Stay in Shape," by F. Skip Latella, Winifred Conkling, and the editors of Consumer Reports Books, offers a wide range of muscle-building and other exercises. It's available at most libraries, or you can order it for $17.45 by calling 800-272-0722.

4. Losing weight

It takes two different kinds of exercise to help you shed pounds and keep them off: one to burn a lot of calories, the other to build muscle.

Burning calories. The more vigorously you exercise, the faster your body will burn calories. However, strenuous exercise is not the best way for the average person to lose weight. That's because most people can sustain regular exercise much longer at a moderate pace—and thus burn many more calories overall—than they could keep going at a strenuous pace. In addition, some evidence suggests that the body consumes mainly carbohydrates during intense workouts, while it relies more on fat to fuel prolonged, moderate exercise.

Building up to a program of workouts lasting at least 45 minutes to an hour, four to five times per week, is generally the most effective exercise strategy for slimming down. Bicycling, brisk walking, and even energetic dancing, for example, are good slimming exercises: They're vigorous enough to burn calories at a reasonable clip; at the same time, they're sufficiently moderate, interesting, and easy on the joints that the average person could do them for an extended period. Exercising on a stationary-cycling, stair-stepping, or cross-country-skiing machine set at a low resistance level also allows you to get a prolonged workout.

Swimming, on the other hand, is not a good way to lose fat, for reasons that aren't clear. Some researchers believe that swimming is simply too easy for overweight people, and doesn't burn enough calories; others speculate that the body responds to the cold water by altering its metabolism to preserve its insulating layer of fat. Aerobic dance routines that mainly feature hand and arm movements won't help you lose much weight either, since those muscles are too small to burn many calories.

More muscle, less weight. Muscle helps you stay slim, because it burns calories faster than fat does, even when you're resting. Lifting weights can

HEALTH BENEFITS OF SELECTED ACTIVITIES

	Disease prevention	Aerobic fitness	Muscular strength	Muscular endurance	Weight loss [1]
Gardening	◓	◒	○	◓	◓
Lawn mowing *(power push)*	◓	◒	○	○	○
Cleaning house	◓	◒	◒	○	◒
Raking leaves	◓	◒	◒	○	○
Shopping	◓	●	○	○	◒
Walking *(leisurely, 2.5 mph)*	◓	◒	●	◒	○
Walking *(brisk, 4 mph)*	◉	◉	◒	○	◉
Jogging *(6 mph)*	◉	◉	○	○	◓
Bicycling *(10 mph)*	◉	○	○	○	◉
Cross country skiing *(slow)*	◉	◉	○	◓	◉
Aerobic dance, low impact *(moderate)*	◉	◉	◒	○	◓
Step aerobics *(moderate)*	◉	◉	○	◓	◉
Tennis *(doubles)*	◓	◒	●	◒	○
Tennis *(singles)*	◉	○	○	○	◓
Golf *(18 holes, with hand cart)*	◓	◒	◒	◒	○
Strength training *(high weight, few repetitions)*	[2]	◒	◉	○	◓ [3]
Strength training *(low weight, many repetitions)*	[2]	○	◓	◉	◓ [3]
Circuit strength training	[2]	◓	◓	◓	◓ [3]

[1] Based on how effectively each exercise would help the average overweight person lose weight or keep it off.
[2] Studies have not determined whether strength training reduces the risk of diseases other than osteoporosis.
[3] These exercises help control weight mainly by building muscle and boosting metabolism.

◉ ◓ ○ ◒ ●
Better ←——→ Worse

EXERCISES FOR SPECIAL AILMENTS

People who have a chronic disorder need a specially tailored exercise program that provides maximal benefit with minimal risk. Here's how to choose the right exercise—and, with your doctor's help, take the right precautions—if you have arthritis, diabetes, or hypertension, three of the most common chronic ailments.

Arthritis

People with arthritis, particularly rheumatoid arthritis, should stretch the affected joints every day, even when those joints are inflamed. It's also important to strengthen the joints: Start with isometric exercises, in which you tense the muscles without moving the joint; if possible, progress to isotonic exercises, such as weight lifting. When you have little or no pain and inflammation, work on improving stamina by doing low-impact aerobic exercises such as walking, cycling, swimming, or dancing.

Two particularly safe and effective workouts are calisthenics in a heated pool and t'ai chi, a relaxing exercise that features slow, sweeping movements. (For more information on exercise and arthritis, see CRH, 9/93; or contact your local chapter of the Arthritis Foundation, or call the national office at 800-283-7800.)

Diabetes

Aerobic exercise can help control diabetes directly, by improving the body's use of sugar, as well as indirectly, by facilitating weight loss. Exercise is safest and most effective for people with type II diabetes (once called "adult-onset" diabetes), the most common form of the disease. But certain precautions are still essential:

- If you're over age 35, ask your doctor for an exercise stress test to check for coronary heart disease, a common complication of diabetes.
- If you have eye or nerve damage, choose low-impact exercises such as cycling or swimming. Jarring exercises like jogging can burst weakened blood vessels in the eye or injure a nerve-damaged foot that no longer sends pain signals to warn of impending damage. Before and after workouts that put stress on your feet, check them for breaks in the skin, blisters, redness, or swelling.
- Monitor your blood-sugar levels carefully before and after exercising.
- Don't lift heavy weights. Straining raises blood pressure and can damage the blood vessels.

Hypertension

Regular aerobic exercise produces temporary and possibly lasting reductions in blood pressure. Moderately intense exercise, between 60 and 70 percent of your maximum heart rate (see story), actually lowers your blood pressure more effectively than intense exercise does. Moreover, strenuous exertion, either from aerobic exercise or from lifting heavy weights, can push blood pressure to dangerously high levels during the workout.

---

build muscle or at least counter the tendency of a low-calorie diet to shrink muscle along with the fat. And since muscle is denser than fat, you can trim your profile without even losing any weight simply by replacing a large amount of body fat with a smaller amount of muscle.

In addition to doing the strengthening exercises described above, overweight individuals may want to focus on two frequently neglected muscle groups—the gluteus maximus and the thigh adductors—that can help improve your appearance by firming up the buttocks and inner thighs:

- **Gluteal lifts.** Crouch down on your hands and knees, with your back straight and your hands directly below your shoulders. Slide one knee straight back. Keeping that knee on the floor, bend it 90° to raise your foot. Now lift that leg as high as possible, keeping the knee bent; hold that position for several seconds, then return your knee to the floor. Repeat with the other leg. To increase the difficulty, wear ankle weights.

- **Inner-thigh lifts.** Lie on your back with your arms by your sides. Lift both legs straight upwards, bending your knees, if necessary, and spread your legs to form roughly a 45° "V." Then separate your legs as wide as possible without discomfort, and slowly bring them back to the original V position. Again, ankle weights will increase the difficulty.

5. Easing stress

Numerous studies have shown that working out reduces anxiety, muscle tension, and blood pressure—three measures of stress—for at least several hours and possibly much longer. Other studies suggest that exercise may ease moderate depression and help people stay calm when they're under pressure.

Aerobic exercise improves mood and eases stress better than strength training and most other nonaerobic exercises. (Yoga and t'ai chi, a martial art that features slow sweeping movements, may also fight stress effectively.) Some people even report that aerobic exercise gives them an exhilarated feeling—the so-called runner's high.

But any exercise that gives you a sense of accomplishment, boosts your confidence, or simply diverts you from your everyday problems can help you feel better—provided you don't turn it into a distasteful chore by pushing yourself too hard. Since the emotional lift may start to fade after several hours, try to exercise often and to time your workouts for maximum impact. If you feel anxious at work, for example, try exercising in the morning; if you have trouble sleeping, exercise in the late afternoon or early evening (though not within three hours of bedtime, which can make it difficult to fall asleep).

LOSING WEIGHT

WHAT WORKS. WHAT DOESN'T.

In the first large-scale survey of the major weight-loss programs, we found that no program is very effective. Here's why diets usually don't work, and how you can manage your weight more wisely.

Fifty million Americans are dieting at any given time, and these days, most of them are thoroughly confused. After decades in which medical authorities, the fashion industry, and most ordinary people agreed that the pursuit of thinness was an unmitigated good, the wisdom of dieting has come into question. Researchers have found that yo-yo dieting, the common cycle of repeatedly losing and regaining weight, may be as bad for you as weighing too much in the first place. Sobered by that research—and by the realization that many dieters become yo-yo dieters—members of a growing antidiet movement have urged people to throw away their calorie counters and eat whenever they're hungry.

Despite those developments, it is still possible and worthwhile for some people to lose weight. But a review of the scientific literature, interviews with experts in the field, and CU's own research show that a major shift in thinking about weight loss is in order. For the typical American dieter, the benefits of weight loss are no longer certain—and the difficulty of losing weight permanently has become all too clear.

Medical researchers have suspected for years that most diets end in failure; studies done at weight-loss clinics in medical centers showed that people almost always regained the weight they lost. But it was never clear whether people at those clinics had an unusually poor success rate because they were "hard cases" who needed special help.

Now CU has undertaken the first large-scale survey of people on ordinary diet programs and shown that they, too, usually fail at losing weight in the long term. We collected information from 95,000 readers who had done something to lose weight over the previous three years, including some 19,000 who had used a commerical diet program. . . . our survey showed that people do lose weight on these programs—but the great majority of them gain back most of that weight within two years.

Although different weight-loss programs use different diets and strategies, none have been able to overcome this basic pattern. The problem is that losing weight is much more than a matter of willpower: It's a process that pits the dieter against his or her own physiology.

Why people get fat

A small number of people have struggled with obesity since childhood and are massively overweight as adults. A greater number are not overweight when they enter adulthood, but become so as they gain 10, 20, or 30 pounds over the course of two or three decades. And about three-quarters of American adults are not overweight at all.

What makes for the difference? Primarily, it's the genes. An individual's body size, studies have conclusively shown, is genetically coded as surely as the shape of a nose. Inheritance overwhelms other factors in determining an individual's normal range of weight, which may be relatively high for one person, low for another. While diet and exercise certainly play a role, they do so within limits set by heredity.

Over and over again, researchers have observed the human body's remarkable resistance to major weight change. Dr. Rudolph Leibel, an obesity researcher at Rockefeller University in New York City, describes how extremely obese people repeatedly enter the university's weight-loss clinic, lose dozens of pounds, go home, and return six months later having regained precisely the amount of weight they lost. Other clinicians have reported similar, if less dramatic, results.

What's less widely known is that the body resists major weight *gain* as much as it resists a major loss. In a classic study conducted in the 1960s by Dr. Ethan Allen Sims of the University of Vermont, a group of 20 prisoners of normal weight volunteered to gain as much weight as possible. Only by forcing themselves to overeat—some by thousands of extra calories a day—were the men able to add 20 percent to their weight and keep it on. Once the study ended, almost everyone returned quickly to his starting weight.

No one knows just how the body keeps weight within a fairly narrow range; researchers posit the existence of some sort of biochemical control system, but they haven't found it. Whatever the mechanism is, however, it allows weight to drift slowly upward as people get older. Two major changes take place with age. People tend to become less physi-

The first modern diet book
In 1863, the Englishman William Banting published his "Letter on Corpulence Addressed to the Public." His advice: Cut back on carbohydrates.

cally active. And, partly as a result of inactivity, people lose lean muscle mass, which burns calories more rapidly than fatty tissue.

No wonder, then, that the prime time for dieting is the mid-40s. "That's when people start to look fat or study a height-weight table and say to themselves, 'Gee, I've crossed over a line,' " says David Williamson, an epidemiologist who studies weight patterns for the Centers for Disease Control and Prevention.

Weight and health

Even if some people are genetically programmed to be fatter than others, their natural body size may not necessarily be a healthy one. Researchers are now struggling with a difficult question: At what point do the risks of overweight make the effort to lose weight worthwhile?

To begin to answer that question, scientists have used a measure called the body mass index, or BMI, which incorporates both height and weight to assess a person's level of fatness. You can find your own BMI by following the instructions on the opposite page. Scientists consider a BMI of 25 or less to be desirable for most people. A BMI between 25 and 30—mild or moderate overweight—carries a slightly increased risk of weight-related health problems such as high blood pressure, high blood cholesterol, heart disease, and Type II (adult-onset) diabetes. At a BMI of 30 or more—considered truly overweight—the risk of developing those conditions and others rises sharply.

There is little doubt that people with a *lifelong* BMI of 25 or less have the lowest risk of disease and premature death (except for cigarette smokers, who are both lean and suffer high rates of cancer, chronic lung disease, and cardiovascular disease). But the benefits of thinness may be greatest for people who have always been thin. Someone who starts out overweight and then slims down is still worse off than someone who never was overweight at all.

The people with the hardest decision to make about their weight are those who are mildly to moderately overweight, with a BMI between 25 and 30. If they have diabetes or cardiovascular risk factors, such as high blood cholesterol or high blood pressure, they may have a medical reason to try to reduce; if not, they may be relatively safe.

Age also affects the risk for this middle group. Americans' median weight rises steadily between the ages of 20 and 55, and a number of studies indicate that isn't necessarily dangerous. The overall risk of moderate overweight apparently diminishes, or even disappears altogether, with advancing age. The reason is not entirely clear, and the data have been the subject of much debate. However, most researchers now accept the phenomenon as fact, as does the U.S. Government. Since 1990, the Government has published weight guidelines for Americans that give different ranges for older and younger adults.

One other critical variable has emerged in the last several years: the waist-to-hip ratio, calculated as the measure of a person's waist at its smallest point divided by the circumference of the hips at their widest point. This ratio distinguishes "apples"—that is, people who carry excess weight above their waist—

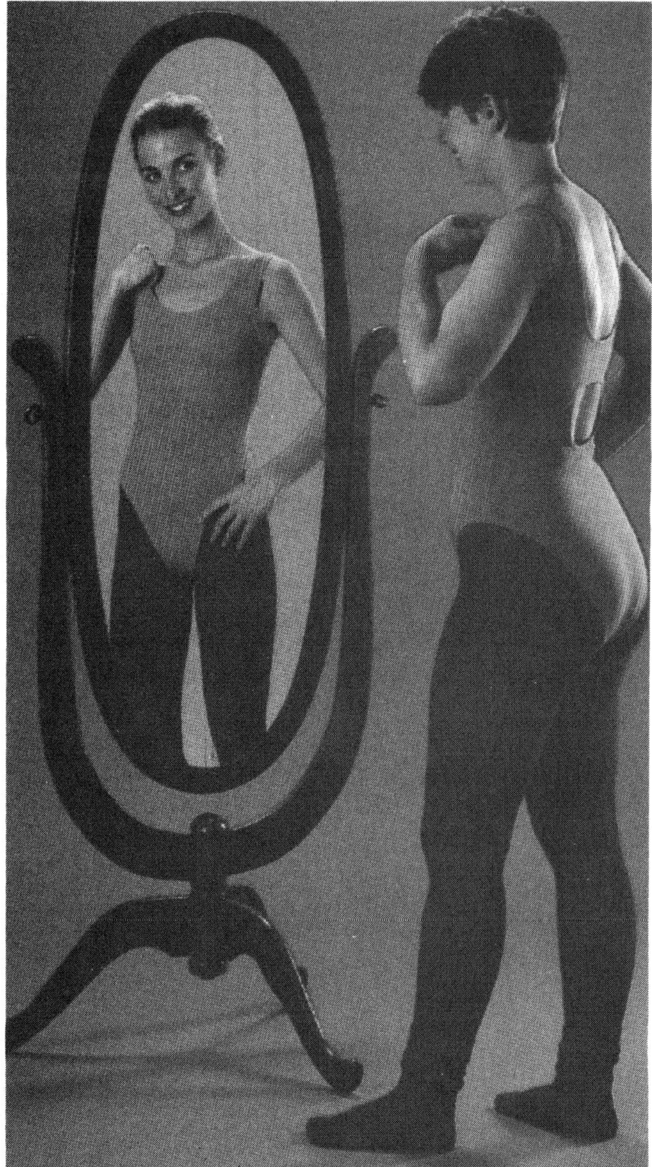

A clash of ideals The woman on the right—5-foot-4 and 130 pounds—has an ideal body type from a health standpoint. But many women her size long to attain a thinner ideal: the super-svelte body, shown in the mirror, that only a tiny fraction of the population can ever match.

from "pears," whose extra fat settles around the hips and buttocks. The higher the waist-to-hip ratio, the more apple-shaped the figure. Most men are apples, with the classic beer belly; most women are pears, although there is a significant minority of female apples.

The correlation between the waist-to-hip ratio and cardiovascular disease has been investigated in at least a half-dozen long-term studies, with consistent results: The higher the ratio, the greater the risk of disease, especially among people who are at least moderately overweight. Many scientists even believe that the waist-to-hip ratio predicts cardiovascular disease better than the degree of overweight. For men, the risk seems to rise above a waist-to-hip ratio of 0.95; for women, the cutoff point is 0.80. Paradoxically, surveys show that overweight men, most of whom are apples, are much less likely to try to lose weight than women, whose fat distribution is more benign.

Scientists think that abdominal fat does its damage because it is more metabolically active than below-the-waist fat. It's also associated with increased insulin resistance (a precursor to diabetes) and may be a cause of hypertension.

Why diets don't work

Even the most optimistic weight-control professionals admit that traditional dieting—cutting calories to lose weight—rarely works in the long term. Clinicians have tried everything to make diets more effective. They've devised ultra-low-calorie regimens that produce fast, large weight losses. They've brought patients in for months, even years, of behavior modification to help them deal with "impulse" eating and distract themselves from hunger pangs. The results are unvarying: When treatment stops, weight gain begins.

IS YOUR WEIGHT BAD FOR YOUR HEALTH?

While being overweight can raise the risk of disease, especially cardiovascular disease, your risk is only partially determined by the number you see on the scale. By completing this worksheet, you can get a fuller picture of how your weight is likely to affect your health. The approach used here is largely adapted from work by Dr. George Bray of the Pennington Biomedical Research Center at Louisiana State University and psychologist Thomas A. Wadden of Syracuse University. To begin, you need to calculate your body mass index (BMI) and your waist-to-hip ratio.

Finding your BMI

Using a calculator, you can calculate your BMI as follows: Multiply your weight in pounds by 700, divide by your height in inches, then divide by your height again.

BMI _______

Finding your waist-to-hip ratio

Using a tape measure, find the circumference of your waist at its narrowest point when your stomach is relaxed.

Waist: _________ in.

Next, measure the circumference of your hips at their widest (where your buttocks protrude the most).

Hips: ________ in.

Finally, divide your waist measurement by your hip measurement.

Waist/hip = _________ Waist-to-hip ratio

Determining your risk

Long-term studies show that the overall risk of developing heart disease is generally related to BMI as follows:

BMI of 25 or less—Risk is very low to low.
BMI between 25 and 30—Risk is low to moderate.
BMI of 30 or more—Risk is moderate to very high.

The BMI determines your likely range of risk. But where you fall within that range depends on the factors at right. The more items you have in the "High-Risk Factors" column, the higher your risk; the more you have in the "Low-Risk Factors" column, the lower your risk. Bear in mind that these factors give you only an approximation of your risk; your physician can give you more precise advice. (It's also possible for someone with a large number of high-risk factors to have a high risk of heart disease at any weight.)

HIGH-RISK FACTORS

- Being male
- Under age 40 with BMI above 25
- Waist-to-hip ratio greater than 0.80 for women or 0.95 for men
- Sedentary life-style
- Smoking
- High blood pressure
- Blood cholesterol of more than 200 mg/dl
- HDL less than 35
- Heart disease or Type II (adult-onset) diabetes—personal or in family history

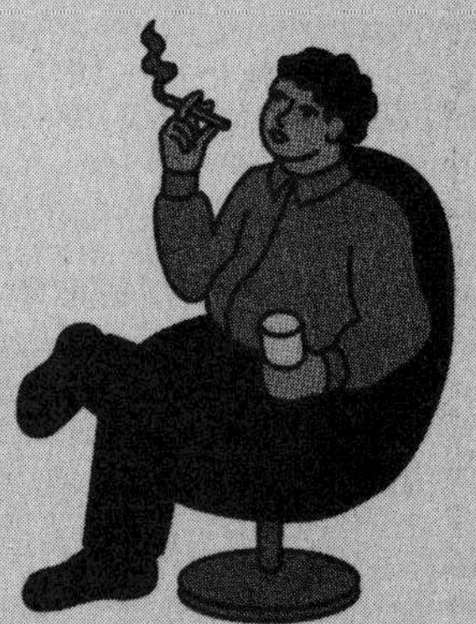

LOW-RISK FACTORS

- Being female
- Waist-to-hip ratio of less than 0.80 for women or 0.95 for men
- Regular exercise
- Normal blood pressure
- Blood cholesterol of less than 200 mg/dl
- HDL more than 45
- No personal or family history of heart disease or diabetes

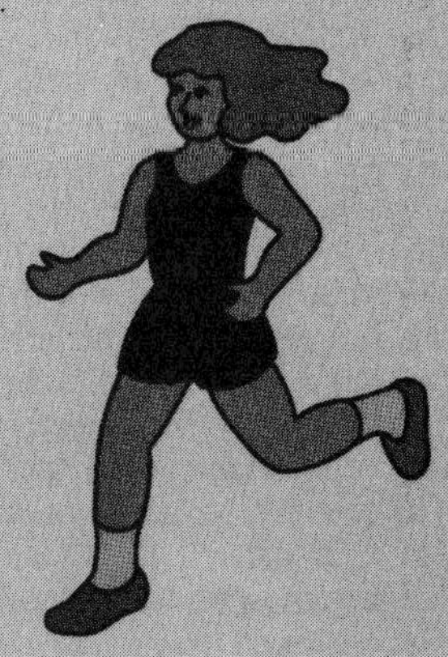

Scientists can't yet fully explain this nearly inevitable pattern, but the explanation may lie in our prehistoric roots. According to one hypothesis, humans evolved under the constant threat of famine. As a result, the human body is programmed by evolution to respond to caloric restriction as if starvation were at hand. After a few weeks on a low-calorie diet, the body goes on a sort of protective red alert. The basal metabolic rate—the speed at which the body burns calories when at rest—begins to decline. In addition, the body uses lean muscle mass as fuel in an effort to preserve fat, which is the major long-term source of energy. Both changes mean that the body burns fewer calories, making it more difficult to maintain a weight loss.

Finally, hunger—true, physiological hunger—increases. And, faced with hunger, "people are not able to keep up with the food restrictions required to maintain a lower weight," says David Schlundt, a psychologist at Vanderbilt University who specializes in obesity. Although the folklore of dieting says that hunger can be overcome by anyone with a decent amount of willpower, this basic biological drive is exceedingly difficult to ignore.

Most obesity researchers now believe that stringent dieting is actually a major trigger for binge eating. This connection was shown vividly in an experiment conducted during World War II by University of Minnesota physiologist Ancel Keys with a group of young, healthy men. Keys put the men on a balanced diet that provided about half their usual caloric intake—a regimen that he called "semistarvation" but that was remarkably similar to the diets prescribed by today's commercial weight-loss programs. When the men were released from the diet after six months, they went on massive eating binges, eating up to five meals and 5000 calories a day until they had returned to their normal weight. The lesson: "Going back to eating after a period of starvation is as natural as taking a breath," says Susan Wooley, a University of Cincinnati psychologist who specializes in obesity and eating disorders.

Is weight loss safe?

In addition to the high physical and emotional cost of dieting, new epidemiological evidence suggests that the practice may actually carry a greater health risk than staying overweight for some people.

For years everyone assumed that if overweight damaged a person's health, losing weight would improve it. That assumption seemed to be well-founded: Many studies have shown that as soon as dieters start to lose weight, their blood cholesterol levels and blood pressure drop and their insulin resistance declines.

Surprisingly, however, not a single long-term epidemiological study has ever proven that losing weight extends life. And over the past year, two important studies have provided evidence to the contrary.

One, headed by Elsie Pamuk of the Centers for Disease Control and Prevention, used the results of the First National Health and Nutrition Examination Survey, a Government survey of the health status of thousands of Americans. When they entered that study in the early 1970s, participants were given a complete checkup that, among other things, recorded what they weighed then and what was the most they had ever weighed. A decade later, the Government scientists tracked the participants to see who had died, and of what causes.

Recently, the CDC team analyzed the records of 5000 men and women who had been between the ages of 45 and 74 when they entered the Government study. The goal was to see whether those who had once been overweight but had lost weight lived longer than peers who had stayed fat. The team eliminated from the analysis anyone who had died within five years of starting the study, to make sure a pre-existing disease had not made them thin. They also adjusted their data to account for the effects of smoking, age, and gender.

The analysis did confirm one piece of conventional wisdom: Maintaining a stable adult weight and avoiding severe overweight is the best possible course. The data also supported the view that moderate overweight is not necessarily detrimental in middle age: Over the period of the study, men and women with a stable BMI between 25 and 30 had death rates as low as those with a stable BMI of 25 or less.

But when the CDC analysts looked at the effect of weight loss, what they found upset all their expectations:

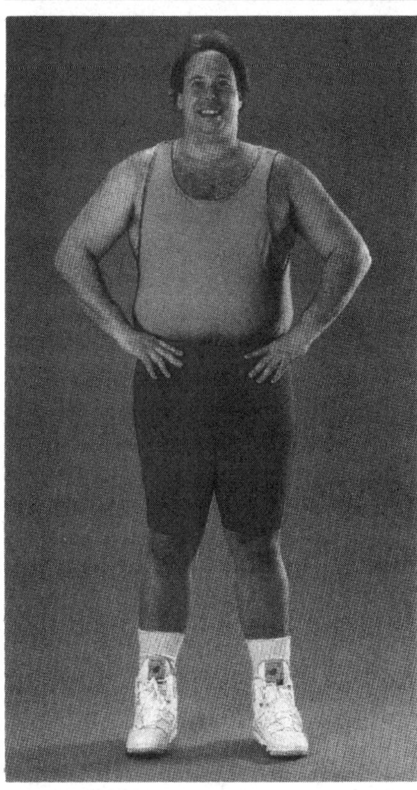

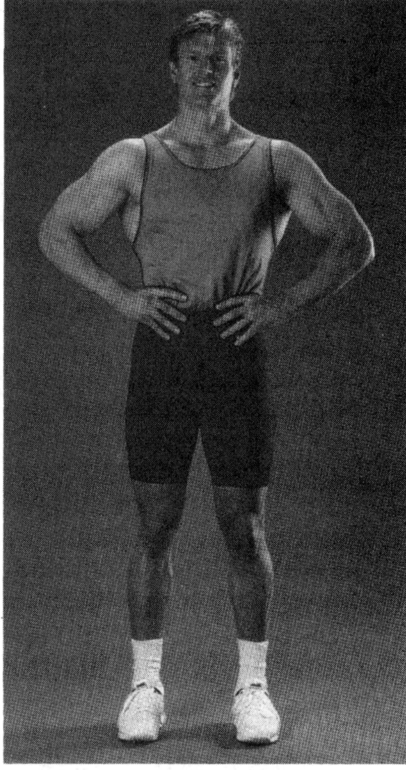

Same weight, different physique Weight is only one determinant of physical health. The man at left is 6 feet tall and weighs 240 pounds; the man at right is almost identical in height and weight, at 6-foot-1 and 230. But the man on the left is a classic "apple," with a high risk of heart disease, while the man on the right is muscular and at low risk.

Instead of improving health, losing weight seemed to do the opposite. Women who lost *any* amount of weight had a higher death rate than those who didn't; the more weight they lost, the higher their risk. Among the fattest group of men, who began with a BMI of 30 or above, those who had a moderate weight loss had a slightly lower than average death rate. But those who lost 15 percent or more had a higher death rate—unless, surprisingly, they were so fat that their weight loss still left them overweight.

The second study was even larger: It included 11,703 middle-aged and elderly Harvard alumni whose weight was recorded in the early 1960s and again in 1977. Like the CDC study, the Harvard study controlled for preexisting disease.

In 1988, the researchers checked alumni records to see who had died. The men whose weight changed least between the 1960s and 1977 had the lowest death rates, whether the researchers looked at deaths from all causes, deaths from cancer, or, especially, deaths from cardiovascular disease. Any significant weight change, whether up *or* down, markedly increased the risk of dying from cardiovascular disease.

Researchers are hard-pressed to explain the findings of the CDC and Harvard studies. The most likely explanation, however, is that people whose weight changed the most over time were more likely to have had cycles of yo-yo dieting in between—especially if they were overweight. Since our culture stigmatizes fatness, anyone who has been overweight for more than a few years has very likely gone through at least one cycle of significant weight loss and regain. Of the 95,000 respondents to our diet survey, 40 percent had had two or more weight-loss cycles within the previous five years; in that survey, overweight people cycled more often than people of normal weight.

Other studies have suggested that repeatedly losing and gaining weight is hazardous to health. One recent analysis used data from the Framingham Heart Study, a long-term study of some 5000 residents of a Boston suburb that began in 1948. Compared with subjects whose weight remained the most stable, those whose weight fluctuated frequently or by many pounds had a 50 percent higher risk of heart disease.

Weighing your options

Studies like those will animate seminars at scientific meetings for years to come. But they're confusing to people who must decide right now what, if anything, to do about their weight.

For some groups, the decision is relatively clear-cut. People who are not already overweight should place top priority on avoiding weight gain through a combination of moderate eating habits and exercise. Most seriously overweight people—those with a BMI of 30 or more—should attempt to lose some weight; for them, the evidence favoring weight loss is greater than the evidence against it. Most adult-onset diabetics should also reduce, since blood-sugar control usually improves with even relatively small amounts of weight loss. Given the possibility that large losses and regains may be hazardous, however, the best strategy is to stay away from quick weight-loss diets and aim instead for slow, modest, but permanent weight loss using the approaches we'll describe below.

The choice for nondiabetic, moderately overweight adults is not so clear. They should do what they can to avoid gaining more weight. But it is not certain that losing weight in and of itself will reduce their risk—especially if they gain it back again.

Fortunately, there is an approach to losing weight through diet and exercise that doesn't involve low-calorie quick-weight-loss plans. It's safer than conventional dieting; it's more likely to be effective; and it can lessen the risk of cardiovascular disease dramatically, even if it doesn't result in a large weight loss.

The importance of exercise

Apart from the risk of developing shinsplints or being chased by a dog, there's almost nothing bad to be said about regular, moderate physical exercise. And a number of studies now show that exercise can be very effective in weight control.

In one recent study, Stanford University researchers put 71 moderately overweight men and women on a low-fat diet for a year, and another, matched group of 71 on a diet with the same kinds of foods—plus a three-day-a-week program of aerobic exercise. After a year, the diet-plus-exercise group had lost more weight overall and more pounds of fat, even though they actually ate more calories per day than the diet-only group. Other studies have shown that exercise can help people lose weight even if they don't change their regular diet at all.

The explanation lies in the nature of human metabolism. More than half the calories we take in are burned up by what's called basal metabolism—the energy expended just to stay alive. In addition to increasing the number of calories burned in activity, exercise increases the basal metabolic rate, so the body burns more calories even at rest. Studies have shown that the basal metabolic rate is closely linked to the amount of muscle on the body, which is built up through exercise.

For most people, exercise alone will be enough to prevent future weight gain; for many, it will enable them to lose weight effectively and safely. In addition, even if exercise doesn't help you lose pounds, it may help you become thinner. A pound of muscle takes up less space than a pound of fat. So as you build muscle and lose fat, you can lose inches even without actually losing any weight.

Exercise plays a critical role not only in burning fat, but in keeping weight off. That was shown dramatically in a study of 184 mildly overweight Massachusetts policemen and civil servants. All were put on a low-calorie diet, and half were also put through three 90-minute exercise sessions per week. After eight weeks, everyone had lost weight. But when the men were re-examined three years later, those who had never exercised—or who had stopped once the study ended—promptly regained all or most of the weight they had lost. In contrast, exercisers who kept at it maintained virtually all their initial weight loss.

The rationale for exercise goes well beyond becoming thinner. "A lot of the health benefits that people are seeking from weight loss can be achieved by exercise, even in the absence of any weight loss," says Steven Blair, director of epidemiology at the Institute for Aerobics Research in Dallas.

In 1970, scientists at that institute began keeping records on more than 13,000 then-healthy middle-aged men and women to determine the effects of physical fitness on cardiovascular risk. The results are now coming in: Exercise seems to protect against disease and death even in people whose risk factors would otherwise put them in danger. Physically fit men in the study who had high blood pressure, insulin resistance, a high BMI, or an unfavorable family history were less likely to die than unfit men with none of those risk factors. Overall, the fittest men in the study had a death rate less than one-third that of the least fit; for women, there was a five-fold differ-

Trading pounds for lung cancer? Smoking tends to make people thinner, and cigarette manufacturers once promoted their products as if they were diet aids. In 1928, the American Tobacco Company introduced the slogan, "Reach for a Lucky instead of a sweet."

ence. The rates for cardiovascular disease were even more dramatically affected by fitness.

This study has now been followed up by a number of others showing that, among people with almost any known cardiovascular risk factor, exercisers do better than nonexercisers. In addition, exercisers develop adult-onset diabetes about 40 percent less often than nonexercisers, according to a study of 21,000 male American doctors.

It may even be that lack of exercise, rather than excess body fat itself, is the true culprit behind many of the ill effects of obesity. Since inactivity often leads to weight gain, overweight may turn out to be more a result of an unhealthful life-style than a cause of ill health.

Despite the evident benefits of exercise, most people with a weight problem still choose dieting instead. One reason has been the exercise community's historic fixation on high-intensity aerobic exercise, with its intimidating target-heart-rate charts and elaborate workout schedules. Most people simply won't attempt such demanding, time-consuming regimens—especially not the sedentary, overweight people who have the greatest need to exercise.

But intense exercise may not be necessary. Blair's study at the Institute for Aerobics Research suggests that the chief benefits of exercise come when people go from a sedentary life-style to moderate activity—not when they move from moderate exercise to intense athletics. In that study, men in the moderate-fitness group had a death rate from all causes nearly 60 percent lower than that of the sedentary group. In contrast, the very fittest men had a death rate only 23 percent lower than that of the moderately fit group. (Moderate exercise was defined as the equivalent of 30 to 60 minutes a day of brisk walking, either in small spurts or all at once.)

Influenced by these findings, Blair has become a prominent advocate of what might be called opportunistic exercise, which is essentially the art of devising an activity plan that can mesh with any schedule, no matter how frenetic. Blair, like many fitness experts, recommends looking for exercise everywhere you can. Park at the far edge of the mall lot instead of next to the front door; get off a bus one stop early and walk the rest of the way; pace the floor while you're on the phone; use an old-fashioned reel-type mower instead of a gasoline-powered one; take the stairs instead of the elevator. Any kind of exercise, however mundane, has potential benefits.

Eat less fat, lose fat

In addition to exercise, changing the kinds of food you eat—even without changing the caloric content—can improve both weight and health. Despite the decades-old wisdom that a calorie is a calorie is a calorie, some recent studies have suggested that calories from fat follow a straighter trajectory to the hips or the belly than calories from other sources. The body can store fat very efficiently. But the body's ability to store carbohydrates is limited, so when people eat more than their bodies can use, the excess is burned.

For that reason, researchers have found that the composition of the diet may be more important than the number of calories in determining who gains and who loses weight. The percentage of fat in the diet was the single strongest predictor of subsequent weight gain, for example, among 294 adults monitored for three years by Memphis State University investigators. By contrast, the total calorie consumption they reported had only a weak relationship to weight gain for women, and none at all for men.

If a high-fat diet can add pounds, a low-fat diet may help take them off. Researchers at the University of Illinois at Chicago switched 18 women volunteers from a diet that derived 37 percent of calories from fat—roughly the fat content of the average American's diet—to a diet that was only 20 percent fat. Over the 20-week experiment, the women lost four to five pounds, even though they increased their caloric intake.

One way to reduce fat intake without feeling chronically hungry is to fill up on something else, namely fruits, vegetables, and whole grains. Those foods are all high in carbohydrates, and a diet rich in fruits and vegetables seems to lower the risk of cancer and cardiovascular disease.

Some high-fat foods are easier to give up than others, as scientists at Seattle's Fred Hutchinson Cancer Research Center found in a study of the relationship between dietary fat and breast cancer. They taught a large group of women simple ways to reduce their fat consumption, and tracked down some of the participants after a year to see if they'd kept up their low-fat habits. The easiest changes to sustain turned out to be those that were least noticeable from a sensory standpoint: switching to

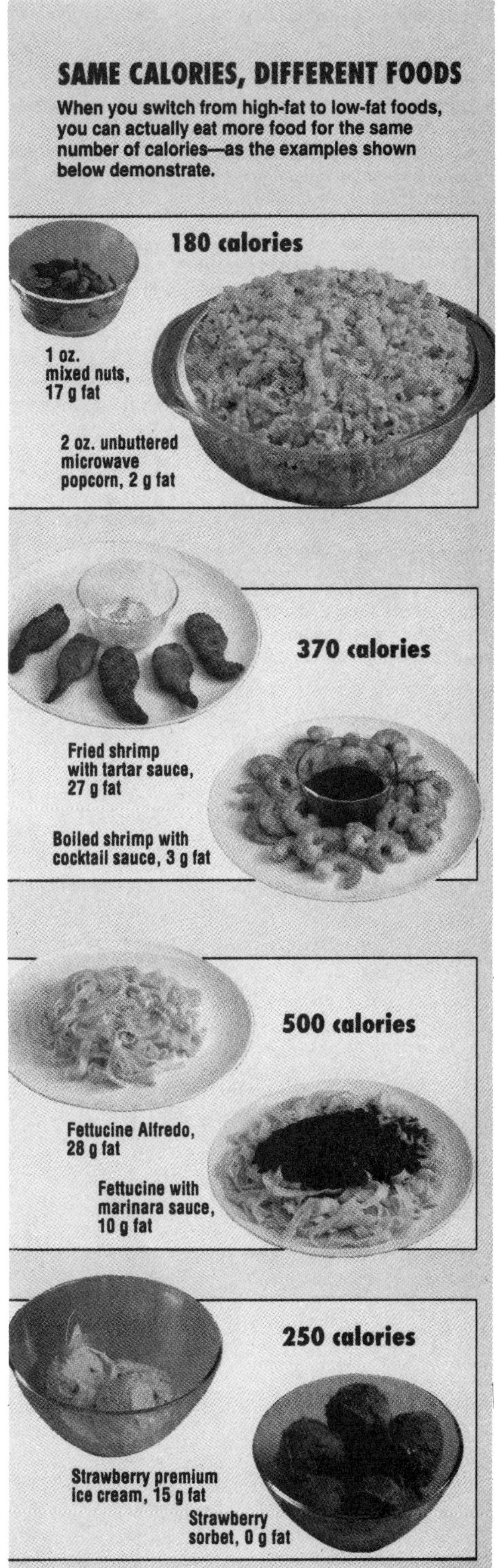
SAME CALORIES, DIFFERENT FOODS
When you switch from high-fat to low-fat foods, you can actually eat more food for the same number of calories—as the examples shown below demonstrate.
180 calories
1 oz. mixed nuts, 17 g fat
2 oz. unbuttered microwave popcorn, 2 g fat
370 calories
Fried shrimp with tartar sauce, 27 g fat
Boiled shrimp with cocktail sauce, 3 g fat
500 calories
Fettucine Alfredo, 28 g fat
Fettucine with marinara sauce, 10 g fat
250 calories
Strawberry premium ice cream, 15 g fat
Strawberry sorbet, 0 g fat

low-fat milk, mayonnaise, margarine, and salad dressing; trimming fat from meats and skin from chicken; having occasional vegetarian meals. Hardest to give up were the foods for which fat was an integral part of the food's appeal: pastries and ice cream, butter, hamburgers, lunch meats, and cheese.

Fortunately, the fat-reducing strategies that are easiest to follow can yield a significant decrease in total fat consumption. A group from Pennsylvania State University calculated the effect of such changes on an average woman's diet. They determined that by substituting skim milk for whole, switching to lower-fat meats and fish (such as skinless chicken and water-packed tuna), and using low-fat dressings and spreads, a woman could cut the fat in her diet from 37 percent of calories to 23 percent.

Your natural weight

Exercising and eating less fat are healthful changes that can benefit anyone, and may lead to weight loss as a bonus. But for many people, especially those who have been overweight all their lives, even faithful adherence to healthful habits won't slim the body to the thin ideal our culture holds dear.

Janet Polivy, an obesity researcher at the University of Toronto, believes that people should learn to be comfortable with their "natural weight"—the body size and shape that results after a person adopts a healthful diet and gets a reasonable amount of exercise. Similarly, Kelly Brownell, a Yale University psychologist who has done extensive research on behavioral obesity treatments, speaks of a "reasonable weight" as an attainable goal. "It's the weight that individuals making reasonable changes in their diet and exercise patterns can seek and maintain over a period of time," he explains. Brownell suggests that people who want to lose weight should start by losing a moderate amount, 10 pounds or so, and should then see how comfortably they can maintain that lower weight before trying to lose a bit more, stabilizing again, and so on.

Accepting the goal of a "natural" or "reasonable" weight may involve giving up long-held fantasies of a slim, youthfully athletic body, and being content with the realities of a middle-aged shape instead. It means accepting a slower rate of weight loss, or none at all. For long-term dieters, many of whom have spent years monitoring everything they put into their mouths and suppressing hunger pangs, it also means learning anew how to eat normally—eating when hungry and stopping when full.

Nevertheless, we believe this moderate approach to weight control is the only one worth trying for most people. It makes sense whether you are trying to maintain your current weight, reverse middle-age spread, or deal with a weight problem that's plagued you all your life. If you change your eating and exercise patterns gradually, and maintain the changes over time, you will almost certainly look and feel better, have more energy, and reduce your risk of cardiovascular disease, whether or not you lose much weight.

THE BEST Shape OF YOUR Life

Here's how to reach your naturally ideal weight—simply, sensibly, and without dieting

Anne Alexander

ANNE ALEXANDER is a senior editor of Walking.

How will we remember 1993? As the year Michael Jordan retired from basketball? Or when Bill and Hillary introduced health care reform? Not those of us who've been dreaming about shedding some extra pounds. We'll remember 1993 as the year diets got officially dissed: when the National Institutes of Health proclaimed that most diets don't work—they might help you lose weight, but it won't stay off.

What does this bode for 1994? Can we forget about calories and retire to our couches with a pint of Ben & Jerry's? Not so fast.

What it *does* do is clear the way for a positive attitude about eating and exercise. It's time to spread the word: You can be perfectly healthy—and look good—without being pencil-thin. You've just got to eat smart, walk regularly, and let your body reach its naturally ideal weight.

The Death of Dieting

"Everyone wants a quick fix to lose weight," says Janet Polivy, obesity and dieting researcher at the University of Toronto. "But the truth is, diets won't lead to permanent weight loss."

Never ever? Not according to the most recent findings. The National Institutes of Health found that with rare exception, people who restricted their overall caloric intake to shed pounds—"dieters"—gain back whatever weight they lost within the first year or two, or at least within five years. Many even add on a few extra pounds along the way.

Why this happens has a lot do with Mother Nature—thanks to the natural selection of our "thrifty genotypes" over thousands of years. That is, humans who could store fat most efficiently survived times when food was scarce. Imagine waif-model Kate Moss trying to survive a paleontologic winter. She'd never last.

These days, radically reducing your caloric intake still trips this ancient "thrifty" switch, sending the body into famine-survival mode. Sensing the threat of starvation, the body spends its fat stores more frugally. Metabolism slows down, enabling you to live on less energy.

"We evolved under circumstances of such deprivation that the ability to store energy was at a premium," explains Dr. Rudolph Leibel, obesity researcher at

Reprinted with permission from *Walking* magazine, January/February 1994, pp. 31-34, 36-38.

Rockefeller University in New York City. "The last 100 to 200 years have been a time of such food abundance and labor-saving devices"— such as cars, prepackaged foods, and elevators—"that we can't change our genetic make-up fast enough to keep up. Since the body keeps conserving energy, people get more and more obese."

Sure enough, despite the fact that 44 million of us go on diets every year, obesity is spreading in America. According to the Centers for Disease Control, 32% of men and 35% of women are obese (defined as 20% over the desirable weight for their height).

Forever Fat?

While your body is anticipating Armageddon, your brain may be wondering how to close the zipper on your pants. They weren't always that tight, you say. It's just those damn thrifty genes. So, are you stuck with well-stocked fat cells forever? Emphatically no. Just because you may have yo-yo dieted in the past doesn't mean you're destined to carry extra pounds forever. Most of us are plumper than need be and are perfectly capable of doing something about it.

Take Gary Ricci, one of the "Heroes on Foot" we profiled in our August 1993 issue (p. 37). Not an obesity researcher per se, Ricci is something of a weight-loss expert. A 38-year-old court officer from West Peabody, Mass., Ricci dallied unsuccessfully for years with every diet under the sun, but none could shrink his 56-inch waist. Then, he stopped dieting. He started walking six days a week and cutting fat from his meals. Before long, Ricci trimmed 210 pounds from his frame. "It's a simple formula of low-fat foods and plenty of walking," says Ricci. These days he's walking about 5½ miles daily, still eating smart, and staying slim.

Like Ricci, we all have a "set point" or "natural" weight lurking somewhere under our skin and waiting to emerge once we switch to a healthier lifestyle. "Your natural weight," according to Polivy, "is the weight that the body naturally adopts when you're eating a healthful diet and getting a reasonable amount of exercise."

Leibel agrees: "Each of us may have a pre-programmed size and shape in our genes." How our bodies actually develop is influenced by environmental, social, cultural, even emotional factors, some of which are under our control. For instance, we can improve our food choices and increase our activity level.

Since our natural shape is as individual as our fingerprints, body weights vary from person to person. In general, most of us should shoot for a weight that is a healthy ratio of body fat and lean body mass (muscle, bone, fluids). Ideally, this means 15% to 20% body fat for men and 19% to 24% for women. A very small number of people have an elevated set point and are naturally obese, but until your doctor tells you that you are in that group, you should probably assume you're not. And those who are can still improve their health by eating low-fat foods and developing a walking program.

Since body types are as individual as our fingerprints, naturally ideal weights vary from person to person.

Cut the Fat

Have you ever joked that fatty foods go straight to your hips? Well, you're right.

Researchers are discovering that all calories are not treated equally by your body. While carbohydrate calories are turned into ready-to-burn energy, fat calories are ushered almost directly to your fat stores, on your hips or around the waist. That's especially true when you eat more calories than you burn off and the body converts the extras into fat for storage. If, for example, you eat 100 extra calories worth of pretzels (carbohydrates), your body burns 25 calories simply processing those carbos for digestion and stores 75. A 100-calorie serving of butter, however, takes only 3

Dump that Scale!

Do yourself a favor. Put this magazine down. Then go to your bathroom, pick up the scale, and drop it in the trash. Better yet, carry it to your backyard garbage can and toss it out there. Cover it with eggshells, coffee grinds, and the remnants of last night's lasagne.

"Scales are good for three things: Weighing vegetables, fruits, and UPS packages," says Rob Sweetgall, *Walking's* contributing editor and co-author of the *Walking Off Weight* workbook. What scales are not good for is measuring your health: Thin doesn't necessarily mean healthy, and a heavier person who walks regularly can improve her health without necessarily seeing a difference on the scale.

But what if you want to slim down and get healthy? Well, tossing out your scale is a great first step. Next, focus on these three important facts:

1 If you want to lose weight for good, diet alone will not work. You must combine a low-fat diet with daily aerobic exercise.

2 A low-fat diet and regular exercise might make you slender. Or they might not. Unfortunately, your genes play a part in whether you are thin, fat, or in between.

"But I'm 20 pounds overweight!" you may cry. "No matter what I eat or how I exercise, I simply can't drop that weight. Am I stuck with it forever?"

Maybe not. Heredity may have determined that you'll never be a size 6 fashion model. But the chances are pretty good that if you're wider than you'd like to be, your lifestyle should share a big part of the blame. That's where fact 3 comes in, and it's the most important one of all.

3 You have to be brutally honest with yourself about what you eat and how much you exercise.

"People say, 'All I eat is salad, and I walk all the time. Why don't I lose weight?'" Sweetgall says. "Then I have

to 5 calories to digest, so 95 to 97 calories are stored as fat.

"You don't get fat without eating it," says Dr. Michael Hamilton, director of the Duke Diet and Fitness Center in Durham, N.C. Learn to recognize low-fat foods—and *eat* them. Also, snack smart. When the munchies strike, try microwaving a cut-up apple sprinkled with cinnamon instead of reaching for a slice of apple pie. Or grab a hard pretzel rather than a bowl of chips.

While some percentage of fat in your diet is necessary, most of us eat way too much. According to U.S. dietary guidelines, we should keep our fat intake under 30% of our total daily calories. Translated into fat grams, that means a woman who weighs 145 pounds and who consumes 1,700 calories per day should limit herself to no more than 57 grams of fat. Translated into food, one plain croissant has about 14 grams of fat—or three pats of butter. For that same 145-pound woman, that croissant delivers one-fourth of her daily fat.

All of the experts suggest limiting your fat intake, but exactly how low to go is controversial. While most recommend eating no more than 30% of calories from fat, some suggest reducing your fat intake to 20% or even less. For example, Dean Ornish's best-selling *Eat More, Weigh Less* advocates eating only 10% of calories from fat. The best advice is simply to keep your fat intake under 30% and to check with your doctor before going much lower.

Loving Low-fat: A True Story

Cutting down on fat has its own delightful advantages. For one thing, you can enjoy much more food on a low-fat diet—as long as it's low-fat or fat-free food.

Too good to be true? Again, listen to Ricci. "I still eat my favorite foods—and *lots* of them," he says enthusiastically, "but I've adapted my recipes to have no or very, very little fat." For example, Ricci makes his family favorite, fettucine Alfredo, with plenty of fat-free cottage cheese and just a dash of Parmesan.

One plain croissant has 14 grams of fat—or three pats of butter. For the average woman, that's one-fourth of her daily fat.

Phyllis Bowen, an associate professor in the department of nutrition and medical dietetics at the University of Illinois at Chicago, is also a staunch supporter of plentiful low-fat meals. During a six-month study, Bowen and her colleagues altered the amount of fat in the diets of six overweight volunteers and adjusted the number of calories they needed to maintain their body weight. For the first month, the volunteers ate a standard American diet with a whopping 38% of calories from fat. Then, they switched to a low-fat diet with just 20% of calories from fat. After five months, the researchers found that the women needed to eat about an extra 680 calories every day just to keep from losing weight.

"By the fourth and fifth month, morale was stupendous," says Bowen. "The women were coming in wearing slacks they hadn't worn in years. They had lost body fat and even increased their lean muscle a little." And that was without increasing their exercise. When you drop the fat in your diet *and* lengthen those daily walks, you'll really be in business.

Walk This Way

Eating less fat will get you halfway to your best shape. You'll have to walk the rest of the way.

Walking works because it burns calories and improves muscle tone—which can make your figure more shapely. What's more, walking revs up your metabolism. Just as carbohydrates raise the rate at which your body burns calories, so do regular brisk walks. Even when just sitting still, in fact, someone who exercises regularly burns more calories than a sedentary person. In addition, walking is critical for maintaining your weight loss.

---

lunch with them, and yes, they do have a salad. But they drench it in oily dressing. They don't even realize it!" Or, Sweetgall will delve into their exercise program and discover they are not walking as much as they think.

You may figure it's OK to nibble a bit of chocolate while you're waiting for your skinless chicken to broil—after all, you walked today. But nibbles add up. "It takes 3 miles of walking to burn off a chocolate bar," Sweetgall says.

So maybe you are being completely honest with yourself: Your diet really is low in fat. You really do exercise regularly. But you still have a thick middle, horsy hips, or gelatinous thighs. What can you do?

You can cheer up, because the best news of all is that even if you aren't as thin as you'd like to be, you can still be healthy. You can still strengthen your heart, reduce your risk of cancer and cardiovascular disease, and keep your arteries clear—all without being a string bean. And you can do it by walking regularly and eating right.

That's where self-acceptance comes in. If you aren't thin, but you are healthy, you need to accept yourself—happily—as a non-thin but healthy person. It's a tough battle, but after you win it you'll feel a lot better about yourself and your body.

Forget about those size 6 fashion models. Sure, many of them are healthy. But some of them, despite their appearance, might be on the fast track to a heart attack. Maybe they get winded walking 25 feet to their limousine. Maybe they live on foie gras and cocktail peanuts and have arteries clogged like storm sewers after a hurricane. If you live right, your 150 pounds can be healthier than someone else's 125. Good health and happiness can't be measured by a scale.

So if you really threw away your scale, congratulations! Celebrate with a long, vigorous walk and a crisp, juicy apple. Then, toss the apple core in the trash can with the scale, the leftover lasagne, and all of the negative behaviors that are standing in the way of your good health and peace of mind.

—Alice Lesch Kelly

Points To Live By

Ever wonder if you're getting enough—exercise and nutritious food, that is? You may walk a few miles during the week, swallow a daily vitamin, and never set foot in a fast food restaurant. But is that enough? Will those concessions to good health keep your waistline—not to mention the Grim Reaper—in check? Or, should you be doing more? To help you find out, we've devised the following point system so that you can analyze your exercise and eating habits. Check your total points on a weekday and on the weekend—you might even want to keep a running score to see how much you're doing on a daily basis.

Look over the following list of activities and foodstuffs. Which of these have you done—or eaten—since waking up this morning and before going to sleep? For every item that applies to you, give yourself the corresponding number of points. Tally up your score and see how your daily routine stacks up.

Fitness Walking

2 points for every mile walked
½ point extra per mile if you're pushing a stroller, carrying groceries, or pulling a sled

Target Heart Rate

1 point total if you reach your THR (or are breathing hard enough to notice and break a sweat)

Warm-Up

1 point for every 10 minutes of strolling you did before walking

Stretching

1 point for 10 or more minutes of stretching after walking

Strengthening

1 point for every 15 minutes of working out with weights

Stairclimbing

1 point for every five flights you walk up
2 points for every 10 minutes on the stairclimber

Maid Service

1 point for 10 minutes of folding clothes or ironing.

Trash Patrol

1 point for 10 minutes of bundling newspapers, crushing soup cans, or carrying out the garbage

Romper Room

2 points for every 10 minutes of playing leapfrog and doing cartwheels

Housekeeping

1 point for 10 minutes of scrubbing the tub, vacuuming the living room, or hanging wallpaper

Green Thumb

1 point for 10 minutes of raking leaves, gardening, or mowing the lawn

Shovelin' It

2 points for every 10 minutes of shoveling snow, hacking ice off the car, or digging ditches

Smart Parking

1 point for every 10 minutes walked to and from your car

Window Shopping

1 point for 20 minutes of stop-and-go strolling

"A lot of the health benefits that people are seeking from weight loss can be achieved by exercise even in the absence of weight loss," says Dr. Steven Blair, director of epidemiology at the Cooper Institute for Aerobic Research in Dallas and former vice president of the American College of Sports Medicine. These benefits include a reduced risk of coronary

Extra Miles

12 points for completing a 10K charity walk or racewalk
50 points for finishing a walking marathon

Couch Potato

-5 points for doing no exercise at all

Casanova

1 point for sex (if you're an active participant)
2 points if it's very vigorous or lasts more than 20 minutes

Food Alert

½ point for thinking about the meaning of low-fat
½ point for knowing your daily limit of fat grams

Cancer Control

5 points for getting your "Five a Day"—eating at least five servings of fruits and vegetables (plus, a pat on the back for each serving over five)

Salad Bar

1 point for eating a salad, period
½ point for selecting spinach leaves over iceberg lettuce
½ point for avoiding the fat sin bins—potato salad, creamy coleslaw, cheddar cheese chunks
½ point for choosing low-fat dressing

Fiber and Fruit

½ point for each serving of pure fruit juice
1 point for eating a piece of fruit
2 points for eating a high-fiber breakfast food (with more than 5 grams of fiber per serving)
1 point for each half-cup serving of cooked legumes

Dining Out

½ point for leaving the butter off your bread
½ point for asking the wait-person to put all sauces and dressings on the side
1 point for ordering pasta with marinara (tomato) sauce rather than meat or cream sauce
1 point for choosing thin-crust pizza over deep-dish (and using a knife and fork)
1 point for ordering chicken or fish broiled with lemon or wine instead of fat
1 point for getting steamed veggies
1 point for taking half your dinner home in a doggy bag

Fat Demerits

-1 point for every 3 grams over your fat limit
-1 point for thinking that a regular bran muffin is low in fat (some muffins can have more fat than a doughnut)
-5 points for a B.L.T. on white bread loaded with mayonnaise
-10 points for eating two helpings of your favorite high-fat food
-15 points for eating a double-bacon cheeseburger, large order of fries, and a chocolate shake

HOW'D YOU SCORE?

All the little things you do all day—both good and bad—accumulate. Here's a key for interpreting your score:

Under 10 points: Your body is begging for some attention. Lavish yourself with exercise and good food in 1994; put on your walking shoes and start to make some inroads into your own good health.

11 to 15 points: You're heading in the right direction, especially if you're earning points in both exercise and eating. Keep up the good work, and you may find your weight stabilize—even drop a bit—in the upcoming year.

16 to 30 points: Bravo! You're A-okay. Reward yourself with flowers, a quiet hour reading the latest Anne Rice novel, or a bubbly soak in the tub. You've earned it.

31 points and over: Give *Walking*'s Mark Fenton a call. You should be on the U.S. racewalking team!

—Anne Alexander

heart disease, high blood pressure, non-insulin-dependent diabetes, osteoporosis, and breast and colon cancer. "For a sedentary person, the adoption of an exercise program appears to be as important in preventing or delaying cardiovascular disease as smoking cessation," says Blair.

It doesn't take a huge amount of time to reap these benefits. The American College of Sports Medicine recommends doing at least half an hour a day of physical activity—particularly walking. When you're walking for weight loss, focus on the amount of time you walk rather than your speed. If you're just starting to walk for exercise, do so gradually—walk a few minutes a day, seven days a week. (If you are obese or suffering from any medical problems, check with your doctor before beginning a walking program.) The most important thing is to get out there regularly—even if you start just by walking to the corner mailbox. As you feel more comfortable, increase the length of your walks and, again, keep at it every day. "I started with just 5 or 10 minutes a day," says Gary Ricci, who weighed 360 pounds when he began to walk for exercise. Ricci's time on the road increased: Some weeks he covered 70 miles, and he now walks 30 miles a week.

In addition, increase your overall level of activity by making small changes in your daily routine. Walk up stairs instead of taking the elevator. Park your car a couple of blocks from work—or get off the bus early—and walk a few extra minutes every day. Also, try to find time for gardening, raking leaves, and shoveling snow. (Remember to warm up to avoid back strain.)

Setting the Ideal Goal

At the Duke Diet and Fitness Center in Durham, N.C., director Dr. Michael Hamilton helps hundreds of patients determine a realistic goal for their natural (or what he calls "healthier") weight. He evaluates each patient according to the following criteria:

1 Examine why you want to slim down. "I've got to know why someone wants to diet," he says, "because so many people diet for the wrong reason." Namely, cosmetic. "I work with those folks who don't have a medical reason to lose weight—but are still trying to—by counseling them to feel better about their bodies."

Does your weight impact your life—psychologically, socially, or physically? If so, it's time to find out why. Look at your eating habits and stress levels. Are they closely linked?

If you find that you turn to food to relieve stress, then your weight could be more of a psychological issue than a physical one, and you might want to consider counseling. If you've dropped activities because your body is too bulky, then exercising and changing your food choices is probably your best choice.

2 Measure your Body Mass Index and waist-to-hip ratio. Hamilton measures patients' BMI and waist-to-hip ratio to find out if they're overweight and at risk for weight-related health problems. Check the box above to determine your BMI and ratio. Scoring high on BMI has been linked to having an elevated risk for developing heart disease. The waist-to-hip ratio test tells if you've got an "apple" or "pear" shaped body. People with a low waist-to-hip ratio are called pears since fat is stored below their waists. Apples, who carry excess fat around their abdomen, have a higher waist-to-hip ratio and are associated with higher blood pressure and increased risk for developing adult-onset diabetes. Losing weight and exercising can reduce an "apple's" risk for both.

3 Think about what has been a realistic weight for you during your adult life. Frequently, middle-age patients tell Hamilton that they hope to look just as they did in high school. "For instance, a 196-pound woman just told me that she wants to weigh 130 pounds" Hamilton says. After learning that she had been 160 for several years and felt good at that weight, he encouraged her to aim for that. "It's not worth it if your life is going to be pure hell just trying to keep your weight down."

4 Consider your family genes. "If both parents of a patient are overweight, then it's probably going to be more difficult to lose weight," says Hamilton. But don't let that discourage you—your parents may have been overweight because of their lifestyle choices, such as not exercising and eating fatty foods. Also, consider your parents' figures—where did each of them stockpile fat? If neither was tall and willowy, your body probably won't look lanky no matter what. But remember, the idea behind reaching your ideal weight isn't to transform yourself into a teen idol, it's to be your healthiest.

Do you need to lose weight?

1. Check your Body Mass Index. Studies show that people with a BMI between 20 and 25 live the longest and have the least risk of developing heart disease. To figure out yours, find a calculator and plug in your weight in pounds. Then, multiply by 700; divide the result by your height in inches; finally, divide by your height again. Your risk for heart disease is related to your score as follows: Under 25, risk is very low; 25–30, risk is low to moderate; over 30, risk is moderate to high.

2. Are you an apple or pear? Check your waist-to-hip ratio. Use a tape measure to find the circumference of your waist. Next, measure your hips at their widest. Divide your waist measurement by your hip measurement. The healthiest ratios are below .80 for women and below .95 for men.

Real Ideals

If 1993 was the year that diets were debunked, maybe 1994 can be the year that we all get real about ideals. Get real about exercise: Start slowly if you need to, building up your time, speed, and exertion. Get real about food: Cut the fat, fill up on carbohydrates, and keep your fridge stocked with fresh fruits and veggies. Get real about your weight and shape: Figure out a sensible, healthy goal and aim for it. Most importantly, get real about your expectations: Don't strive to whittle yourself down to what you weighed when you were 17. Instead, get real about your resolutions, and promise yourself that when 1994 rolls into 1995, you'll be fitter and healthier and stronger than you are today—*without* dieting.

Body Mania

After a lifetime of work on the body-image front, one of the country's leading experts reveals her insights into the dilemma—and offers a way out

Judith Rodin, Ph.D.

Judith Rodin, a professor of psychology, medicine, and psychiatry at Yale University, is the author of more than 200 articles and papers as well as Breaking the Body Traps *(William Morrow, 1992). She is codirector of the Yale Center for Eating and Weight Disorders and past president of the Society for Behavioral Medicine.*

If *Pygmalion* were written today it would not be a story about changing Eliza Doolittle's speech, clothing, or manners, but rather about changing her face and body. Using methods from face-lifts to miracle diets to liposuction, women in increasing numbers are striving—with a degree of panic and, more often than not, to their own detriment—to match the ultimate template of beauty.

Has the situation worsened in the past few decades? The answer is undeniably yes. Since beginning this research 20 years ago, I have witnessed growing concern with appearance, body, and weight among women of all ages. Men, too, no longer seem immune.

In 1987, PSYCHOLOGY TODAY published the results of a survey of readers' feelings about appearance and weight. Only 12 percent of those polled indicated little concern about their appearance and said they didn't do much to improve it. The results of this survey are similar to those of many studies where the participants are selected at random: People feel intense pressure to look good.

An earlier survey on body image was published in PSYCHOLOGY TODAY in 1972. The 1970s respondents were considerably more satisfied with their bodies than were the 1980s respondents. The pressure to look good has intensified for both sexes in the last two decades. As the table below shows, our dissatisfaction has grown for every area of our bodies.

Unhappy Bodies

THE SURVEY ALSO SHOWS HOW IMPORTANT weight has become to body image; it is the focus of dissatisfaction in both studies and the area showing the greatest increase. I recently evaluated a survey for *USA Today* which also showed identical results. People today are far more critical of themselves for not attaining the right weight and look.

Body preoccupation has become a societal mania. We've become a nation of appearance junkies and fitness zealots, pioneers driven to think, talk, strategize, and worry about our bodies with the same fanatical devotion we applied to putting a

People Dissatisfied With Body Areas or Dimensions

1972	MEN	WOMEN	1987	MEN	WOMEN
Height	13%	13%	Height	20%	17%
Weight	35	48	Weight	41	55
Muscle Tone	25	30	MuscleTone	32	45
Overall Face	8	11	Face	20	20
Breast/Chest	18	26	Upper Torso	28	32
Abdomen	36	50	Mid Torso	50	57
Hips and Upper Thighs	12	49	Lower Torso	21	50
Overall	15	25	"Looks As They Are"	34	38

From *Psychology Today,* January/February 1992, pp. 56-60. Excerpt from Breaking the Body Traps. © 1992 by Judith Rodin. Reprinted by permission of William Morrow & Company, Inc.

man on the moon. Abroad, we strive for global peace. At home, we have declared war on our bodies.

It is a mistake to think that concern with appearance and weight is simply an aberration of contemporary Western culture. Generations of ancient Chinese women hobbled themselves by binding their feet in order to match the beauty ideal of the time. And we all remember Scarlett O'Hara in search of the 17-inch waist. What *Gone With The Wind* did not show us was that tight corseting induced shortness of breath, constipation, and, occasionally, uterine prolapse. But if we moderns are following a tradition hallowed by our forebears, the industrialization of fitness and beauty is conspiring with other trends to raise the stakes to their highest point in history.

Of all the industrial achievements of the 20th century that influence how we feel about our bodies, none has had a more profound effect than the rise of the mass media. Through movies, magazines, and TV, we see beautiful people as often as we see our own family members; the net effect is to make exceptional beauty appear real and attainable. Narcissus was lucky: He had only to find a lake. The modern woman has television, in which she doesn't see herself reflected.

In my experience as a researcher and clinician, I have found that many women avoid the mirror altogether; those who do look may scrutinize, yet still fail to see themselves objectively. Most of us see only painful flaws in exquisite detail. Others still see the fat and blemishes that used to be there in the teenage years, even if they're no longer there.

Like a perverse Narcissus, a woman today looks at her reflection in a mirror and finds it wanting—and then is consumed by a quest to make herself fit the reflection the media has conditioned her to expect is possible. She works harder and harder to attain what is, as I will explain, most likely impossible. Ignoring the hours movie stars spend on makeup and hair, forgetting how easily and well the camera can lie, she aspires to a synthetic composite of what she thinks her reflection should be.

It is also likely that she is unaware of what other research shows: Such detailed attention has a negative influence on self-esteem. It makes us feel that many features of ourself are flawed, even those having little to do with weight or appearance.

Many of us have traveled through the looking glass with Alice into a world where what is and what might be blur and confuse us. We may be thin and think we are not. We may be heavy and think that life isn't worth living because we do not match our culture's physical ideal. Our self-image has become far too plastic, too malleable. It depends too much on transitory moods, on what we feel is expected of us and how we feel we are lacking. It is not dependent enough upon a stable internal sense of ourself. We grow larger or smaller, in our mind's eye, in response to the image of woman modern society has encouraged us to idealize.

Unlike Alice, however, we have not returned. We are stuck there in a world of obsessional self-criticism, where what we see is not at all what we really are. The mirror is woman's modern nemesis.

Some call such obsession with appearance vanity—but that misses the point. We are responding to the deep psychological significance of the body. Appearance does indeed affect our sense of self and how people respond to us; it always has, always will. What's different today is that the body and how it looks has become a significant component of our self-worth.

Why Now?

WHY DO WEIGHT AND APPEARANCE MATTER so much? And why now? What is occurring at this particular moment in time?

Our society has changed dramatically in this century. There are few remaining hierarchies or social structures based on religion, parentage, money, or education. Society has become more egalitarian, but intrinsic to human nature is the desire to judge, evaluate, and compare ourselves to others. If class and lineage no longer provide the tools for measuring ourselves against our neighbors, what are the new social standards? It is my premise that they are the more visible, tangible, observable aspects—first among these, the physical self.

Our bodies have become the premier coin of the realm. Appearance, good looks, and fitness are now the measure of one's social worth. How closely we can approximate a perfect body has also unfortunately become a sign of how well we're doing in life.

Not only is how we look suddenly of the utmost importance, but we have also come to accept and idealize a single image of beauty—slim but fit. The media now expose us to this single "right" look, and the beauty industry promises it is attainable by all. When the prescription for how we should look is so well-defined, deviations are all the more noticeable.

What's more, our culture holds out the lure of an easy fix for all corporeal dissatisfactions. The goal of looking good is attainable by anyone, as long as he or she works out hard enough, exercises long enough, and eats little enough.

Beauty, health, diet, and fitness have become very big businesses. But they weren't always. During the late 1950s and early '60s—when models and Miss Americas wore girdles, did a little exercise just for their thighs and hips, and wore a size 10—only overweight women dieted. A survey of *Ladies Home Journal* issues from the 1960s showed an average of only one diet article every six months. But by the mid-'70s almost every woman in America had tried some kind of diet, and losing weight was a national obsession.

Because we sincerely believe that the perfect body is attainable by anyone, Americans spend more on beauty and fitness aids than they do on social services or education. Such distribution of a primary resource is a shocking revelation of our true priorities.

Yet another reason appearance is everything today hinges on the blurring of traditional definitions of female and male. Our view of the differences between the sexes is in flux, as women move into such traditionally male domains as the office and men become more involved in the household. In many ways our bodies remain our most visible means of expressing the differences between the sexes. Having the right body may be a way for women who have moved into male occupations to declare their feminine identity without compromising their professional persona.

Asked to make it in a man's world, they are, like the rest of society, still confused about women's roles. Internalizing society's ambivalence, they succeed in one domain and fall back in the other, reverting to the traditionally feminine arena of competition over thinness and beauty.

In addition, the fitness movement, taken to extremes, has fostered the notion that a "good" physique not only equals a healthy body but a healthy soul. Getting in shape has become the new moral imperative—an alluring substitute for altruism and good work, the desire to look good replacing the desire to do good. In this new secular morality, values and ideals of beauty and appearance supplement moral and religious standards.

Today's moral transgressions involve eating something we feel we shouldn't have or feeling we don't look good enough or haven't tried hard enough to look good.

If our current self-absorption has its reasons, it also has its comforts. The quest for physical perfection is the up-to-date way we barter with the uncertainty of life. Like a set of worry beads, we always have our calories to count, our minutes of aerobics to execute. If everything else in our lives seems out of control, we at least have our diet and exercise regimens. In the chaos called modern life, ordering the body to do what we want it to may give us a much-needed illusion of control.

Where we differ, too, from our forebears is that the body today is no longer considered a finished product, a fait accompli. It is strictly a work in progress. And we devote ourselves to perfecting it with the dedication of the true artist. According to the American Society of Plastic and Reconstructive Surgeons, "aesthetic" surgeries are up 61 percent over the past decade. A marketing research firm in New York calculates that Americans spent $33 billion on diets and diet-related services in 1990, up from $29 billion in 1989. By the turn of the century we will be spending $77 billion to lose weight—just slightly less than the entire gross national product of Belgium.

Social Attitudes Scale

Please read the following statements and indicate how strongly you agree or disagree with each.

1. A man would always prefer to go out with a thin woman than one who is heavy.

Strongly Agree	Agree Somewhat	Agree	Neither Agree nor Disagree	Disagree	Disagree Somewhat	Strongly Disagree
☐	☐	☐	☐	☐	☐	☐

2. Clothes are made today so that only thin people can look good.

Strongly Agree	Agree Somewhat	Agree	Neither Agree nor Disagree	Disagree	Disagree Somewhat	Strongly Disagree
☐	☐	☐	☐	☐	☐	☐

3. Fat people are often unhappy.

Strongly Agree	Agree Somewhat	Agree	Neither Agree nor Disagree	Disagree	Disagree Somewhat	Strongly Disagree
☐	☐	☐	☐	☐	☐	☐

4. It is not true that attractive people are more interesting, poised, and socially outgoing than unattractive people.

Strongly Agree	Agree Somewhat	Agree	Neither Agree nor Disagree	Disagree	Disagree Somewhat	Strongly Disagree
☐	☐	☐	☐	☐	☐	☐

5. A pretty face will not get you very far without a slim body.

Strongly Agree	Agree Somewhat	Agree	Neither Agree nor Disagree	Disagree	Disagree Somewhat	Strongly Disagree
☐	☐	☐	☐	☐	☐	☐

6. It is more important that a woman be attractive than a man.

Strongly Agree	Agree Somewhat	Agree	Neither Agree nor Disagree	Disagree	Disagree Somewhat	Strongly Disagree
☐	☐	☐	☐	☐	☐	☐

7. Attractive people lead more fulfilling lives than unattractive people.

Strongly Agree	Agree Somewhat	Agree	Neither Agree nor Disagree	Disagree	Disagree Somewhat	Strongly Disagree
☐	☐	☐	☐	☐	☐	☐

8. The thinner a woman is, the more attractive she is.

Strongly Agree	Agree Somewhat	Agree	Neither Agree nor Disagree	Disagree	Disagree Somewhat	Strongly Disagree
☐	☐	☐	☐	☐	☐	☐

9. Attractiveness decreases the likelihood of professional success.

Strongly Agree	Agree Somewhat	Agree	Neither Agree nor Disagree	Disagree	Disagree Somewhat	Strongly Disagree
☐	☐	☐	☐	☐	☐	☐

These items test how much you believe that appearance matters. Score your responses as follows:

For items 1, 2, 3, 5, 7, and 8, give yourself a zero if you said "strongly disagree"; a 2 for "disagree"; up to a 6 for "strongly agree."

Items 4, 6, and 9 are scored in reverse. In other words, give yourself a zero for "strongly agree" and a 6 for "strongly disagree."

Add together your points for all nine questions. A score of 46 or higher means that you are vulnerable to being influenced by the great importance that current society places on appearance.

The Limits of the Body

THERE IS AN OVERRIDING FALLACY IN THIS view of ourselves. The body is not infinitely malleable in the way that advertisers with a product to sell would have us believe. Despite wide dissemination of news about great advances in science and medicine, the individual American remains virtually unaware of the role that physiology plays in body weight, in determining how quickly we lose or gain weight and in how our general health and appearance respond to exercise and diet. Most of us are exposed to and accept a staggering amount of misinformation.

Genes play a major role in setting metabolism as well as body shape and size; they determine how much fat we burn, how much we can store easily, and where it's distributed on our bodies. One of our clinic patients came from a family where everyone had thick, solid legs and big thighs. For years she tried every diet that became popular. No matter how much she lost, no matter how thin she became, she couldn't change the size of her legs and thighs nearly as much as the rest of her body. "My greatest goal in life," she admitted, "is to have thin legs.... I know why women have liposuction. It's the ultimate solution. I used to dream about a big vacuum cleaner sucking out the fat—it was my constant childhood wish—but I just can't afford it yet."

The Pursuit Is Costly

THE QUEST FOR THE PERFECT BODY IS, LIKE most wars, a costly one—emotionally and physically, to say nothing of financially. It leaves most of us feeling frustrated, ashamed, and defeated. Yet we keep at it, wearing down our bodies and our optimism while narrowing the focus of our lives.

In addition, as a society obsessed with a set standard of beauty, we have become intolerant of and sometimes cruel to those who do not meet it, especially the overweight. We learn early in life that there is something shameful about obesity. And the obese are painfully stigmatized. Even children with a life-threatening chronic illness would rather be sick than fat.

We learn these antifat attitudes in childhood, and they figure strongly into why normal-weight people greatly fear becoming overweight. In our research, we hear many people state that they would kill themselves if they were fat. While this is just a figure of speech, some overweight people are so unhappy about their appearance that they *do* contemplate suicide. A few follow through.

The accompanying test will give you an idea of how much you subscribe to society's standards of beauty.

The vast majority of American women have accepted at face value the message we have been continually exposed to: that beauty and physical perfection are merely a matter of personal effort and that failure to attain those goals is the result of not doing enough. Consequently, we are now subjecting ourselves and even our children to an ever more complicated regimen of diet, exercise, and beauty. We have come to believe in what I see as the "techno-body," shaped by dieting and surgical techniques.

Humans appear to be the only animals who decline to eat when hungry, who willingly starve the body. Occasionally they do it to feed the soul. Many religions have institutionalized fasting as a way of asking for redemption. But in the more modern version of these self-denial rituals, people fast and starve, purge and renew in search of a better self.

It has become fashionable, even politically correct, to worry about the environment. We rally to plant trees to save the Earth without even realizing that at the very same moment in history we are defacing and dehumanizing our bodies by using chemical peels, dermabrasion, hair dye, synthetic diet foods, and fake fats and sweeteners. Where is our concern for the human part of our environment?

What Is the Problem?

My studies show that surgery, diet, and exercise are only symptoms of the real problem: body preoccupation and an obsessive concern with body image. In accepting the quick fix as a solution, we are overlooking the depth and complexity of the problem we are facing. Shedding pounds, counting calories, and pumping iron—manifestations of body preoccupation—are only a reflection of the fact that we now believe the body is the window to the self, perhaps even the soul.

The psychological self is fundamental to our preoccupation with the physical self. Of all the ways we experience ourselves, none is so primal as the sense of our own bodies. Our body image is at the very core of our identity. Our feelings about our bodies are woven into practically every aspect of our behavior. Our bodies shape our identity because they are the form and substance of our persona to the outside world. Appearance will always be important because we are social beings. How we look sends messages, whether we want it to or not, and people respond to us accordingly.

The old saw cites death and taxes, but in fact we have one other nonnegotiable contract in life: to live in and with our bodies for the duration. People must learn to treat the issue of body image seriously and validate their concerns about their bodies. In my clinical experience, people find that hard to do because admitting how deeply we anguish about our bodies often leads to a profound sense of shame.

In an era of acid rain, AIDS, nuclear disaster, and poverty, we are embarrassed by our body preoccupation—but that, of course, does not stop it.

In an era of acid rain, AIDS, nuclear disaster, and poverty, we are embarrassed by our body preoccupation—but that, of course, does not stop it.

Getting Out of the Body Trap

Recognizing the problem is the first step to solving it. Our work has shown that people do better when they are nonjudgmental about their concerns with body, diet, and exercise patterns. These are not trivial worries and complaints, but painful experiences and issues deserving attention. It is crucial to acknowledge the scope and depth of what you are feeling. No one is alone in their body concerns. All women share them to some extent—as do many men these days, as well.

If you treat your body with more respect, you will like it better. What your body really needs is moderate exercise, healthy foods, sensual pleasures, and relaxation. Give it those, and it will respond by treating you better. Not everyone can afford expensive trinkets or clothes, but everyone can afford small indulgences—a long, warm bath, a half-hour of time off, a new haircut. Some of you will be amazed at how hard it is to do something nice for yourself. But treating your body better will make you feel better about yourself.

To break the body-image barrier, we must bring self-image into focus. When people worry about how they look, they are worrying about who they are. That's not necessarily good, but we need to acknowledge that there is a deep connection between the two. In my work with patients, I strive to help them overcome the feeling that their happiness rises or falls depending on what the scale said that morning.

We must also look at what we really want and need from our lives and pursue those goals; it is not wise to continue expending so much of our creative energy on thinness and appearance. Since our bodies are not infinitely plastic, it may be easier to add other joys to life than to subtract pounds. Increasing and nurturing self-complexity by expanding the number of roles we value may boost health in many ways. Current research suggests that multiple roles are typically health enhancing. Varying our routines and adding new interests to our lives will help broaden our horizons so that how we look is not the sum of what we are.

As a character in Henry Jaglom's movie *Eating* says, "Twenty or thirty years ago, sex was the secret subject of women. Now it's food." In fact, sex and food have become interchangeable. "I like the feel of food. I don't like knives and forks because I like to touch it all over," says one woman. Another: "I think it is erotic. It's the safest sex you can have, eating." Food. It is comfort, balm for a trying day in a trying world, sometimes even more. Moderation is the best advice. It is the key to body sanity.

Whether we want to value, accept, or change our bodies, we need first to change our minds. We have to relearn how we observe ourselves. Instead of searching for flaws, we must attempt to see ourselves objectively. We must scrutinize our appearance less.

Caring about our bodies is normal, but how we look has become far too significant. Women have become martyrs to their appearance, slaves of that impossible master, perfection. Men go through life judged mostly on their achievements; women bear the burden of society's image. Although the effort is exhausting and painful, the deep, psychological significance of the body has made it seem worthwhile.

The burden of maintaining a perfect body image is far too costly. Women are crippled by a tragic degree of self-consciousness that limits other aspects of their lives—friendships, careers, even families.

One of the most important steps toward changing your body image is to have compassion for the millions of women struggling with their own body-image problems—especially for yourself. It is time to face the person you see in the mirror with profound new insight: She hasn't been worrying about nothing. In fact, she hasn't been taking the real problem, body preoccupation, seriously enough. Neither has society. It's time to understand the price she has been paying and help her shed that burden.

Current Killers

Over the past 30 years, Americans have witnessed remarkable scientific achievements in medical technology. Today not only are organ transplants a common occurrence, but human organs are even being replaced with artificial substitutes. While these medical marvels are a testament to America's technological sophistication, they have done little to prevent the ravages associated with cardiovascular disease and cancer—the leading killers in this country. These diseases that are termed chronic illnesses are most likely to afflict those who have made lifestyle choices that disregard their genetic predisposition toward these illnesses. Even if you are conscientious about trying to live a healthy lifestyle, it is not always possible to prevent these illnesses. Your chances of success are much greater, however, if you are aware of any genetic predispositions that you may have inherited. While we cannot change our genetic predispositions, we can modify our lifestyles to compensate for them. "Trace Your Family Tree" by Ruth Papazian discusses how an awareness of the medical histories of your ancestors can be used to promote and safeguard your health.

Of all the diseases in America, coronary heart disease is the nation's number one killer. Frequently, the first and only symptom of this disease is sudden death. While medical science has been unable to prevent this disease, epidemiological studies have revealed a number of risk factors that increase one's likelihood of developing it. These risk factors include hypertension, a high serum cholesterol level, diabetes, cigarette smoking, obesity, a sedentary lifestyle, a family history of heart disease, age, sex, race, and stress. Research further indicates that as the numbers of risk factors increase, the risk of developing premature coronary heart disease rises dramatically. The article "Rating Your Risks for Heart Disease" examines all the known risk factors and predictors of coronary heart disease and presents a brief discussion of nine intervention strategies that can reduce one's risk of developing this deadly disease.

While the link between high serum cholesterol levels and premature cardiovascular disease is irrefutable, the connection between dietary fat and elevated serum cholesterol is embroiled in controversy. The controversy surrounding this connection is not whether dietary fat can raise one's serum cholesterol level, but what percentage of the population is susceptible to this cholesterol elevating effect. Over the past few years, A. E. Harper, Ph.D., professor of nutritional sciences and biochemistry at the University of Wisconsin, has been a vocal opponent of the National Research Council's (NRC) recommendation concerning dietary fat. Briefly stated, the NRC recommends that dietary fat should constitute less than 30 percent of one's total caloric intake, and saturated fats should be replaced with monounsaturated and polyunsaturated fats whenever possible. Dr. Harper has argued that while this recommendation is valid for those individuals that test high for blood cholesterol, it is inappropriate and unnecessary for the majority of Americans. In the past, Dr. Harper has been criticized for his position on the dietary fat issue, but new scientific findings provide strong evidence that Dr. Harper is correct in his assertions. The medical community has been taken aback by the discovery that very low blood cholesterol levels, while reducing one's risk of heart disease, increase one's risk of dying from suicide, stroke, certain cancers, liver disease, and lung disease. Most striking is the finding that the mortality rate is the same for those with either high or low blood cholesterol levels. The article "Cholesterol," published in the Mayo Clinic Health Letter, provides the reader with a comprehensive look at cholesterol.

Cardiovascular disease may be America's number one killer, but cancer takes top billing in terms of the "fear factor." This fear of cancer stems from an awareness of the degenerative and disfiguring nature of this deadly disease. Today cancer specialists are employing a variety of complex agents and technologies, such as monoclonal antibodies, interferon, and immunotherapy, in their attempts to fight it.

What can individuals do to reduce their risk of cancer? Lung cancer, colon cancer, and skin cancer have been linked to lifestyle patterns. Lung cancer, associated with cigarette smoking, is the most common form of cancer among men, and has overtaken breast cancer as the most common form of cancer among women. While this type of cancer is the most deadly, it is also almost entirely preventable by eliminating smoking. Non-melanoma skin cancer, which is the most common form of cancer for both sexes across all age groups, is fortunately the easiest to prevent. Most authorities agree that the best way to prevent this type of cancer is to minimize the skin's exposure to the damaging effects of ultraviolet radiation.

Recent discoveries in the area of cell biology have started to unlock the mysterious behavior of cancer cells. Scientists now believe that cancer cells are simply normal cells that have become defective in very specific and correctable ways. This knowledge regarding the transformation from a normal cell to a cancerous cell has provided scientists with information that may eventually be used to halt or even reverse the process. In "Stopping Cancer in Its Tracks," J. Madeleine Nash discusses several recent scientific breakthroughs in the area of cancer research

Unit 7

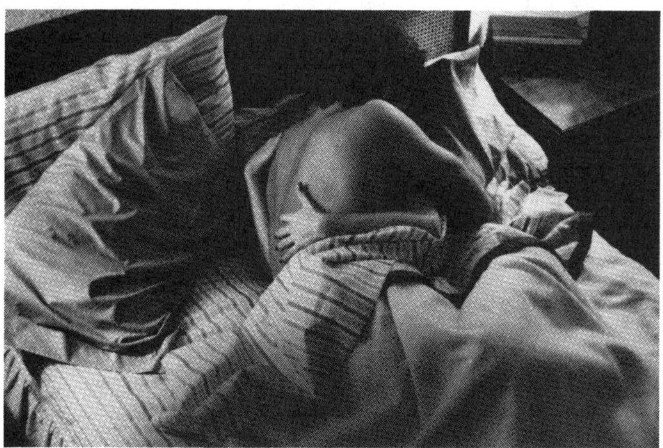

AIDS

If you think you can't get it, you're dead wrong.

that may yield therapeutic interventions that can actually cure this horrendous disease.

Of the three diseases discussed in this unit, AIDS has the potential to become the worst epidemic of this century. As medical researchers intensify their search for an effective AIDS vaccine, the disease continues to spread and infect countless people. This disease has already been diagnosed in over 80,500 individuals. Of those diagnosed, half have already died. Conservative estimates indicate that by the year 2000, between 30 and 110 million people will be infected with the AIDS virus. The World Health Organization estimates that there are already 5 million people carrying the virus with no apparent symptoms. One of the problems with trying to estimate the exact number of potential AIDS victims is the fact that this disease has an incubation period that may be as long as 10 years.

What is known about AIDS? Researchers have been able to identify the virus that causes AIDS. This virus, termed the HIV virus, has been found in both the blood and body fluids of infected persons, and case studies have documented that the disease can be transmitted through intimate sexual contact and the mixing of blood products. To date there have been no documented cases of AIDS being spread through casual social contact, and most experts do not believe that the viral content of saliva is sufficient to spread the disease. Currently there is no vaccine available to protect one from this dreaded disease, and there are no antiviral drugs available that can cure it. The only bright spot in this regard are the drugs AZT and DDI. Recent findings have revealed that while AZT has been shown to prolong the life of some AIDS patients, it is particularly effective in slowing the progress of this disease if taken prior to the appearance of symptoms. Unfortunately, researchers are also finding that the HIV virus in individuals receiving AZT for prolonged periods of time is capable of mutating to AZT-resistant strains. AZT may also produce side effects serious enough to preclude its use for certain individuals. These limitations have prompted the FDA to relax its testing and approval procedures for the drug DDI, so that it may also be used to treat AIDS patients. At the time of this writing, little is known regarding its therapeutic effectiveness or potential side effects. Until such time that there is a safe and effective vaccine against AIDS, our best defense against this killer is education. "Confronting the AIDS Pandemic" discusses the current state of the AIDS pandemic and speculates on how it will grow and the economic impact it will have on the world economy by the year 2000.

While coronary heart disease, cancer, and AIDS are all deadly diseases, the good news is that many of the risk factors associated with each of them can be controlled through lifestyle choices. This fact, coupled with the need to curb the high cost of U.S. health care, may be just what it takes to elevate the role of primary prevention to the forefront of health care where it belongs.

Looking Ahead: Challenge Questions

Should doctors and other medical personnel be required to submit to AIDS testing? If so, how often should they be tested?

Do doctors have a right to know if their patients are infected with AIDS? If so, how would you secure this information?

What role can and should education play in combating the spread of AIDS?

What lifestyle changes could you make that would reduce your risk of developing cardiovascular disease, cancer, and AIDS?

What dietary advice would you give someone to reduce their risk of cancer?

To what extent should the government be involved in promoting preventative medicine?

Assuming that you live long enough, which chronic disease do you think you are most likely to contract, based on your family history and lifestyle?

TRACE YOUR FAMILY TREE

Charting your relatives' medical history can save your life

RUTH PAPAZIAN

Ruth Papazian, a New York City-based writer specializing in health and medicine, is constructing a family tree for herself and her niece and nephew.

When it comes to health, the apple doesn't fall far fom the family tree: Research suggests that an astonishing number of diseases—from rare to common—have some sort of hereditary link.

That is why constructing a family health tree can offer life-saving glimpses into your future. If you're at risk of inheriting a serious disease, you can get regular checkups to spot early symptoms and increase the chances for a cure. You may also want genetic counseling, to learn the risk of passing a disease on to your children.

Aside from health problems caused by accident or infectious disease, you can assume that most every disease in your family's background has some sort of genetic basis. These can be divided into two classes: *susceptibility diseases,* in which genes don't cause the problem but influence your risk of becoming ill; and *purely genetic diseases,* which people almost invariably develop if they inherit the requisite genes.

Susceptibility diseases typically occur later in life and include major ailments such as heart disease, diabetes (especially the non-insulin-dependent type) and several types of cancer, including breast, lung, colorectal (colon and rectal), prostate, ovarian and skin. The inherited tendency to develop a disease probably results from complex interactions among several genes. Also on the list of disorders with a genetic component: rheumatoid arthritis, allergies, asthma, glaucoma, Alzheimer's disease, osteoporosis, glaucoma and behavioral and emotional problems including schizophrenia, alcoholism and depression. ("Hereditary Risk" lists for several diseases the increased risk faced by someone with an afflicted parent.)

Although genes set the stage for these disorders, the actual illness is usually caused in part by some environmental factor—cigarette smoke in the case of lung cancer, for example, or high-fat diets in heart disease and non-insulin-dependent diabetes, as well as prostate, colorectal and perhaps ovarian cancer. Luckily, people who know that a susceptibility disease lurks in their family tree may be able to control those nongenetic risk factors, or at least be on the alert for early symptoms.

For example, if your mother or sister developed breast cancer before menopause, your lifetime risk would be as

From *American Health,* May 1994, pp. 80-84. © 1994 by Ruth Papazian. Reprinted by permission.

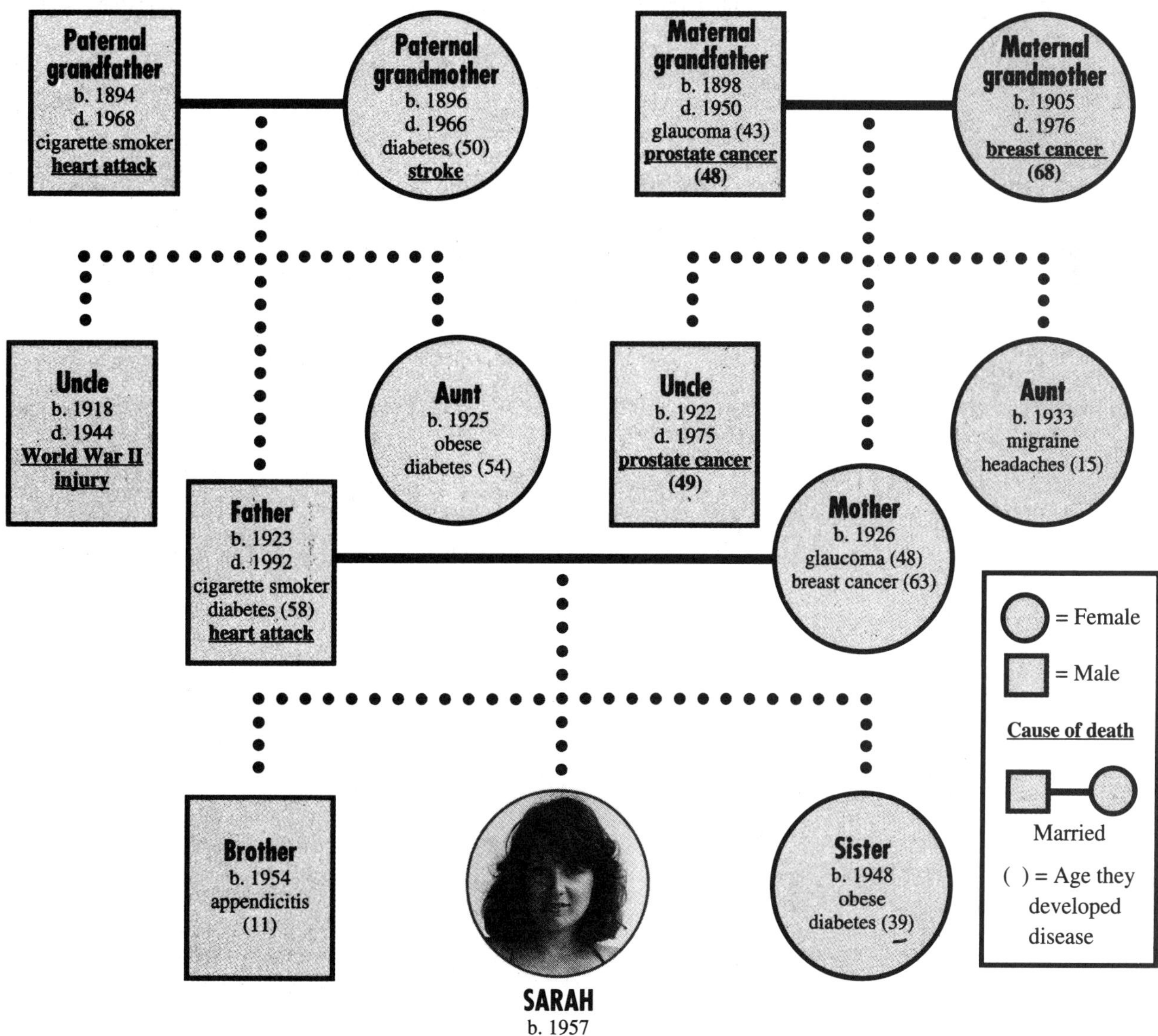

SARAH'S FAMILY MEDICAL HISTORY

Sarah risks inheriting non-insulin-dependent diabetes from her father's side of the family and breast cancer and glaucoma from her mother's side. But the two fatal heart attacks on her father's side shouldn't cause concern; both occurred relatively late in life and probably stemmed from major risk factors—smoking (her grandfather) and both smoking and diabetes (her father).

Diabetes: Sarah's sister already has it. Sarah and her brother should have their blood sugar monitored regularly; they can help ward off the disease by exercising and adopting a prudent diet.

Glaucoma: Sarah and her two siblings should have yearly eye exams to detect glaucoma at its early stages.

Breast cancer: Sarah and her sister face a higher than normal risk, since their mother and maternal grandmother developed it. Both sisters should have a baseline mammogram between the ages of 30 and 35, and yearly mammograms after 35; her sister should lose weight, since obesity adds to her risk.

Finally, Sarah should alert her brother to the fact that he's at increased risk for *prostate cancer.* His maternal grandfather and uncle both developed it early in life. He needs regular screening: each year, a digital rectal exam, plus a PSA (prostate-specific antigen) test.

great as one in three, vs. one in nine for other women. (Early onset of any disease increases the probability that heredity played a role.) A family history of breast cancer means you should get annual mammograms beginning at age 35, plus frequent professional exams.

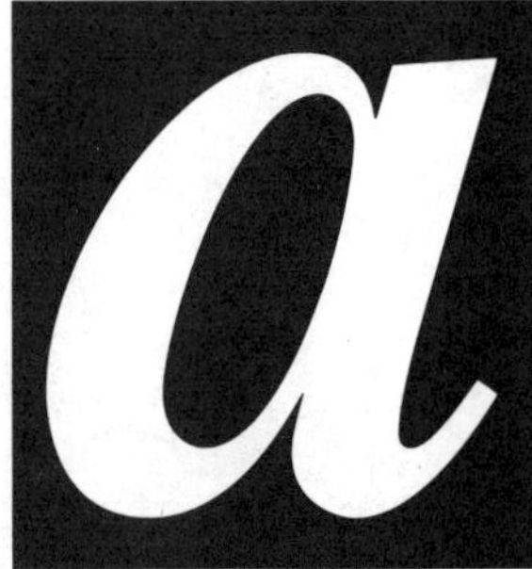

s for purely genetic diseases, there are more than 4,000—most of them rare—that result from defects in single genes. If you have such a disorder in your family tree, your chance of inheriting it depends on the nature of the gene responsible.

For instance, if one of your parents died of a heart attack before age 60, there's a one-in-five chance that he or she had familial hypercholesterolemia (an inherited extremely high cholesterol level); if so, there's a 50-50 chance you have it too. The gene responsible for familial hypercholesterolemia is "dominant": Inherit a defective version from one parent and you'll get the disease, even if your other parent gave you a normal copy.

Familial hypercholesterolemia, which affects one in every 500 people, can clog arteries and lead to a heart attack at an early age. If you have a family history of heart disease, be sure to get your cholesterol level measured. Once detected, an abnormally high cholesterol level can often be controlled with a lowfat diet and cholesterol-lowering drugs.

Familial adenomatous polyposis, another inherited disorder, afflicts one in 8,000 people and almost always results in intestinal cancer. ("Surviving a Family Curse," below, describes a family coping with this dominant-gene problem.) Other dominant diseases include Huntington's disease (the degenerative nervous-system disorder that killed singer Woody Guthrie), adult polycystic renal disease (a kidney disorder) and Marfan's syndrome (characterized by abnormally long limbs and heart problems). Diseases controlled by a dominant gene rarely skip a generation, so you've probably been spared if neither of your parents had the disease, even if a grandparent did.

Fortunately, most purely hereditary diseases are "recessive": that is, they afflict only those unlucky enough to inherit two copies of a defective gene—one from each parent. The most common of these recessive diseases seem to target certain ethnic groups.

For example, about one in 25 white Americans carries the gene for cystic fibrosis (CF), one of the most common lethal hereditary diseases (for those of northern European descent the risk is somewhat higher). The gene defect in CF results in a thick, sticky mucus in the lungs; the mucus encourages severe respiratory infections that usually prove fatal by age 30.

A CF carrier—with one abnormal and one normal gene—will be healthy. But if someone with the gene marries another carrier, their offspring will have a one-in-four chance of inheriting two defective copies of the gene and being born with CF. Following the discovery in 1989 of the gene that causes CF, a blood test became available that can tell whether a person is a carrier and whether a couple's fetus will develop the disease. ("Family Roots" lists several ethnic groups, the diseases to which they're susceptible, and how common those diseases are.)

Purely hereditary diseases (or disorders) that usually affect only men are called X-linked recessive diseases. The best known are hemophilia, color blindness and Duchenne muscular dystrophy. An X-linked disorder is transmitted from mother to son by a gene on one of her two X chromosomes. Each son has a 50-50 chance of getting the disease, from inheriting just a single copy of the recessive gene.

Mom may be a healthy carrier, since her other X chromosome carries a normal copy of the gene, which masks the defective one. But her son, with his X chromosome paired with a Y from his father, isn't as lucky. A woman should suspect she may be a carrier of an X-linked disorder if the disease has shown up in a male relative.

Virtually every month, researchers identify a gene linked to yet another hereditary disease; these findings are leading to increasing numbers of blood tests to identify people who carry these genes or who are destined to develop the diseases. ("Testing for Risk" lists some of these diseases.) To take advantage of these advances, you must first learn whether you or other family members are at risk.

Surviving a Family Curse

Larry Howard* had considered his family's medical history a curse, but knowing about it probably saved his life.

Larry's mother, three brothers and a sister all had been diagnosed with familial adenomatous polyposis, a disease in which thousands of polyps—tiny wartlike growths—sprout from the lining of the large intestine (colon). People with this condition (about one in 8,000) almost always develop colon cancer from polyps that turn malignant.

Larry's mother and his four affected siblings had to have their colons removed to prevent cancer from taking hold—the treatment reserved for severe cases. But Larry and his other sister, Mary, thought they had been spared.

Since early adolescence, when the polyps generally arise, Larry and Mary had taken part in the Johns Hopkins University familial polyposis study, undergoing annual sigmoidoscopies (visual examination of the lower third of the colon) and receiving clean bills of health. Ten years ago, when Larry was 32, he was told he didn't need any more checkups, since his risk of having inherited the disease seemed minimal.

Then last year he and Mary were given a new blood test, developed at Johns Hopkins, that identifies the gene that causes familial polyposis. The test determined that Mary did not carry the defective gene, but Larry did. Sure enough, a subsequent exam revealed sprouting polyps.

Larry plans to have his colon removed later this year. His three children have taken the blood test too: One of the three has tested positive.

**Not his real name.*

Gathering information about illnesses that run in your family is not as daunting as it may seem—especially if you ask relatives for help. Here is a guide for constructing your medical family tree:

1. Make a list of your first-degree relatives (parents, siblings and children) and second-degree relatives (grandparents, aunts and uncles). Adding more peripheral branches to your tree usually isn't worthwhile: The more distant the relative, the less relevant his medical fate is to you (you and your second cousin, for example, inherit only about 3% of the same genes). A possible exception: when you need more evidence to confirm a pattern involving a serious health problem such as cancer or heart disease.

2. Construct your family tree, using the sample as a guide. Your name and the names of your siblings go on the bottom row. On the row above, put the names of your parents, along with the names of their brothers and sisters. The names of all four grandparents go on the top line. It's customary to put male relatives in squares and female ones in circles and to indicate marriages by connecting relatives with horizontal lines.

3. Record the following information for each relative:

- *Date of birth, date of death and cause of death.* If necessary, you can usually obtain this information from the death certificate. To get a copy, contact the department of vital records in the state where the relative lived. (Be sure to check the family Bible first—birth and death certificates are often tucked inside the covers.)
- *All known illnesses and major surgeries, including the age when they occurred.* This information could be more relevant than the cause of death—if an uncle had a heart attack at age 40 but died 20 years later from an automobile accident, for example. Medical records are the most reliable sources for this information.

Ask relatives who are still living either to give you copies of their medical records or to sign a consent form allowing their doctors to give you this information. To obtain a deceased relative's records, contact the doctor or hospital that treated him; those names should be on the death certificate. You may have to provide a letter of consent from your relative's next of kin, as well as a copy of the death certificate.

- *Lifestyle factors that may have contributed to illness.* For instance, heart disease would be less of a genetic threat if you found that the uncle who suffered the heart attack at age 40 was a chain smoker. Most every family has a self-appointed "historian" who is the repository of family lore. You may be able to learn about relatives' lifestyles by talking to that person.
- *Occupation (optional).* This information may be important if there were job-related factors (such as exposure to toxic chemicals) that may have contributed to illness, miscarriage or birth defects.
- *Unusual physical characteristics.* Prominent features or chronic skin rashes could hint at certain medical conditions or birth defects (but you'll want to corroborate your hunches with medical records or other documents). Again, the family historian may be a good source. Family photo albums can also be revealing: A grandmother's "dowager's hump," for example, probably indicates that she had osteoporosis.

As you research your family medical tree, be prepared for difficulties. Information may be unavailable (some family

TESTING FOR RISK

The genes responsible for more than 300 diseases, most of them rare, can now be identified through blood tests. In some cases, these tests detect the gene itself; in others, they identify DNA "markers" that suggest the gene is present.

- **Cystic fibrosis**
- **Familial hypercholesterolemia**
- **Duchenne muscular dystrophy**
- **Fragile-X syndrome** (the most common inherited form of mental retardation)
- **Huntington's disease**
- **Neurofibromatosis** (a nerve disease characterized by dozens of skin tumors all over the body)
- **Retinoblastoma** (an eye tumor that usually occurs in childhood)
- **Sickle-cell anemia**
- **Tay-Sachs disease**
- **Thalassemia** (a blood disorder that occurs most often in people of Mediterranean descent)
- **Wilms' tumor** (a malignant kidney tumor that usually occurs in childhood)

Source: *Heredity and Your Family's Health,* by Aubrey Milunsky, M.D. (Johns Hopkins University Press, 1992)

FOR MORE HELP

Free pamphlets

- **"Genetic Counseling,"** GC Pamphlet, March of Dimes, 1275 Mamaroneck Ave., White Plains, NY 10605.
- **"Genetic Counseling: Valuable Information for You and Your Family,"** the National Society of Genetic Counselors, 233 Canterbury Dr., Wallingford, PA 19086-6617.
- **"Where to Write for Vital Records,"** Superintendent of Documents, U.S. Government Printing Office, Washington, DC 20402.

Books

- **Heredity and Your Family's Health** by Aubrey Milunsky, M.D. (Johns Hopkins University Press, 1992).
- **How Healthy Is Your Family Tree? A Complete Guide to Creating a Medical and Behavioral Family Tree** by Carol Krause (Collier Books).

Organizations

- **The Hereditary Cancer Institute,** Creighton University School of Medicine, 2500 California Plaza, Omaha, NE 68178.
- **Gilda Radner Familial Ovarian Cancer Registry,** Roswell Park Cancer Institute, Elm and Carlton streets, Buffalo, NY 14263.
- **University of Utah Cardiovascular Genetics Research Clinic,** 410 Chipeta Way, Room 161, Research Park, Salt Lake City, UT 84108.
- **The Hereditary Disease Foundation,** 1427 Seventh St., Suite 2, Santa Monica, CA 90401.

Family Roots

Risk of certain genetic diseases in specific races or ethnic groups.

Racial or ethnic background	Diseases	Carriers	Afflicted
Italian or Greek	Thalassemia	1 in 10	1 in 400
African	Sickle-cell anemia	1 in 12	1 in 650
Caucasian	Cystic fibrosis	1 in 25	1 in 2,500
Eastern or Central European Jewish (Ashkenazic), Cajun American or French Canadian	Tay-Sachs disease*	1 in 30	1 in 3,600
Mediterranean Jewish (Sephardic) or Armenian	Familial Mediterranean fever**	1 in 45	1 in 8,000

*Neurological disorder invariably fatal within the first five years of life. **Repeated bouts of fever and abdominal pain.
Adapted from *Choices, Not Chances: An Essential Guide to Heredity and Health,* ©1977 by Aubrey Milunsky, M.D.
By permission of Little, Brown and Company.

Hereditary Risk

Estimated risk for some common disorders that are influenced by inherited genes but not directly caused by them. Risks are for people with one parent who had the disease. The risk would be greater if a second parent or a sibling also had the disease.

Disease	General population	One parent with condition
	Lifetime risk	
Alcoholism	5%	10% to 20%
Alzheimer's disease	2% to 5%	19%
Asthma	4%	26%
Cancer, breast	11%	22%*
Cancer, colon	4%	10%
Cancer, ovarian	1%	5%
Cancer, uterine	3%	9%
Diabetes (non-insulin-dependent)	2%	5% to 10%
Duodenal ulcer	10%	30%
Glaucoma	2%	4% to 16%
Manic depression	1%	25%
Migraine	5% to 10%	45%
Schizophrenia	1%	8% to 18%

*The risk may be three times as great as in the general population if the mother was premenopausal when her cancer was diagnosed.

members may not cooperate, for example), or it may not exist (as when a child died and no diagnosis was ever made) or it may not be accurate (family legend, for example, may attribute an aunt's pregnancy loss to a miscarriage when in fact she had an abortion).

A little tact goes a long way. Family members may not want to talk about sad events or what they consider to be the family's dirty laundry. A good approach: "My doctor is interested in Cousin Bobby's condition because it could affect the children I may have. Can you tell me about his problem so that we can calculate the risks?" Offer to share your completed tree with relatives, along with the opinions of medical or genetic experts you consult.

Now that you've constructed your family tree, here are some tips on interpreting it:

- Your tree's two most important "branches" are your mother and father: Each gave you half your genetic inheritance, so their diseases will be most relevant to you and your siblings.
- The earlier a disease develops, the more likely that heredity played a role in it (except for ailments with obvious nongenetic causes such as infections).
- A disease that strikes two or more relatives at the same age is likely to be strongly influenced by heredity.
- A clustering of cases of the same disease on one side of the tree is more likely to suggest that genes play a strong role in causing it than a similar number of cases scattered on both sides. On the other hand, your risk of inheriting a purely hereditary disease like cystic fibrosis would actually be greater when it's present on both your mother's and father's side.

If you have questions about your family tree, you should show it to your doctor. If the doctor suspects a genetic problem, you will probably be referred to a genetic counselor, who can assess your risk of developing the diseases you're worried about, and of passing them on to a child. A counselor can also tell prospective parents if a fetus can be tested for conditions of concern.

Genetic counselors typically have a master of science degree in genetics and are certified by the American Board of Medical Genetics. Your family doctor, obstetrician or pediatrician can probably refer you to one, or you can contact a major hospital or medical school in your area or your local chapter of the March of Dimes for referrals (for further information, see "For More Help").

Your medical family tree should be a living, growing document. As you and your brothers and sisters get married and have children, keep adding to it: It can contribute to your health today and to the health of future generations.

Cholesterol

Put knowledge behind your numbers to lower your confusion level

"My doctor just gave me the results of my cholesterol test. He said, 'Your good cholesterol is low—that's bad, and your bad cholesterol is high—that's bad too. You need to raise your good and lower your bad—that would be good.' "

Confusing? You bet it is.

Chances are you know your cholesterol level is important and that it shouldn't be too high. But beyond that you may be unsure exactly how cholesterol fits into the cardiovascular disease puzzle.

Maybe you're too concerned about your cholesterol. Maybe you're not concerned enough.

In the following pages, we answer common questions, such as:

- What exactly is cholesterol?
- How can cholesterol be both good and bad?
- What does cholesterol do in your body?
- What is an elevated cholesterol level?
- When should you be concerned?
- What can you do about your concerns?

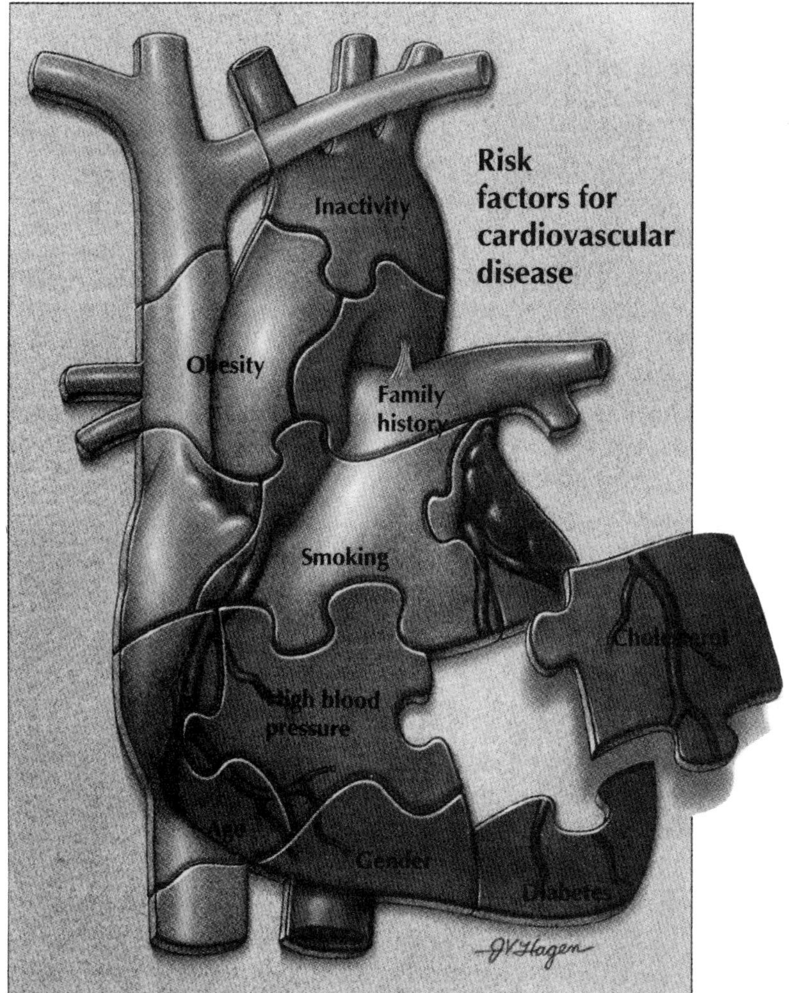

This puzzle includes nine major risk factors for cardiovascular disease, the nation's No. 1 killer. Cholesterol is among the most complex and important of all risk factors.

Why all the fuss about cholesterol?

Your blood cholesterol is important. Heart and blood vessel (cardiovascular) disease is the No. 1 killer of Americans, and study after study points to elevated cholesterol as a major contributor to the problem.

In general:

- The higher your cholesterol level, the greater your risk of cardiovascular disease.
- The higher your cholesterol level, the greater your chances of dying of cardiovascular disease.
- You can lower your risk of cardiovascular disease by lowering your cholesterol level.

Cholesterol and cardiovascular disease

The good news . . . Deaths from cardiovascular disease continue to fall. This encouraging trend is due to improved treatment and modification of cardiovascular disease risk factors, including cholesterol.

In 1980, heart attacks accounted for 163 deaths per 100,000 people. By 1990, this number had dropped to 112 people per 100,000.

The numbers for stroke are improving, too. In 1980, strokes claimed 41 people per 100,000. By 1990 this figure was down to 28.

The bad news . . . Far too many people still die from cardiovascular disease. The American Heart Association reports that cardiovascular disease still kills almost 1 million Americans each year. This is more than all cancer deaths combined.

Many of these deaths occur because of narrowed or blocked arteries (ath-

From *Medical Essay,* supplement to *Mayo Clinic Health Letter,* June 1993, pp. 1-8. © 1993 by Mayo Foundation for Medical Education and Research, Rochester, MN 55905. Reprinted by permission.

erosclerosis). Cholesterol plays a significant role in this largely preventable condition.

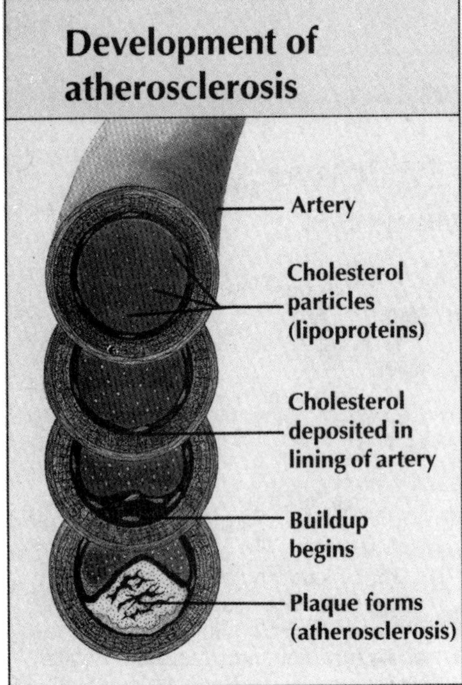

A high number of cholesterol particles (lipoproteins) in your blood increases your risk for a buildup of cholesterol within the wall of your artery. Eventually, bumps called plaques may form, narrowing or even blocking your artery.

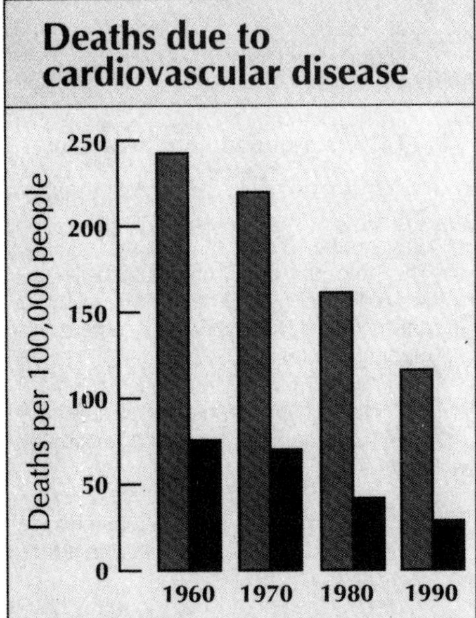

Deaths from heart attacks (gray bars) and stroke (black bars) are declining. This encouraging trend is due to improved treatment and modification of cardiovascular disease risk factors, including cholesterol.

(Sources: National Center for Health Statistics and American Heart Association.)

Atherosclerosis (ATH-ro-scler-OH-sis) is a silent, painless process in which cholesterol-containing fatty deposits accumulate in the walls of your arteries. These accumulations occur as bumps called plaques. (See illustration.)

As plaque builds up, the interior of your artery narrows. This reduces the flow of blood. If reduced flow occurs in your coronary (heart) arteries, it can lead to a type of chest pain called angina pectoris.

As a plaque enlarges, the inner lining of your artery becomes roughened. A tear or rupture in the plaque may cause a blood clot to form. Such a clot can block the flow of blood or break free and plug an artery downstream.

If the flow of blood to a part of your heart is stopped, you'll have a heart attack. If blood flow to a part of your brain stops, you'll have a stroke.

Many factors influence the clogging of arteries. Cholesterol is important in the process, but it's not the only piece of the puzzle.

What is cholesterol?

Cholesterol is a waxy, fat-like substance (lipid). Although it's often discussed as if it were a poison, you can't live without it. Cholesterol is essential to your body's cell membranes, to the insulation of your nerves and to the production of certain hormones. It's used by your liver to make bile acids, which help digest your food.

The confusion that clouds cholesterol is partly due to the way some people use the word. "Cholesterol" is often a catch-all term for both the cholesterol you eat and the cholesterol in your blood.

- *Your dietary cholesterol*—Cholesterol exists in your food as a dietary lipid. You'll find cholesterol only in animal products, such as meat and dairy foods.
- *Your blood cholesterol*—Cholesterol also exists in a different way as a natural component of your blood lipids.

The cholesterol in your blood comes both from your liver and from the foods you eat. Your liver makes about 80 percent of your blood cholesterol. Only about 20 percent comes from your diet.

The amount of fat and cholesterol you eat may influence all levels of your blood lipids, including your blood cholesterol levels.

Blood cholesterol—the good, the bad and the ugly

To be carried in your blood, your body coats cholesterol with proteins called apoproteins (AP-oh-PRO-teens). Once coated, they form a package called lipoproteins (LIP-oh-PRO-teens).

Lipoproteins carry both cholesterol and triglycerides (another blood lipid) in your blood.

Some of your lipoproteins are called low-density lipoproteins (LDLs). They contain lots of cholesterol. Others are called high-density lipoproteins (HDLs). They contain mostly protein.

A third type of lipoprotein is called a very-low-density lipoprotein (VLDL). This type contains cholesterol, triglycerides and protein.

Some people call LDL "bad cholesterol" and HDL "good cholesterol." Here's why:

Cholesterol serves as a building material in cells throughout your body. LDL particles, which carry cholesterol, attach themselves to receptors on cell surfaces and are then received into your cells.

If there are too many LDL particles in your blood, if your liver cells (LDL receptors) do not receive LDL particles normally, or, if there are too few LDL receptors in your liver, your body's cells become saturated with cholesterol from the LDL particles. Cholesterol is then deposited in your artery walls.

At this point your high-density lipoproteins (HDLs) play their "good" role. They actually pick up cholesterol deposited in your artery walls and transport it to your liver for disposal.

The situation can turn ugly if too much cholesterol from LDL particles remains deposited in your artery walls. Your arteries will develop plaques and begin to narrow. This is atherosclerosis.

This is why a high HDL level relative to an LDL level is good. It can help protect you from developing atherosclerosis.

What's to blame?

Why do some people have high cholesterol? High levels result from genetic makeup or lifestyle choices, or both. Your genes can give you cells that don't remove LDL cholesterol from your blood efficiently, or a liver that produces too much cholesterol as VLDL particles, or too few HDL particles.

Lifestyle choices such as smoking, diet and inactivity can also cause or contribute to high cholesterol levels, leaving you at risk for atherosclerosis.

The cholesterol test

The only way to find out if your blood lipids are in a desirable range is to have them tested. The test is done by taking a blood sample after you have fasted overnight. You should have this test every three to five years—more often if you have a problem with your cholesterol level.

How much fat is that?

Limit fat to "30 percent of daily calories." Good advice. But what does it really mean?

This table converts this recommended guideline into the actual amount of fat you should limit yourself to daily.

If you eat . . .	Allow yourself this much fat daily . . .
1,400 calories	47 grams
1,600 calories	53 grams
1,800 calories	60 grams
2,000 calories	67 grams
2,200 calories	73 grams
2,400 calories	80 grams
2,600 calories	87 grams
2,800 calories	93 grams

Note: 1,400 calories is the minimum you should eat if you're trying to lose weight. 1,600 calories is about right for many inactive women and some older adults. 2,200 calories is about right for many sedentary men, most children, teenage girls and active women. 2,800 is about right for teenage boys, many active men and some very active women.

Calorie allowances are based on recommendations of the National Academy of Sciences and on calorie intakes reported by people in national food consumption surveys.

The test should measure your total cholesterol, HDL cholesterol and triglycerides. (Total cholesterol is made up of your LDL, HDL and other blood cholesterol particles.)

Some laboratories measure LDL directly, as part of the blood test. However, if your triglycerides are normal, your doctor can calculate your LDL level using the following formula:

$$\text{Total cholesterol} - \left(\text{HDL} + \frac{\text{triglycerides}}{5}\right) = \text{LDL}$$

In addition to your LDL level, your doctor might calculate the ratios between your LDL and HDL cholesterol, or between your total cholesterol and HDL.

Today, physicians pay more attention to your HDL number. Studies show that even with a desirable total cholesterol level, if you have a low HDL level, you may be at risk for cardiovascular disease.

It's critical to realize that numbers in the table on this page are only guidelines. If your numbers stray from the desirable ranges, your physician will counsel you.

Remember this too: Each number takes on greater meaning when you look at it in relation to the other numbers on your test and in relation to your other cardiovascular disease risk factors.

Other cardiovascular risk factors—the remaining puzzle pieces

To make the picture of your cardiovascular health more complete, you must consider your other risk factors for cardiovascular disease. (See illustration.) Each risk factor may influence your lipid levels.

The more risk factors you have, in combination with undesirable lipid levels, the greater your risk of developing cardiovascular disease. If you have several risk factors, their effects don't simply add up, they amplify each other.

For example, if you have high total cholesterol and you smoke, you're at much greater risk than a nonsmoker with the same cholesterol level.

However, you can make this amplifying effect work for you. Eating a diet low in fat, combined with exercise, can help you lose weight. At the same time, you can reduce your risk of high blood pressure, heart attack and stroke.

Risk factors for cardiovascular disease are divided into those you can change and those you can't. Consider

Your blood test: What do those numbers mean?

Your lipid levels can tell your doctor whether you're a candidate for cardiovascular disease. As you compare your numbers with these, remember: Numbers alone don't tell the whole story. Rely on your physician to interpret your test results.

Test	Your level (in mg/dl)*		
	Desirable	*Borderline*	*Undesirable*
Total cholesterol	Below 200	200-240	Above 240
HDL cholesterol	Above 45	35-45	Below 35
Triglycerides	Below 200	200-400	Above 400
LDL cholesterol	Below 130	130-160	Above 160
Cholesterol/HDL	Below 4.5	4.5-5.5	Above 5.5
LDL/HDL	Below 3	3-5	Above 5

* *For people without known heart disease*

Note: The numbers in this table represent a compilation of informed medical opinions from a variety of sources.

how each risk factor affects your blood cholesterol and triglycerides.

Here are factors you can change:

■ *Smoking*—Smoking cigarettes damages the walls of your blood vessels, making them prone to accumulate fatty deposits. Smoking may also lower your HDL by as much as 15 percent. If you stop smoking, your HDL may return to its higher level.

■ *High blood pressure*—By damaging the walls of your arteries, high blood pressure can accelerate the development of atherosclerosis. Some medications for high blood pressure increase LDL and triglyceride levels and decrease HDL levels. Other medications don't.

■ *Inactivity*—Lack of physical exercise is associated with a decrease in HDL. Aerobic exercise is one way to increase your HDL. Aerobic activity is any exercise that requires continuous movement of your arms and legs and increases your breathing. Even 30 to 45 minutes of brisk walking every other day helps protect your cardiovascular system.

■ *Obesity*—Excess weight increases your triglycerides. It also lowers your HDL and increases your VLDL cholesterol. Losing just five or 10 pounds can improve your triglyceride and cholesterol levels.

■ *Diabetes*—Diabetes can increase triglycerides and decrease HDL in many people. Diabetes accelerates the development of atherosclerosis which, in turn, increases the risk for heart attack, stroke and reduced circulation to your feet.

If you have diabetes, have your total cholesterol, triglycerides and HDL tested at least annually. Keep your weight and blood sugar under control. Still, complications may develop. Diabetes is not a risk factor you can always change. (See *Mayo Clinic Health Letter* Medical Essay on diabetes, June 1992.)

These are risk factors you can't change:

■ *Age*—As you age, your level of LDL cholesterol usually increases. Researchers aren't sure why. The increase could be caused by aging or by an increase in your body fat.

■ *Gender*—Until age 45, men generally have higher total cholesterol levels than women. Also, up to about this age, women tend to have higher HDL levels. However, after menopause, women's total cholesterol rises and the protective HDL drops.

Caution: Don't think of cardiovascular disease as mainly a man's disease. Cardiovascular disease is also the No. 1 killer of women, claiming almost 500,000 women each year. Cancer kills fewer than 220,000 women. Women get cardiovascular disease as often as men; it just happens later in life.

■ *Family history*—If members of your family have undesirable lipid levels and cardiovascular problems, your risks for these problems are increased.

Your first lines of defense against high cholesterol

Diet and exercise are your first lines of defense against undesirable lipid levels. Changes in your diet, along with exercise, can reduce your blood cholesterol level by up to 15 percent. However, some people have genetically determined lipid problems (especially LDL) that don't respond to diet and require medication.

Making diet changes to improve your blood cholesterol levels involves three steps:

■ *Reduce your weight by reducing your total fat*—Limit all types of fat, saturated, polyunsaturated and monounsaturated, to no more than 30 percent of your total daily calories. Because all foods with fats contain a combination of these fats, it's important to reduce total fat.

Don't assume each food you eat must have less than 30 percent of its calories from fat. Use the guideline as a daily average. By balancing occasional high-fat foods with low-fat choices, your fat intake should average 30 percent of your daily calories.

■ *Reduce saturated fat*—No more than one-third of the fat you eat should be saturated. Major sources of saturated fat are butter, cheese, whole milk, cream, meat, poultry, chocolate, coconut, palm and palm kernel oil, lard and solid shortenings.

■ *Reduce dietary cholesterol*—Your daily limit for dietary cholesterol is 300 milligrams. A good way to accomplish this goal is to avoid dairy products made with whole milk and cream, and organ meats such as liver and tongue.

These limits on fat and cholesterol can also help you lose weight, which can improve your blood lipid levels. . . .

Exercise enhances the benefits of diet

A low-fat, low-cholesterol diet can improve your VLDL cholesterol level. If you also exercise and lose excess weight, you may see even greater improvements in your triglyceride and cholesterol levels.

Exercise helps you lose excess weight and reduces your chances of gaining weight as you get older.

For these benefits, set up your program using these guidelines and your doctor's advice:

■ *Choose aerobic activity*—Get involved in brisk walking, jogging, bicycling or cross-country skiing.

■ *Build up time and frequency*—Gradually work up to exercising for 30 to 45 minutes at least three times a week. If you're severely overweight or have been inactive for many years, take several months to gradually work up to this level. The higher the level of your activity, the greater your rate of weight loss.

■ *Keep it up*—Schedule a regular time for exercise. Make exercise fun. If it's not enjoyable you'll have difficulty exercising regularly, year in and year out.

Find a friend, or join an exercise group, to keep you motivated and committed to exercise. Or take up an activity that keeps you active.

Unless you stay with your program, you may not be able to keep off the pounds exercise helped you lose. Staying active also may prevent a gain in weight that often accompanies age. This, in turn, may help maintain lower levels of blood fats.

When are medications necessary?

Often changes in diet, exercise and smoking habits will improve your VLDL cholesterol and triglyceride levels. But if you've carried out these important lifestyle changes and your total cholesterol, especially your LDL level, remains high, your doctor may recommend a medication.

Before recommending a medication, your doctor will use careful judgment and weigh many variables—your changeable risk factors, your age, your current health, and the drug's side effects. If you need a medication to lower your cholesterol, chances are you will need it for many years.

Your LDL cholesterol level is usually the deciding factor. If you have no risk factors for cardiovascular disease, an LDL level over 190 generally requires medication. With two or more risk factors, an LDL level over 160 may require medication.

And remember . . .

The issue of cholesterol and cardiovascular health is important, but by no means simple. Just knowing your total cholesterol level is not enough. Understanding how your other blood fat levels and your cardiovascular disease risk factors influence this number is essential.

Only with this knowledge can cholesterol assume its proper place in the cardiovascular disease puzzle.

Rating your risks for heart disease

Since 1960, the mortality rate from heart attack in the U.S. has dropped by half, according to the National Center for Health Statistics—and since 1980 alone, by one-third. This success has been due not only to improved medical treatment of coronary artery disease (CAD), but also to preventive steps people have taken. Heart attack is still the leading killer of American men and women, however, accounting for about 500,000 deaths every year—about 20% in people under age 65. Most of these deaths, too, could be avoided or at least postponed if everyone paid attention to the risk factors for CAD and took preventive measures to counter them.

Just how far we have to go in preventing this disease can be seen in a recent report from the CDC that showed that only 18% of adults are free of the six major coronary risk factors. And among those over 50, only about 10% report that they are free of the major risk factors. Many people don't even know what these factors are, except perhaps high blood cholesterol. The other five proven risks—smoking, obesity, high blood pressure, diabetes, and being sedentary—are as bad, or even worse, for the heart.

The pillars of prevention

Scientists now know far more about the major controllable risk factors for CAD than for most other diseases. A risk factor merely increases the probability that you will develop CAD; it doesn't guarantee that you will develop it, nor does its absence (or even the absence of all risk factors) guarantee that you won't have a heart attack. If you have more than one CAD risk factor, the combined impact is greater than it would be if you added the individual risks together.

Most of the risk factors can be countered by relatively simple preventive measures. In 1992 Dr. JoAnn Manson and her colleagues from Harvard reviewed nearly 200 studies on CAD to evaluate the role of the known preventive measures; the results were published in the *New England Journal of Medicine (NEJM)*. Some of the details are as follows:

1. Quit smoking. This is perhaps the single most effective step you can take. Anywhere from 20 to 40% (100,000 to 200,000 every year) of all CAD deaths are still directly attributable to smoking. It more than doubles your chance of eventually having a heart attack and increases the chance of dying from it by 70%; it is also the leading cause of sudden cardiac death. Low-tar, low-nicotine cigarettes are not significantly safer for your heart than regular brands. Smoking even a few cigarettes a day can endanger your heart. In addition, it's estimated that more than 35,000 nonsmoking Americans die each year from heart disease because of long-term exposure to other people's smoke. The good news is that quitting smoking quickly reduces your CAD risk: within five to ten years, your risk of heart attack declines to a level similar to that of people who never smoked.

2. Reduce cholesterol. For every 1% reduction in blood cholesterol, there's a 2 to 3% decline in the risk of heart attack. Since 1960, the average blood cholesterol level in the U.S. has declined from 220 to 205 mg/dl (a "desirable" level is below 200), a 7% decline. That's a significant decline, but still leaves 20% of American adults with high cholesterol levels (above 240) and another 30% with borderline-high levels (200 to 239). For information on the government's new guidelines on cholesterol and for advice on how to lower total cholesterol and raise protective HDL cholesterol, see *Wellness Letter,* December 1993.

3. Avoid or control hypertension. About 50 million Americans have high blood pressure, which is a risk factor for stroke and heart attack. For every 1 point drop in diastolic blood pressure, there's a 2 to 3% drop in the risk of heart attack. If you can reduce your blood pressure by making the life-style changes—including limiting intake of sodium, calories, and alcohol—the coronary benefits are likely to be particularly great.

4. Stay active. Dozens of studies have shown that exercise protects against CAD. The *NEJM* report estimated that sedentary people who begin a regular program of exercise reduce their risk of a heart attack by 35 to 55%. And yet it is estimated that more than 60% of Americans are sedentary, and there has been little improvement in decades. Even low-intensity activities, such as

Risk factors you can't change

These should serve as an incentive to address the factors that *can* be changed.

Heredity. People with a parent or sibling who had a premature heart attack (before age 55 in a man or 65 in a woman) are at increased risk of CAD.

Race. African-Americans, for example, have an elevated risk of CAD, primarily because they have a higher risk of hypertension and diabetes than whites.

Increasing age. About 55% of all heart attacks, and more than 80% of fatal ones, occur after age 65.

Sex. Before age 55, men have a much higher rate of CAD than women. By the time they reach 60, women develop CAD at the same rate as men at 50—and this 10-year gap prevails until about the age of 75 or 80, when the differences disappear and the rates become similar. Women who have a heart attack, especially at older ages, are more likely to die from it than are men.

Reprinted with permission from the *University of California at Berkeley Wellness Letter,* May 1994, pp. 4-5.

gardening or walking, if done regularly and over the long term, can decrease the risk of heart attack. Exercise helps the heart work more efficiently, reduces blood pressure, decreases the tendency of blood to form clots, moderates stress, helps the body use insulin, helps people maintain a healthy weight, and may boost HDL ("good") cholesterol.

5. Maintain a healthy weight. About one in three American adults is seriously overweight or obese, which doubles the risk for CAD at a given age. And the more overweight you are, the greater the effect on CAD risk. Obesity also increases the risk for diabetes, hypertension, and high blood cholesterol, which further worsen CAD risk. How fat is distributed on the body also affects the risk. People who put weight on around the waist (apple-shaped or pot-bellied body) have a greater chance of CAD than those who accumulate weight on the hips (pear-shaped).

6. Avoid or control diabetes. Non-insulin-dependent diabetes (also called adult-onset diabetes), which afflicts about 12 million Americans, is an important risk factor for both CAD and hypertension. Diabetes increases the risk of CAD in men two- to three-fold, but in women three- to seven-fold. Even people who merely have slightly elevated blood sugar levels but no detectable diabetes are at increased risk. Weight control and exercise can improve the utilization of blood sugar and prevent or slow the onset of diabetes.

Mind/body: stress and anger

Until recently, people with so-called Type A personality (aggressive, competitive, tense) were considered coronary-prone. But studies largely failed to confirm this notion. Some researchers therefore shifted their focus to various components of Type A—notably anger or hostility. Most studies have indeed found a link between anger or hostility and CAD risk. People who suppress their anger appear to be at greatest risk for CAD and other illness, though some studies have found that venting anger isn't necessarily better.

Some of the best research on stress has involved the workplace. A worker's sense of control, or lack thereof, is perhaps the major determinant of how he reacts to stress and of the effect stress has on health. Studies have consistently shown that people in high-strain jobs (heavy pressure to perform but little sense of control), such as bus drivers, have the highest rates of hypertension and heart attacks. Stereotypical "high-stress" jobs such as manager, engineer, and doctor tend to have the lowest rates, because these professionals have a greater sense of control. Even when such risk factors as age, race, education, and smoking are statistically eliminated from the equation, people in the bottom 10% of the job echelon have four to five times the risk of heart attack as those at the top 10% of the ladder.

Additional steps

7. Consider hormone therapy after menopause. Estrogen therapy raises HDL cholesterol and also lowers the risk of heart attack in other ways. It also decreases the risk of osteoporosis and perhaps stroke. Today hormone replacement therapy, or HRT, usually includes progestin (a synthetic form of the hormone progesterone) along with estrogen. Recent studies suggest that the combined estrogen-progestin therapy also protects against heart disease. HRT is not appropriate for all women, so talk to your doctor about it.

8. Consider a drink a day. There's a growing consensus that light to moderate alcohol consumption—that is, two drinks or less a day for a man, one drink for a woman (a drink is defined as 12

Separating the wheat from the chaff

Frequent media reports of new risk factors for CAD and new potential protectors—often trivial and sometimes contradictory—may distract people from the truly significant risk factors. These scientific tidbits usually come from single studies or preliminary research and were never intended to guide personal behavior. Some are based on tenuous statistical associations; many will inevitably turn out to be false leads. Here are just four factors that have received much attention recently:

Baldness. Last February a study in the *Journal of the American Medical Association* claimed that white men under age 55 with a bald spot on top of the head are substantially more likely to suffer a heart attack than those with a full head of hair or a receding hairline. One theory: the male sex hormones that cause this type of baldness may also endanger the heart. But most researchers believe that if this type of baldness does pose a risk, it is minor when compared to, say, smoking or hypertension. In any case, if you're bald you can't do anything about the slightly increased risk, except to be diligent about controlling the known, modifiable risk factors.

Shortness. Several studies have found that women less than 5 feet tall and men less than 5 feet 6 inches have an elevated risk of heart attacks. But researchers have pointed out that the increased risk is comparatively minor. In addition, other researchers have suggested the shorter people in the studies may have been more likely to come from disadvantaged backgrounds (with poor childhood diets and health habits), which might account in part for their increased health risks.

Earlobe crease. As strange as it seems, most studies on the subject have found that men (and sometimes women) who have a crease across the earlobes are at increased risk for CAD.

Iron level in the body. In 1992 a Finnish study made headlines when it suggested that a high level of iron in the body dramatically increases the risk of a heart attack. At the time, we concluded that the study raised more questions than it answered (*Wellness Letter,* December 1992). Recently, three newer studies, which received far less media attention, disputed the results of the Finnish study. More research will need to be done. Meanwhile, continue to eat foods that supply your daily requirement of iron.

ounces of beer, four ounces of wine, or 1.5 ounces of 80-proof spirits) has a minor beneficial effect for the heart. However, drinking more than that is a good way to *increase* the risk of heart attack and stroke, as well as cirrhosis, cancer, and car crashes. As the *NEJM* report put it, "the difference between drinking small-to-moderate quantities of alcohol and drinking large amounts may mean the difference between preventing and causing disease."

9. Consider aspirin. Low-dose aspirin—usually half an aspirin (160 milligrams) a day—can lower the risk of heart attack by about one-third by reducing the ability of platelets in the blood to stick together and thus form a clot. Aspirin therapy is particularly advisable if you have an elevated risk of CAD. The research has focused mostly on men so far, but at least two encouraging studies have suggested that women benefit, too. Aspirin can have side effects and isn't right for everyone, so don't start aspirin therapy on your own—ask your doctor about it.

What about diet?

Although a healthful, low-fat diet is not generally considered a separate preventive measure against CAD, it clearly plays a role in many of the steps listed above, such as controlling cholesterol and body weight. In addition, there has been accumulating evidence that a high intake of antioxidant vitamins (usually supplements of C, E, and beta carotene) helps reduce the risk of CAD—see our January 1994 issue.

STOPPING CANCER IN ITS TRACKS

New discoveries about wayward genes and misbehaving proteins show how cells become malignant—and perhaps how to bring them under control

J. Madeleine Nash
/Chicago

Stealthy as a pirate slipping from a cove, the cancer cell severs the moorings that attach it to surrounding tissue. Slowly it extends one, two, three fingerlike probes and begins to creep. Then it detects the pulsating presence of a nearby capillary and darts between the cells that compose the blood-vessel wall. It dives into the red river that courses through lung and liver, breast and brain. An hour or so later, it surfaces on some tranquil shore, settles down and—at the expense of its hapless neighbors—beings to prosper.

Gradually the cancer cell invades the turf occupied by its normal counterparts, killing all those in its path. It tricks nearby cells into forming food-bearing blood vessels, then compels them to churn out growth-spurring chemicals. To shield itself from patrolling immune cells, the cancer cell sprouts spiny armor like a sea urchin's. To expel the agents physicians send to kill it, the cancer cell deploys along its membrane a battery of tiny pumps. Is there a way to fight such a foe?

Until now, medicine has tried to overwhelm the cancer cell with brute force, slicing it out with surgery, zapping it with radiation or poisoning it with chemotherapy. All too often, however, a few cells managed to survive the onslaught and germinate, sometimes years later, into tumors that are impervious to treatment. The ability of the cancer cell to outmaneuver its attackers has long been reflected in mortality statistics. Despite gains made against cancers such as childhood leukemia and Hodgkin's lymphoma, the overall death rate remains dismally high. This year more than half a million Americans will succumb to cancer, making it the nation's second leading killer after cardiovascular disease.

Yet despite the continuing casualties, there is reason to believe the war against cancer has reached a turning point. During the past two decades, a series of stunning discoveries has pried open the black box that governs the behavior of the cancer cell and revealed its innermost secrets. Now the insights gleaned from basic research are being translated into novel approaches to cancer therapy. It still looks difficult to eradicate malignant cells, but scientists are exploring ways to tame them, to make them behave and thus greatly prolong the lives of people with the disease. The new therapies carry the promise of being not only more effective than the current slash-and-burn strategy but also much gentler to the patients who must endure the treatment. Exclaims Dr. Dennis Slamon, a UCLA cancer specialist: "This is the most exciting time imaginable!"

The excitement was running especially high last week, as encouraging news poured out of several labs all at once. From Thomas Jefferson University in Philadelphia came word that an experimental vaccine had given patients unusually long remissions from advanced melanoma, a deadly form of skin cancer. From Canada's McMaster University came a report identifying a telltale enzyme found in cancer cells—but conspicuously absent from most normal cells. If cancer researchers can find a way to deactivate this enzyme, known as telomerase, they may at last have the magic bullet they have long been seeking. Equally tantalizing was the article published in *Science* by molecular biologist Alexander Kamb and his colleagues at Myriad Genetics, a Salt Lake City, Utah, biotech firm. A majority of cancer cells, they found, lack functioning copies of a gene that serves as a circuit breaker and shuts down the abnormal cell growth that causes malignancy. Already Kamb is dreaming up ways to fix this seemingly simple glitch. "The route to therapy," he says, "seems surprisingly clear."

GOOD GENES GONE BAD The conceptual revolution that is just now sweeping into the clinic began in the 1960s, when researchers started to realize that cancer is a disease of DNA, the master molecule that

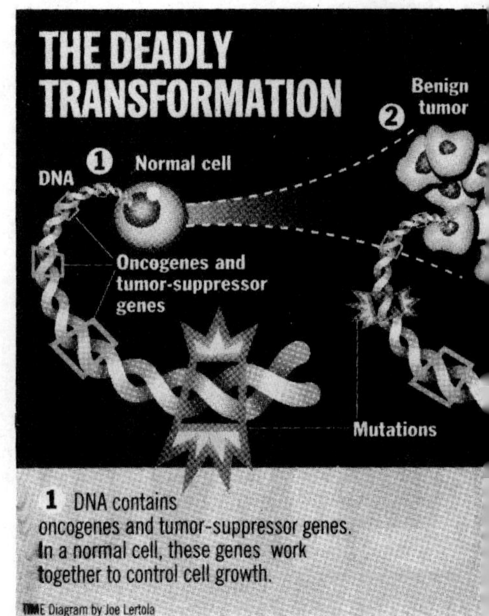

1 DNA contains oncogenes and tumor-suppressor genes. In a normal cell, these genes work together to control cell growth.

TIME Diagram by Joe Lertola

encodes the genetic script of life. One of DNA's most important jobs is to govern cell division, the process by which a cell makes a copy of itself and splits in two. Ordinarily, cell division is tightly regulated, but a cancer cell divides uncontrollably, pushing into surrounding tissue.

A pivotal discovery came in 1976, when Drs. J. Michael Bishop and Harold Varmus at the University of California, San Francisco, made a startling observation. They saw that a viral gene known to cause cancer in chickens was practically a carbon copy of a normal gene found in animal and human cells. The virus had somehow stolen a perfectly good gene and put it to bad use. This finding helped lead to a general conclusion: cells become cancerous because their normal genetic machinery goes awry. The culprits that initiate the damage can be viruses, radiation, environmental poisons, defective genes inherited from parents—or a combination of all of the above.

By last week researchers had found perhaps 100 cancer genes, at least three dozen of them important in human tumors. Some, known as oncogenes, turn on cell division, whereas others, called tumor-suppressor genes, are responsible for switching the process off. In their normal form, both kinds of genes work as a team, enabling the body to perform such vital tasks as replacing dead cells or repairing defective ones. But mutations in the chemical makeup of these genes, whether inherited or acquired later in life, can disrupt these finely tuned checks and balances. A cell containing a faulty oncogene is often likened to a car with a stuck accelerator, a cell with a damaged tumor-suppressor gene to a car with no brakes.

Scientists have thus stripped away cancer's mystery and revealed the malignant cell for what it is: not an intrinsically evil villain but an ordinary machine that has broken down in very specific, and potentially reparable, ways. They have studied the life history of a cancer cell and found errant genes at almost every step of the way, from the initial formation of a tumor to the advanced stages of metastasis, the lethal spread of the disease through the body.

FATAL FLAWS Cancer is not a modern disease. Some of our apelike ancestors undoubtedly suffered from it; so did the dinosaurs. In fact, says Robert Weinberg, a molecular biologist at the Massachusetts Institute of Technology, "it is a risk all multicellular organisms run." Each time a human cell divides, it must replicate its DNA, a biochemical manuscript some 3 billion characters long. In the course of transcribing such a lengthy document, even a skilled typist could be expected to make mistakes, and cells, like typists, occasionally err. More often than not, the mistakes they make are minor and quickly repaired by proteins that serve as miniature mechanics. Occasionally, though, cells with defects in their DNA will continue to divide, eventually forming small growths. The more cell-division cycles an organism undergoes, the more likely it is to accumulate colonies of abnormal cells, each the offspring of a single progenitor. By the time humans reach middle adulthood, then, their bodies contain millions of cells that have taken at least one step toward cancer.

EVEN SO, CANCER IS HARDLY INevitable. For example, 50% of Americans will develop at least one precancerous polyp in their colon at some point, but only a fraction of such polyps will develop into aggressive tumors. Why? Usually it takes so long for colon cancer to unfold that most people end up dying of other causes. Indeed, contrary to popular perception, getting cancer is not at all easy. To begin with, a cell must accumulate mutations not in just one or two genes but in several. In the case of colon cancer, Dr. Bert Vogelstein and his colleagues at Baltimore's Johns Hopkins Oncology Center have shown that a cell must sustain damage to at least three tumor-suppressor genes and one oncogene. The first mutation spurs the growth of the cell, triggering the formation of a benign polyp. Later changes cause the polyp to expand and become increasingly irregular in shape. By the time a cell in this growing mass suffers a final, fateful hit to its DNA, many decades may have gone by.

Clearly, however, some people are at a much higher risk of developing cancer than others, and at an earlier age. For them, heredity plays a major role. Over the past five months, competing teams at Johns Hopkins and Boston's Dana-Farber Cancer Institute have identified four new genes associated with a form of early onset colon cancer known to afflict particular families. These genes are carried by as many as 1 in every 200 Americans, making them the most common cause of cancer susceptibility yet discovered. In their normal form, these biological versions of computerized spelling checkers produce pro-

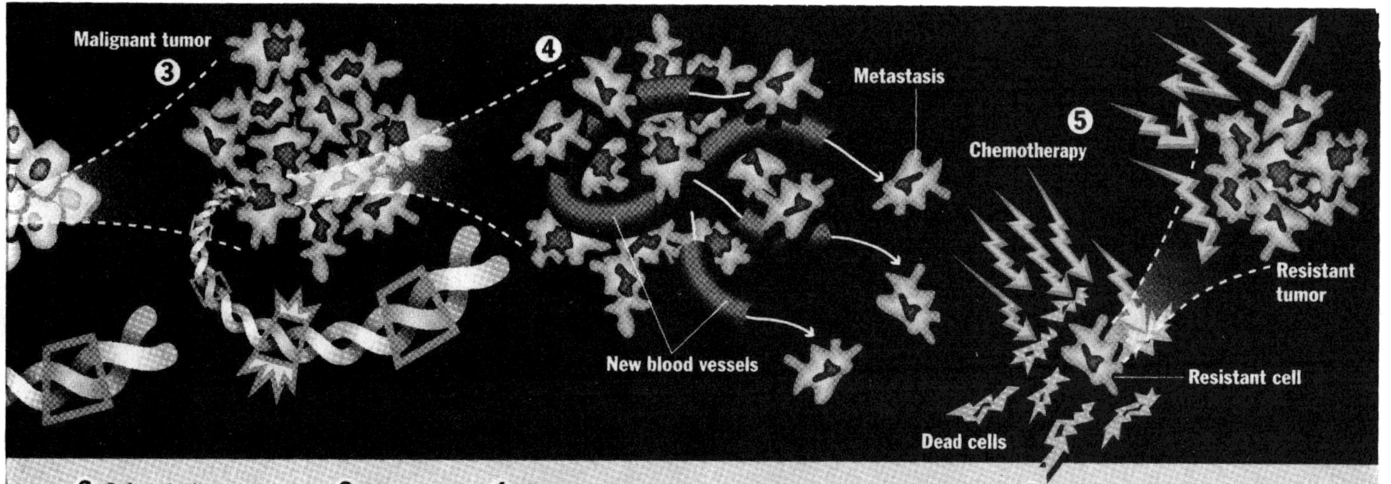

2 Defects in these genes, either inherited or caused by radiation, chemicals or viruses, eventually let the cell grow into a tumor.

3 More mutations may cause the cells to become malignant.

4 The malignant cells stop producing a chemical that prevents blood vessels from forming. New capillaries then grow into the tumor, providing it with nutrients. This also creates a route for malignant cells to break away from the main tumor mass and travel to other parts of the body, where they start new cancers.

5 Chemotherapy can kill the malignant cells, but if there is even one cancer cell that is resistant to the treatment, it will survive and grow into a new tumor. This new cancer will be impervious to the treatment.

teins that scoot along strands of replicating DNA, searching for tiny typos. When a protein finds an error in one of the words spelled out by DNA's four-letter chemical alphabet, it flashes an alarm. A person born with only one good copy of any of these genes is fine, until some cell in his or her colon loses or mutates its backup copy. Without a spelling checker, mutation piles upon mutation, telescoping the time it takes for cancer to develop.

BENT OUT OF SHAPE Cancer-causing mutations can occur quite by accident. But chronic exposure to carcinogens—chemicals whose by-products bind to DNA and damage it—greatly accelerate the rate at which dividing cells make errors. Proven carcinogens include asbestos, benzene and some ingredients of cigarette smoke. Many carcinogens, it turns out, are not blunderbusses but leave highly individualized fingerprints in the DNA they touch. At the National Cancer Institute, Dr. Curtis Harris, a molecular epidemiologist, has been examining cells from liver- and lung-cancer patients, searching for mutations in a tumor-suppressor gene known as p53 (p stands for the protein the gene makes and 53 for the protein's molecular weight). Smokers who develop lung cancer, Harris has found, show tiny alterations in the p53 gene that differ from those in nonsmokers. They also vary from the changes found in Chinese liver-cancer patients. In the latter group, aflatoxin, a fungal contaminant of food, is the carcinogen, and it alters DNA in an exquisitely precise way, substituting in a single location a *T* (thymine) for a *G* (guanine) in DNA's four-letter chemical alphabet.

How can such a small mistake—the equivalent of changing the spelling of Smith to Smyth—have such an impact? Each three-letter "word" of a gene "sentence" spells out the instructions for producing 1 of 20 amino acids, compounds that in turn link to form proteins. A change in just one letter can result in the substitution of one amino acid for another. The new amino acid will be larger, smaller, stiffer or more elastic than the correct one. In ways radical and subtle it will affect the shape of the protein and its activity. For if a cell is like a factory, then a protein is a cog in a machine that may have as many as 50 components. "If one of them develops a kink in its structure," says Harris, "then the machine doesn't fit together as well."

Kinks is proteins that form the nuclear matrix—a dynamic scaffold to which DNA is attached—may be particularly diabolical. The reason cancer cells typically have a swollen and misshapen nucleus, believes Johns Hopkins molecular biologist Donald Coffey, is that the proteins that form the nuclear matrix are misaligned in some fashion. Inside the matrix, notes Coffey, 50,000 to 100,000 loops of DNA are coiled like a Slinky, but the length of the loops, and where they begin and end, varies from tissue to tissue. The genes closest to the matrix are those that a particular cell intends to have turned on. Genes meant to stay inactive are much farther away. The conclusion is inescapable: a mutation in a gene that changes the architecture of the nuclear matrix could wreak havoc by turning the wrong genes on or off.

YEARNINGS FOR IMMORTALITY Normal cells do not live forever. Under certain circumstances, cells are actually programmed to die. One of the most fascinating features of early development, for example, is the explosive proliferation of certain types of cells, followed by mass suicide. Human embryos start with paddles for hands; it is cell death that gives them fingers. Neurons also expire by the billions as the brain refines its circuitry during development. In adults, the cell-death program serves as a stern disciplinarian. Cells that become irreparably damaged are expected to fall on their swords for the greater good of the organism. "For an animal to live," says Dr. Samuel Broder, director of the National Cancer Institute, "it must contain within its cells the knowledge that they have to die. But the cancer cell divides at all cost. It's forgotten how to die."

The tumor-suppressor gene p53 is often described as "the guardian of the genome" because it keeps watch over DNA during cell division. When damage occurs, p53 commands other genes to bring cell division to a halt. If repairs are made, then p53 allows the cell cycle to continue. But in some cases, if the damage is too serious to be patched, p53 activates other genes that cause the cell to self-destruct. Mutations in p53, which have been detected in more than 50% of all human cancers, are thus extremely dangerous. In laboratory cultures, some cancer cells that possess mutant versions of p53 do not die when challenged by antitumor agents, while those that have normal p53 genes go belly-up.

Healthy cells apparently have a precise system for ensuring their mortality; short strips of DNA known as telomeres seem to provide a molecular clock. When a cell is young, it has more than a thousand telomeres strung along the ends of chromosomes like beads in a necklace. Each time a cell divides, 10 to 20 telomeres are lost, and the necklace grows shorter. Eventually, after many cell divisions, the necklace becomes so short that the cell fails an internal health check designed to keep old, possibly damaged cells from reproducing. Result: cell division stops, the cell begins to age rapidly, and eventually it dies. Cancer cells, in contrast, have learned to stop the ticking of the telomere clock. According to research published last week in the *Proceedings of the National Academy of Sciences* by Calvin Harley and colleagues at McMaster University in Hamilton, Ontario, malignant cells foil the clock by producing an enzyme—telomerase—that protects the length of the telomere chains. In essence, telomerase makes the cancer cell immortal.

A CALL FOR BLOOD Perhaps the most critical stage in the life of a tumor comes after it expands to about a million cells. At this point, it is "much smaller than a BB," says Dr. Judah Folkman of Harvard Medical School. This tiny mass—known as a carcinoma in situ, literally cancer in place—is malignant, but not yet dangerous. Why? Because the cells at the center of the tumor are too far from the bloodstream to obtain essential nutrients, they are less vigorous. Like a society with zero population growth, a carcinoma in situ adds about as many new cells as it loses old ones.

Months, years, even decades may pass. Then an ominous transition occurs. Some cells in the tumor begin secreting chemicals that attract endothelial cells—the key components of blood vessels. These cells form capillaries that grow into the tumor. They also pump out molecular messengers called growth factors that stimulate the tumor to divide more quickly.

What triggers blood-vessel formation, or angiogenesis, as the process is known? A major factor, scientists believe, is a sudden drop in the cancer cell's production of thrombospondin, a protein that inhibits the growth of new blood vessels. In the normal adult, angiogenesis is not only a rare event, but one cells strive to prevent, save for special circumstances like wound healing. For blood vessels invading joints can cause arthritis, and those invading the retina of the eye can cause blindness. To prevent such damage, cells keep blood vessels at bay by pumping out thrombospondin. At a recent scientific conference, Noel Bouck, a molecular biologist from Northwestern University Medical School, stunned her colleagues by presenting preliminary data suggesting that thrombospondin production may be regulated by that ubiquitous gene, p53.

PULLING UP STAKES Angiogenesis is the harbinger of metastasis. The same vessels that feed the tumor also provide it with avenues of escape. Not all the myriad cells shed by tumors survive the turbulent voyage through the bloodstream, notes experimental oncologist Ann Chambers of the London Regional Cancer Centre in Ontario. But those that do eventually slip through blood-vessel walls with ease. Using a video camera attached to a microscopic lens, Chambers has watched in wonder as melanoma and breast-cancer cells, injected into mice, become lodged in capillary walls, then crawl out into the liver. Three days later, her camera resolves the spidery shapes of tiny metastatic growths. The lesson, Chambers believes, is depressingly clear. Cancer cells zip in and out of blood vessels so readily that, once angiogenesis occurs, they should be presumed to have already spread around the body.

Metastasis is an event of awesome complexity, one that requires multiple genes to cooperate as closely as musicians in an orchestra. Some of these genes code for chemical solvents that enable the advancing cell to dissolve surrounding tissue. Others order up the production of adhesion molecules that, like treads under a tank, move the cell forward. Why would genes do that? The answer, notes Patricia Steeg of the National Cancer Institute, is that while the genes important to metastasis are abnormally turned on, they are not necessarily abnormal themselves. A cancer cell, in many ways, is not that different from an embryonic cell on its way to becoming a patch of skin or a bundle of nerves. Both embryonic and cancer cells divide and form ill-defined clumps. Both get up and move around. Both migrate and populate new areas. But while an embryonic cell stops proliferating and matures into adult tissue, the cancer cells just keep dividing.

One reason for the difference may lie in a gene known as nm23, first identified by Steeg in 1988. It seems to help mature cells stop dividing and arrange themselves in an orderly fashion. Steeg's research suggests that in cancer cells this crucial gene often malfunctions. When she introduced a normal nm23 gene (nm stands for nonmetastatic) into highly malignant human breast cells, then injected these cells into mice, their tendency to form metastases dropped as much as 90%.

THE BIG KILLERS

Estimates in the U.S., 1994

Cancer		Deaths	New cases	Five-year survival rate	Risk Factors
Lung		153,000	172,000	13%	Cigarette smoking; exposure to asbestos, chemicals, radiation, radon
Colon/Rectum		56,000	149,000	58%	Family history; high-fat, low-fiber diet
Female Breast		46,000	182,000	79%	Age; family history; no pregnancies; late menopause; early menarche
Prostate		38,000	200,000	77%	Age; family history; possibly fat intake
Pancreas		25,900	27,000	3%	Age; smoking; fat intake
Lymphoma	Hodgkin's Non-Hodgkin's	22,750	52,900	78% 52%	Reduced immune function; exposure to herbicides, solvents, vinyl chloride
Leukemia		19,100	28,600	38%	Genetic abnormalities; exposure to ionizing radiation, chemicals; viruses
Ovary		13,600	24,000	39%	Age; family history; genetic disorders; no pregnancies
Kidney		11,300	27,600	55%	Smoking
Bladder		10,600	51,200	79%	Smoking
Uterus	Cervical Endometrial	10,500	46,000	67% 83%	Intercourse at an early age; multiple sex partners; smoking Early menarche; late menopause; obesity
Oral		7,925	29,600	53%	Smoking; excessive use of alcohol
Skin Melanoma		6,900	32,000	84%	Sunburn; fair complexion; exposure to coal tar, pitch, creosote, arsenic, radium

Source: American Cancer Society

GUARDING THE MASTER SWITCH Until last week, p53, the subject of some 1,000 scientific papers in 1993 alone, was considered the most important cancer gene. The journal *Science* even named it Molecule of the Year. But now there is a new contender for notoriety—MTS1, as Alexander Kamb and his colleagues refer to the multiple tumor-suppressor gene they have just discovered. "Multiple" refers to the fact that defects in this gene can cause many kinds of cancer, including melanoma, lung, breast and brain tumors. In fact, functional copies of MTS1 may be missing in more than 50% of all human cancers.

What makes MTS1 so significant is its clear role in the cell-division cycle. A cell divides not at will but in response to specific signals, such as growth factors produced by white blood cells rushing to repair a wound. These signals are picked up by receptors on the membrane of the cell and passed along—like batons in a high-speed relay—through the interior, all the way to a master "on" switch positioned deep in the nucleus. Not surprisingly, many oncogenes, including one called ras, the first human cancer gene ever identified, are involved in this type of signaling pathway. But there are other molecules that determine whether the cell should heed these signals. And the small protein produced by MTS1 appears to be among the most important inhibitors of cell division. Last year researchers at New York's Cold Spring Harbor Laboratory discovered that a protein they called p16 stifled an enzyme that is a growth promoter. Last week it became clear that p16 and the MTS1 protein are one and the same.

TARGETS FOR CANCER FIGHTERS Theoretically, any gene that goes awry in a cancer cell offers a way to attack the problem. But those that directly influence a cell's decision to divide are spurring particular interest. The protein made by the MTS1 gene seems exceptionally promising, for it has characteristics suggesting it may be easily fashioned into a drug, which then might be able to stop tumor cells in their tracks. "In terms of therapeutic potential," declares Kamb, "MTS1 may be the most important tumor-suppressor gene yet discovered."

Still, as pharmaceutical companies well know, many surprises can pop up on the way to developing a new drug, and other approaches to cancer therapy may win out in the end. Among the possibilities are anticancer vaccines designed to stimulate the immune system to combat tumors. Currently being tested in the U.S. and Canada is a vaccine that spurs an assault on the weirdly configured carbohydrates that protrude from tumor cells like spikes on a medieval ball and chain. At the meeting of the American Society for Cancer Research last week, Dr. David Berd of Thomas Jefferson University presented the most encouraging evidence to date that the vaccine strategy may work. Berd told of inoculating 47 melanoma patients with a vaccine made of their own tumor cells inactivated by radiation. Three years later, 60% remained tumor-free, compared with 20% in the unvaccinated control group. The approach works best, apparently, in patients who have tumors small enough to be surgically removed but whose disease shows signs of spread.

The discovery announced last week that cancer cells rely on the enzyme telomerase to stay alive opens up a different attack strategy. The leader of that research team, Calvin Harley, has taken a leave from McMaster University to work at Geron Corp. in Menlo Park, California. The company is trying to craft a drug that will block the action of telomerase. "The cancer cell," explains Harley, "is already very old. If we can inhibit telomerase, we might cause the tumor to die after a few doublings." Even better, the fact that cancer cells produce telomerase and that normal cells (save for sperm) don't, says Harley, "gives us hope that we may be able to develop a drug without serious side effects."

The formation of blood vessels in a tumor through angiogenesis is another promising target for an anticancer drug—

because the process is so rare in normal cells. Clinical trials have begun on several compounds that interfere with angiogenesis. One such compound comes from a fungus that was accidentally discovered in 1989 when it contaminated cultures of endothelial cells in Judah Folkman's Harvard laboratory, dramatically curtailing their growth. This drug, says Folkman, is aimed not at curing cancer but at prolonging the period of time colonies of tumor cells missed by conventional therapy remain in place without spreading. "Suppose we prolong this period of dormancy for 10 years, and then another 10 years," muses Folkman. "Why, now we're beginning to compete with the normal life span."

Indeed, what seems most significant about all the new therapies, what joins them together, is not their power, for this has yet to be proved. Rather, it is the seismic shift in strategy they collectively represent. Increasingly, researchers speak not of slaughtering the cancer cell but of tricking it into dying naturally, perhaps of old age, as other cells do. They also talk of reining in the cancer cell, even rehabilitating it, a task that demands the development of less toxic drugs that can be tolerated over a lifetime. The model for cancer therapy of the future already exists. "After all, we don't cure diseases like diabetes and hypertension," says Dr. Lance Liotta, the National Cancer Institute's leading metastasis expert."We control them. Why can't we look at cancer that way?"

By this reasoning, even metastatic cancer may eventually be brought to heel. Squeezed into a tiny cubicle day after day at the National Cancer Institute, Patricia Steeg stares at colonies of aggressive breast-cancer cells that have shut down the protective nm23 gene. Soon she will squirt over these colonies newly identified antitumor compounds. Among them she hopes to find one, maybe more, that interferes with metastatic growth. A total of 14 of these compounds are already sitting in a freezer in her lab—white crystals that cluster like snowflakes in the bottom of test tubes. If these fail to have an effect, Steeg has a list of more than 30 others that might. Like many cancer researchers, she conveys, through her own personal enthusiasm, a sense that an immense psychological barrier has been breached. No, Steeg has not yet found a drug that cures cancer or even controls it. But, she exclaims, "I'm beginning to like the odds."

ANALYSIS

Confronting the AIDS Pandemic

Daniel J. M. Tarantola and Jonathan M. Mann

Daniel J. M. Tarantola, M.D., is a lecturer in international health at the Harvard School of Public Health. Jonathan M. Mann, M.D., is director of the International AIDS Center of the Harvard AIDS Institute.

In 1986, the world undertook to mobilize against the AIDS pandemic in an effort that continued to grow until the beginning of this decade, when it began to stall. Today, the global HIV/AIDS pandemic is spinning out of control—its broad course has yet to be influenced in any substantial way by policies and programs mounted against it.

In 1991–1992, the Harvard-based Global AIDS Policy Coalition undertook a review of the state of the AIDS pandemic. The findings of this review, which appear in our new book *AIDS in the World* (Harvard University Press, December 1992), raise the alarm and call for an urgent revival of the response to AIDS.

The magnitude of the pandemic has increased over 100-fold since AIDS was discovered in 1981. From an estimated 100,000 people infected with HIV worldwide in 1981, it is estimated that by early 1992, at least 12.9 million people around the world (7.1 million men, 4.7 million women, and 1.1 million children) had been infected with HIV. Of these, about one in five (2.6 million) have thus far developed AIDS, and nearly 2.5 million have died.

The spread of HIV has not been stopped in any community or country. In the United States, at least 40,000 to 80,000 new HIV infections were anticipated during 1992; in 1991, more than 75,000 new HIV infections occurred in Europe. In just five years, the cumulative number of HIV-infected Africans has tripled, from 2.5 million to over 7.5 million today. HIV is spreading to new communities and countries around the world—in some areas with great rapidity. An explosion of HIV has recently occurred in Southeast Asia, particularly in Thailand, Burma, and India, where, within only a few years, over one million people may have already been infected with HIV. HIV/AIDS is now reported from areas that, so far, had been left relatively untouched, such as Paraguay, Greenland, and the Pacific island nations of Fiji, Papua New Guinea, and Samoa. The global implications are clear: During the next decade, HIV will likely reach most communities around the world; geographic boundaries cannot protect against HIV. The question today is not *if* HIV will come, but only *when*.

INCREASED COMPLEXITY

The pandemic becomes more complex as it matures. Globally it is composed of thousands of separate and linked community epidemics. Every large metropolitan area affected—Miami, New York, Bangkok, London, Amsterdam, Sydney, Rio de Janeiro—contains several subepidemics of HIV going on at the same time. The impact on women is increasing dramatically, as heterosexual transmission accounts for almost 71 percent of HIV infections. Worldwide, the proportion of HIV infected who are women is rising rapidly, from 25 percent in 1990 to 40 percent by early 1992. The epidemic also evolves over time: In Brazil, the proportion of HIV infections linked with injection

This article appeared in *The World & I*, January 1993, pp. 80-87. Reprinted with permission from *The World & I*, a publication of The Washington Times Corporation. © 1993.

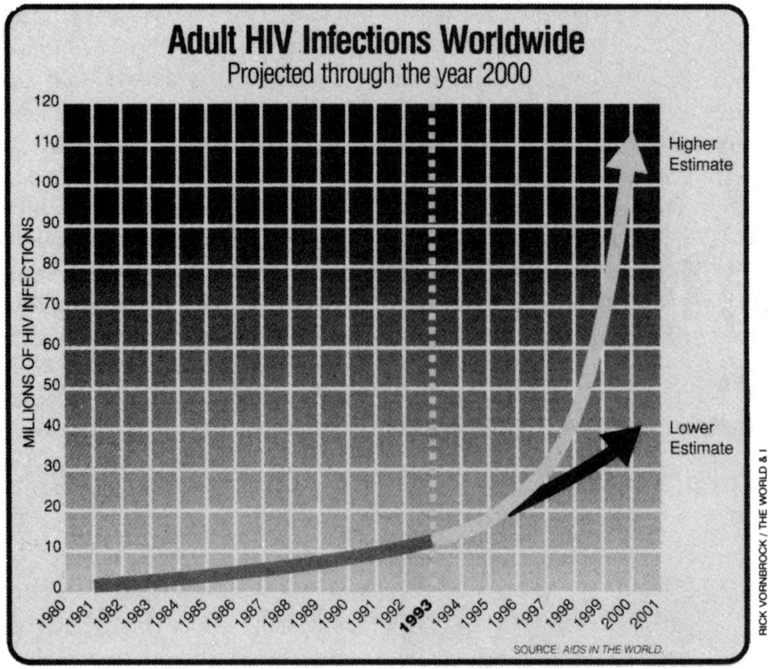

drug use has increased over tenfold since the early 1980s; in the Caribbean, heterosexual transmission has now replaced homosexual transmission as the major mode of HIV spread.

The pandemic's major impacts are yet to come. During the period 1992–95 alone, the number of people developing AIDS—3.8 million—will exceed the total number who developed the disease during the pandemic's history prior to 1992. The number of children orphaned by AIDS will more than double in the next three years: from approximately 1.8 million today to 3.7 million by 1995. The pandemic has not peaked in any country—no community or country can claim "victory" against HIV/AIDS. By 1995, an *additional* 5.7 million adults will become infected with HIV. Thus, from 1992 to 1995, the total number of HIV-infected adults will increase by 50 percent. During the same period, the number of children infected with HIV will more than double, from 1.1 million to an estimated 2.3 million.

By the year 2000, the Global AIDS Policy Coalition has projected that between 38 million and 110 million adults—and over 10 million children—will become HIV infected. The largest proportion of HIV infections will be in Asia (42 percent), surpassing sub-Saharan Africa (31 percent), Latin America (8 percent), and the Caribbean (6 percent). By the end of this decade, 24 million adults and several million children may have developed AIDS—or up to 10 times as many as today.

Only a few years ago, tuberculosis was considered a stable problem that was endemic mostly in the developing world. If it was also prevalent in certain socioeconomic groups in industrialized countries, there was a common belief that the situation was largely under control. This general sense of complacency, denounced by many who had been fighting the disease, led to a decline in resources allocated to surveillance, prevention, and treatment services. When HIV came on the scene, it found a vulnerable population.

There is a dangerous synergy between HIV and tuberculosis that makes the combined effects of both worse than their separate effects added together. HIV makes individuals and communities more vulnerable to tuberculosis; it increases the rate of reactivation of tuberculosis infection, shortens the delay between TB infection and disease, and reduces the accuracy of diagnostic methods. Recent outbreaks of multiple-drug resistant tuberculosis have occurred in New York City and in Miami, especially in hospitals and prisons. Combining its projections with estimates made by the World Health Organization, *AIDS in the World* estimates that, by early 1992, there were more than 4.6 million people with both TB and HIV infection worldwide, 81 percent of them in Africa.

Geographic boundaries cannot protect against HIV. The question today is not *if* HIV will come, but only *when*.

TAKING STOCK

Confronting the growing pandemic are national AIDS programs. These actions may involve governmental institutions and agencies, nongovernmental organizations, and the private sector.

Almost invariably overseen by ministries of health, they are generally implemented through government agencies and health services.

The success of a national AIDS program involves the extent to which it helps curb the course of the HIV epidemic and provides quality care to those already affected. On this basis, no program in the world can yet claim success.

Of the 38 countries surveyed by the Global AIDS Policy Coalition, 24 reported having conducted an evaluation since the inception of their national program. In general, the evaluation findings can be summarized as follows:

- Once created, programs become operational rapidly.
- They were successful in raising public awareness on AIDS issues although they did not always prevent (and at times they even generated) misperceptions among certain communities.
- They raised appropriate human rights issues and in some instances managed to prevent violations of these rights.
- They exchanged information—and in some cases made funds and skills available—at the international level.

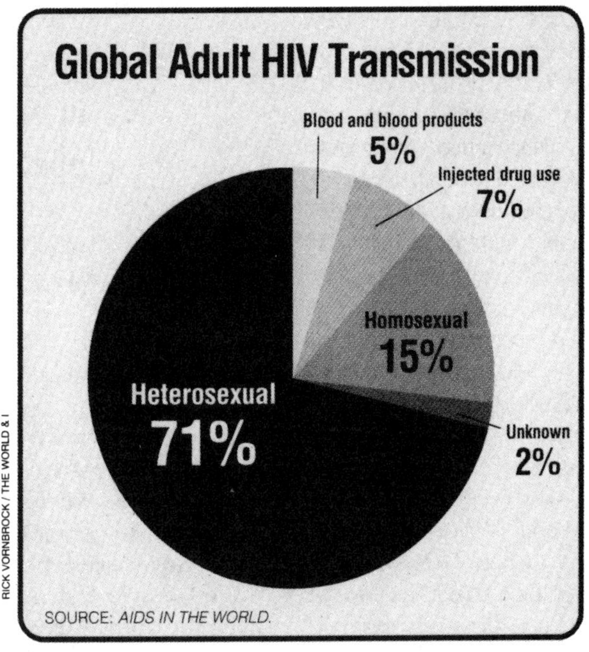

SOURCE: *AIDS IN THE WORLD.*

Industrialized countries were generally able to secure the financial, human, and technological resources required to increase drastically the safety of blood and blood products, and establish diagnostic and treatment schemes reaching most (but not all) people in need. The same could not be said, however, about developing countries, which are constrained by lack of resources, weak infrastructures, and multiple developmental or even survival issues.

Common criticisms of these programs are their lack of focus and priority setting, their weak management, their lack of integration with existing disease prevention and control services, and their inability to actively involve other health programs, sectors, and nongovernmental organizations. Denial persists about the pandemic's impact upon women; prevention and research efforts worldwide still inadequately involve them.

In its report, the Global AIDS Policy Coalition suggests indexes that can be applied at the national or regional levels. Similar indexes are being developed for the assessment of community vulnerability.

THE COST OF AIDS

AIDS policies and programs used to be guided by two motives misperceived by many as antagonistic: a human rights/humanitarian approach and a public health perspective. The economic argument was seldom raised because it was not politically advantageous to make the cost of AIDS a major public issue. It did not conform to the humanitarian agenda (cost is secondary to human rights) nor to the public health perspective (the population must be protected). But with the rising number of people and communities affected by the pandemic, the cost of prevention and care and the general economic impact of AIDS have become critical issues.

The economic perspective considers the impact of AIDS in a decade that began in a worldwide recession. It can be argued that the impact of HIV/AIDS on young, productive adults and their children will jeopardize the national development of many countries. In July 1992, a study conducted by an American team estimated the economic impact of the pandemic by feeding epidemiological projection data into a computer model of the global marketplace. It concluded that by the year 2000, the pandemic could drain between $356 billion and $514 billion from the world's economy, and developing countries are expected to be the hardest hit.

The Global AIDS Policy Coalition estimated that money spent on AIDS in a one-year period during 1990–91 was in the range of $1.4–$1.5 billion for prevention, approximately $3.5 billion for adult AIDS care alone, and $1.6 billion for research, for an adjusted total of $7.1 to $7.6 billion (including costs for treating those persons with HIV before AIDS occurs). Interestingly, about 95 percent was spent in industrialized countries that have less than 25 percent of the world's population, 18 percent of the people with AIDS, and 15 percent of HIV infections worldwide.

For HIV prevention activities in 1991, about $2.70 was spent *per person* in North America and $1.18 in Europe. In the developing world, spending on prevention amounted to only $0.07 per person in sub-Saharan Africa and $0.03 per person in Latin America. Of the $5.6 billion spent on AIDS research since the discovery of AIDS in 1981, $5.45 billion, or 97 percent, has been spent in industrialized countries. The United States is the biggest contributor to global AIDS research spending, with $4.8 billion, or 86 percent of the world total. Domestic and international research have led to a considerable advancement of knowledge. Research funds benefited from annual increases in the late 1980s, but resources supporting this research are reaching a plateau.

The United States is the biggest contributor to global AIDS research spending, with 86 percent of the world total.

For AIDS care, 89 percent of world spending in 1990 was used to help less than 30 percent of the world's people with AIDS—those living in North America and Europe. And yet, the cost of medical care for each person with AIDS—roughly equivalent to annual per capita income in developing countries—is overwhelming individuals and households everywhere. Inequities in treatment and prevention are growing. The cost of one year's treatment with AZT is about $2,500, while per capita income in all developing countries averages $700—in sub-Saharan Africa the figure is $470—or less than one-fifth the cost of AZT for one year. Individual studies have indicated that the annual cost of care for an adult with AIDS varied in 1990–91 from $32,000 in the United States to $22,000 in western Europe, $2,000 in Latin America, and a mere $393 in sub-Saharan Africa.

These figures translate into the harsh reality of length of survival and quality of life of people with AIDS. The need for AIDS care and the inequity in access to quality services will continue to grow: The number of AIDS treatment years for adults alone will increase from an estimated 433,000 in 1992 to 619,000 in

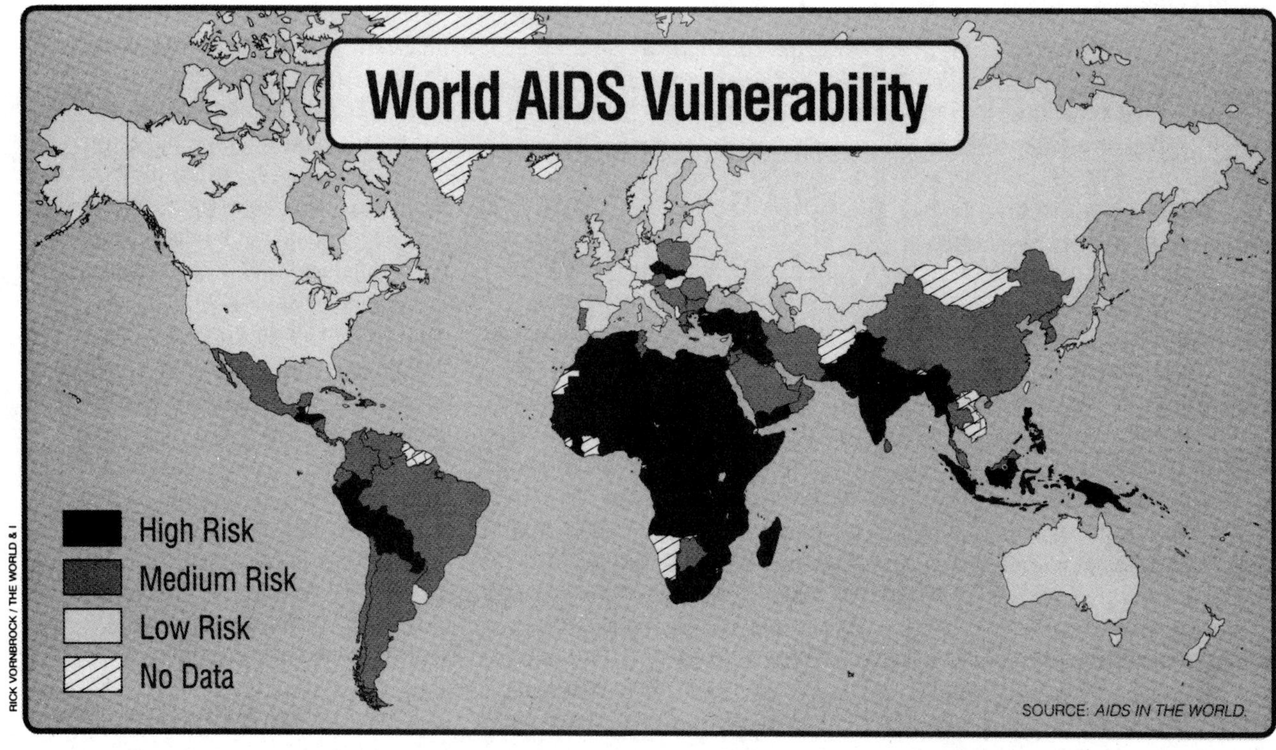

1995; almost 60 percent of these will be in Africa and 26 percent in the industrialized world. Built into these estimates, however, is the average duration of survival of an adult with AIDS, which in Africa is estimated at about one year after diagnosis, less than half of the survival duration of an adult with AIDS in the industrialized world.

Despite the introduction of HIV diagnostic tests over seven years ago, unscreened blood is currently responsible for at least 5 percent of global HIV infections. Most sub-Saharan African countries still cannot afford a safe blood supply. And even if an AIDS vaccine became available today, its impact on the world would be limited by inequities in access to it.

NEED FOR A GLOBAL VISION

Where efforts have been made to provide a coordinated response to the growing crisis, there are clear signs of positive individual responses. But where programs are confronted with weak national commitment, declining resources, and a growing sense of complacency, national AIDS programs are in jeopardy and, together with them, the people they are intended to serve. Many governments, constrained by their lack of resources, continue to avoid the reality of the pandemic: More people become infected because they do not have sufficient access to information and services; more individuals require care that they cannot afford; more families and communities are affected by the impact of a pandemic that has only begun.

Industrialized nations are turning away from coordinated efforts, showing a growing preference to work independently, on a bilateral basis, with chosen developing countries. Fragmentation of efforts by industrialized countries has led to competition among donors in some countries. It is clear that as the pandemic continues to worsen, AIDS programs will be forced to struggle with insufficient funds.

Global efforts have failed to motivate low-prevalence countries to act before the epidemic reaches them in force. India, Burma, and the Sudan are examples of a delayed response and a failure to learn from the experience of heavily affected countries.

Overall, the world has become more vulnerable to HIV and AIDS. On the basis of the societal factors that create vulnerability to spread of HIV, *AIDS in the World* has identified 57 countries as *high risk* for HIV spread—including countries that have thus far escaped the brunt of the pandemic, such as Indonesia, Egypt, Bangladesh, and Nigeria. An additional 39 countries are considered to be at *substantial* risk of a major HIV epidemic, including 11 Latin American countries, 8 in the southeast Mediterranean, 7 in Asia (including China), 4 in the Caribbean, and 9 in other regions.

We *are* at a critical juncture in the confrontation with AIDS, but we are not helpless. By revitalizing leadership, by addressing prevention and the needs of the affected, by formulating clear, international strategies, by accelerating effective, safe, and affordable treatments and vaccines, it *is* possible to stall the future spread of the pandemic.

At a time when many countries are undergoing major geopolitical transitions and are facing severe economic recessions, HIV/AIDS is not simply fading away. The world will continue to experience a rapid increase in the number of people developing AIDS until there is a cure. In the meantime, a troubled world population can unite together to fairly and equitably make available prevention and treatment programs until that day comes.

Human Sexuality

Sexuality is one of the most basic aspects of self-awareness. How sex differences affect the behavior of human beings is a topic that scientists and lay persons have been considering for quite some time. That women and men do differ, behaviorally, cognitively, and biologically, cannot be disputed. Why they differ and whether or not these differences matter are questions that remain unanswered.

One area in which men and women differ is in the area of sexuality and mating. Evolutionary psychologists who have studied mating behaviors contend that men and women are as different psychologically as they are biologically. For example, women are attracted to men based on their status, ambition, and resources, whereas men are attracted to women based on their youthful appearance and attractiveness. Cross-cultural studies have validated the universality of these preferences, and evolutionary psychologists have theorized that these preferences evolved in response to the differing biological demands faced by men and women in the process of having children. These psychologists say that even behaviors such as infidelity and jealously are still being shaped by the mating concerns of our ancient ancestors. "The Mating Game" examines various contemporary mating behaviors of both men and women and explains how these behaviors are an evolutionary throwback to our ancient ancestors.

While sex is an important component of intimacy between a man and a woman, it is by no means the most significant or the best predictor of a lasting relationship. Most people will admit that love tops their wish list, but statistics indicate that nearly 50 percent of all marriages fail, and intimate relationships without the marital trappings fare even worse. This high rate of divorce has prompted research efforts designed to understand why some marriages succeed while others fail. The results of these studies suggest that there are indeed certain factors that are vital to the success of lasting relationships. In "The Indispensables: 10 Key Reasons Why Love Endures," Catherine Houck examines 10 factors that make some intimate relationships, lasting relationships.

Three topics in human sexuality that have received considerable media attention are teenage pregnancy, abortion, and AIDS. The one thing that all of these topics have in common is that they deal with reproduction. As a result, the standard approach for dealing with them has been to provide students with contraceptive-based sex education. How successful has this approach been? If statistics regarding the incidence of pregnancy, abortions, and AIDS among teenagers indicates the effectiveness of this approach to sex education, then we certainly must consider some alternative strategies. Critics of contraceptive-based sex education argue that not only has this approach failed to reduce teenage pregnancies, abortions, and the spread of AIDS, but it may actually be contributing to the problem by fostering the expectation that it is normal for teenagers to experiment sexually. This assertion is supported by a 1986 Harris poll that found teenagers who received contraceptive-based education were 53 percent more likely to have intercourse than those whose sex education did not include information on contraceptives. What is even more distressing is the fact that the majority of the teens choosing to become sexually active do not even use the contraceptives they have learned about. This poor showing on the part of contraceptive-based sex education has prompted a growing movement within this country that thinks it is time to try abstinence-based sex education. William Bergman, in "It's Not Just AIDS," discusses why contraceptive-based sex education is failing and suggests that perhaps the time is right to try teaching our teens the value of virginity and abstinence.

Birth control itself has been a source of controversy and confusion. In the 1970s one of the most popular contraceptive devices was the IUD. This form of birth control was very effective and convenient to use. This all changed rather abruptly in the 1980s as it fell victim to legal and medical issues. An IUD called the Dalkon Shield was linked to pelvic inflammatory disease, infertility, and, sometimes, death. The litigation that ensued prompted several other manufacturers to remove their IUDs from the market for fear of staggering lawsuits. The impact of this incident had a chilling effect on the entire contraceptive industry. Research and development into new birth control technologies was put on hold, and some manufacturers abandoned the contraceptive market altogether. It now appears that the fallout from the Dalkon Shield has finally ended as new contraceptive choices are once again starting to appear in the marketplace. Depo-Provera, Norplant, and the female condom are the first wave of new contraceptive devices to enter the U.S. market in more than a decade. In addition to these newly approved products, several others are currently under development. They include contraceptive vaccines, a male birth control pill, more comfortable male condoms, a two-capsule version of the Norplant device, creams and gels with anti-HIV and spermicidal properties, and barrier methods that release spermicides. "Choosing a Contra-

Unit 8

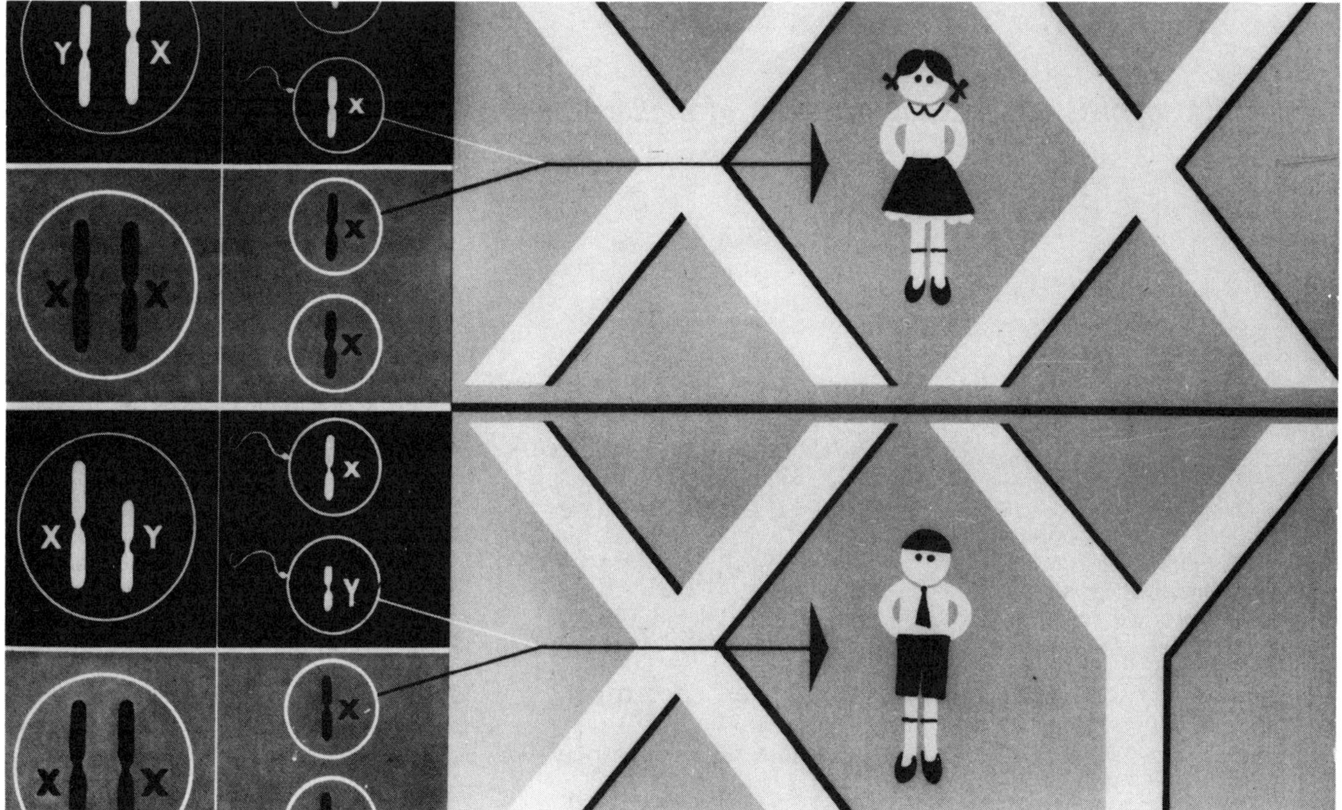

ceptive" by Joseph Anthony examines the contraceptive choices currently available and compares them on the basis of their cost, failure rate, and ability to prevent sexually transmitted diseases.

Clearly the most controversial issue in the area of human sexuality is that of abortion. The abortion issue involves an emotionally charged debate between pro-choice advocates, who defend individual freedom, and pro-life advocates, who defend the right to life—both of which are constitutional rights. Most pro-choice supporters feel that abortion should not be used as a form of birth control, but as an option to preserve the individual rights of a woman if birth control efforts fail and an accidental pregnancy results. The pro-life advocates argue that once the egg has been fertilized, a life has been created, and any action on the part of the woman to terminate the pregnancy is tantamount to murder. This debate between pro-choice and pro-life supporters has cooled off considerably since Bill Clinton was elected president, but the debate may heat up once again as this country prepares to legalize the abortion pill RU 486. Jill Smolowe, in "New, Improved and Ready for Battle," discusses how changes in the political climate could make the abortion pill RU 486 widely available to all Americans within the next three years.

Looking Ahead: Challenge Questions

Do you feel that birth control has contributed to increased promiscuity and the rapid spread of sexually transmitted diseases? Why or why not?

What approach to sex education do you think would be most effective in reducing teenage pregnancies, abortions, and the spread of AIDS?

Do you feel at risk of contracting AIDS? If not, why not? If you do, what are you doing to reduce your risk?

Do you think a female version of the condom would do much to slow the spread of AIDS?

Do you think it would be a good idea to have a compatibility assessment done prior to marriage?

THE Mating GAME

The sophisticated sexual strategies of modern men and women are shaped by a powerful Stone Age psychology.

It's a dance as old as the human race. At cocktail lounges and church socials, during office coffee breaks and dinner parties—and most blatantly, perhaps, in the personal ads in newspapers and magazines—men and women perform the elaborate ritual of advertisement and assessment that precedes an essential part of nearly every life: mating. More than 90 percent of the world's people marry at some point in their lives, and it is estimated that a similarly large number of people engage in affairs, liaisons, flings or one-night stands. The who, what, when and where of love, sex and romance are a cultural obsession that is reflected in everything from Shakespeare to soap operas and from Tristram and Isolde to 2 Live Crew, fueling archetypes like the coy ingénue, the rakish cad, the trophy bride, Mrs. Robinson, Casanova and lovers both star-crossed and blessed.

It all may seem very modern, but a new group of researchers argues that love, American style, is in fact part of a universal human behavior with roots stretching back to the dawn of humankind. These scientists contend that, in stark contrast to the old image of brute cavemen dragging their mates by the hair to their dens, our ancient ancestors—men and women alike—engaged in a sophisticated mating dance of sexual intrigue, shrewd strategizing and savvy negotiating that has left its stamp on human psychology. People may live in a thoroughly modern world, these researchers say, but within the human skull is a Stone Age mind that was shaped by the mating concerns of our ancient ancestors and continues to have a profound influence on behavior today. Indeed, this ancient psychological legacy influences everything from sexual attraction to infidelity and jealousy—and, as remarkable new research reveals, even extends its reach all the way down to the microscopic level of egg and sperm.

How we choose

Women are more concerned about whether mates will invest time and resources in a relationship; men care more about a woman's physical attractiveness, which in ancient times reflected her fertility and health.

These new researchers call themselves evolutionary psychologists. In a host of recent scientific papers and at a major conference last month at the London School of Economics, they are arguing that the key to understanding modern sexual behavior lies not solely in culture, as some anthropologists contend, nor purely in the genes, as some sociobiologists believe. Rather, they argue, understanding human nature is possible only if scientists begin to understand the evolution of the human mind. Just as humans have evolved specialized biological organs to deal with the intricacies of sex, they say, the mind, too, has evolved customized mental mechanisms for coping with this most fundamental aspect of human existence.

Gender and mind. When it comes to sexuality and mating, evolutionary psychologists say, men and women often are as different psychologically as they are physically. Scientists have long known that people typically choose mates who closely resemble themselves in terms of weight, height, intelligence and even earlobe length. But a survey of more than 10,000 people in 37 cultures on six continents, conducted by University of Michigan psychologist David Buss, reveals that men consistently value physical attractiveness and youth in a mate more than women do; women, equally as consistently, are more concerned than men with a prospective mate's ambition, status and resources. If such preferences were merely arbitrary products of culture, says Buss, one might expect to find at least one society somewhere where men's and women's mating preferences were reversed; the fact that attitudes are uniform across cultures suggests they are a fundamental part of human psychology.

Evolutionary psychologists think many of these mating preferences evolved in response to the different biological challenges faced by men and women in producing children – the definition of success in evolutionary terms. In a seminal paper, evolutionary biologist Robert Trivers of the University of California at Santa Cruz points out that in most mammals, females invest far

From *U.S. News & World Report*, July 19, 1993, pp. 57-63. © 1993 by U.S. News & World Report. Reprinted by permission.

more time and energy in reproduction and child rearing than do males. Not only must females go through a long gestation and weaning of their offspring, but childbirth itself is relatively dangerous. Males, on the other hand, potentially can get away with a very small biological investment in a child.

Human infants require the greatest amount of care and nurturing of any animal on Earth, and so over the eons women have evolved a psychology that is particularly concerned with a father's ability to help out with this enormous task–with his clout, protection and access to resources. So powerful is this psychological legacy that nowadays women size up a man's finances even when, as a practical matter, they may not have to. A recent study of the mating preferences of a group of medical students, for instance, found that these women, though anticipating financial success, were nevertheless most interested in men whose earning capacity was equal to or greater than their own.

Healthy genes. For men, on the other hand, reproductive success is ultimately dependent on the fertility of their mates. Thus males have evolved a mind-set that homes in on signs of a woman's health and youth, signs that, in the absence of medical records and birth certificates long ago, were primarily visual. Modern man's sense of feminine beauty–clear skin, bright eyes and youthful appearance–is, in effect, the legacy of eons spent diagnosing the health and fertility of potential mates.

This concern with women's reproductive health also helps explain why men value curvaceous figures. An upcoming paper by Devendra Singh of the University of Texas at Austin reveals that people consistently judge a woman's figure not by whether she is slim or fat but by the ratio of waist to hips. The ideal proportion – the hips roughly a third larger than the waist – reflects a hormonal balance that results in women's preferentially storing fat on their hips as opposed to their waists, a condition that correlates with higher fertility and resistance to disease. Western society's modern-day obsession with being slim has not changed this equation. Singh found, for instance, that while the winning Miss America has become 30 percent thinner over the past several decades, her waist-to-hip ratio has remained close to this ancient ideal.

Women also appreciate a fair face and figure, of course. And what they look for in a male's physique can also be explained as an evolved mentality that links good looks with good genes. A number of studies have shown that both men and women rate as most attractive

WHOM WE MARRY

More than 90 percent of all people marry and, they typically choose mates who closely resemble themselves, from weight and height, to intelligence and values, to nose breadth and even earlobe length.

faces that are near the average; this is true in societies as diverse as those of Brazil, Russia and several hunting and gathering tribes. The average face tends to be more symmetrical, and, according to psychologist Steven Gangestad and biologist Randy Thornhill, both of the University of New Mexico, this symmetry may reflect a person's genetic resistance to disease.

People have two versions of each of their genes–one from each parent–within every cell. Sometimes the copies are slightly different, though typically each version works just as effectively. The advantage to having two slightly different copies of the same gene, the researchers argue, is that it is harder for a disease to knock out the function of both copies, and this biological redundancy is reflected in the symmetry in people's bodies, including their faces. Further evidence for a psychological mechanism that links attractiveness with health comes from Buss's worldwide study of mating preferences: In those parts of the world where the incidence of parasites and infectious diseases is highest, both men and women place a greater value on attractive mates.

Some feminists reject the notion that women should alter physical appearance to gain advantage in the mating game. But archaeological finds suggest that the "beauty myth" has been very much a part of the human mating psychology since the times of our ancient ancestors—and that it applies equally to men. Some of the very first signs of human artistry are carved body ornaments that date back more than 30,000 years, and findings of worn nubs of ochre suggest that ancient humans may have used the red and black chalklike substance as makeup. These artifacts probably served as social signs that, like lipstick or a Rolex watch today, advertised a person's physical appearance and status. In one grave dating back some 20,000 years, a male skeleton was found bedecked with a tunic made from thousands of tiny ivory beads—the Stone Age equivalent of an Armani suit.

Far from being immutable, biological mandates, these evolved mating mechanisms in the mind are flexible, culturally influenced aspects of human psychology that are similar to people's tastes for certain kinds of food. The human sweet tooth is a legacy from a time when the only sweet things in the environment were nutritious ripe fruit and honey, says Buss, whose book "The Evolution of Desire" is due out next year. Today, this ancient taste for sweets is susceptible to modern-day temptation by candy bars and such, though people have the free will to refrain from indulging it. Likewise, the mind's mating mechanisms can be strongly swayed by cultural influences such as religious and moral beliefs.

Playing the field. Both men and women display different mating psychologies when they are just playing around as opposed to searching for a lifelong partner, and these mental mechanisms are also a legacy from ancient times. A new survey by Buss and his colleague David Schmitt found that when women are looking for "short term" mates, their preference for attractive men increases substantially. In a study released last month, Doug Kenrick and Gary Groth of Arizona State University found that while men, too, desire attractive mates when they're playing the field, they will actually settle for a lot less.

Men's diminished concern about beauty in short-term mates reflects the fact that throughout human evolution, men have often pursued a dual mating strategy. The most successful strategy for most men was to find a healthy, fertile, long-term mate. But it also didn't hurt to take advantage of any low-risk opportunity to sire as many kin as possible outside the relationship, just to hedge the evolutionary bet. The result is an evolved psychology that allows a man to be sexually excited by a wide variety of women even while committed to a partner. This predilection shows up in studies of men's and women's sexual fantasies today. A study by Don Symons of the University of California at Santa Barbara and Bruce Ellis of the University of Michigan found that while both men and women actively engage in sexual fantasy, men typically have more fantasies about anonymous partners.

Surveys in the United States show

that at least 30 percent of married women have extramarital affairs, suggesting that, like men, women also harbor a drive for short-term mating. But they have different evolutionary reasons for doing so. Throughout human existence, short-term flings have offered women an opportunity to exchange sex for resources. In Buss and Schmitt's study, women value an "extravagant lifestyle" three times more highly when they are searching for a brief affair than when they are seeking a long-term mate. Women who are secure in a relationship with a committed male might still seek out attractive men to secure healthier genes for their offspring. Outside affairs also allow women to shop for better partners.

Sperm warfare. A woman may engage the sexual interest of several men simultaneously in order to foster a microscopic battle known as sperm competition. Sperm can survive in a woman's reproductive tract for nearly a week, note biologists Robin Baker and Mark Bellis of the University of Manchester, and by mating with more than one man within a short period of time, a woman sets the stage for their sperm to compete to sire a child—passing this winning trait on to her male offspring as well. In a confidential survey tracking the sexual behavior and menstrual cycles of more than 2,000 women who said they had steady mates, Baker and Bellis found that while there was no pattern to when women had sex with their steady partners, having sex on the side peaked at the height of the women's monthly fertility cycles.

Since in ancient times a man paid a dear evolutionary price for being cuckolded, the male psychology produces a physiological counterstrategy for dealing with a woman's infidelity. Studying the sexual behavior of a group of couples, Baker and Bellis found that the more time a couple spend apart, the more sperm the man ejaculates upon their sexual reunion—as much as three times higher than average.

This increase in sperm count is unrelated to when the man last ejaculated through nocturnal emission or masturbation, and Baker and Bellis argue that it is a result of a man's evolved psychological mechanism that bolsters his chances in sperm competition in the event that his mate has been unfaithful during their separation. As was no doubt the case in the times of our ancient ancestors, these concerns are not unfounded: Studies of blood typings show that as many as 1 of every 10 babies born to couples in North America is not the offspring of the mother's husband.

Despite men's efforts at sexual subterfuge, women still have the last word on the fate of a man's sperm in her reproductive tract—thanks to the physiological effects of the female orgasm. In a new study, Baker and Bellis reveal that if a woman experiences an orgasm soon after her mate's, the amount of sperm retained in her reproductive tract is far higher than if she has an earlier orgasm or none at all. Apparently a woman's arousal, fueled by her feelings as well as her mate's solicitous attentions, results in an evolutionary payoff for both.

JEALOUS PSYCHE

Men are most disturbed by sexual infidelity in their mates, a result of uncertainty about paternity. Women are more disturbed by emotional infidelity, because they risk losing their mate's time and resources.

Cads and dads. Whether people pursue committed relationships or one-night stands depends on their perceptions of what kind of mates are in the surrounding sexual environment. Anthropologist Elizabeth Cashdan of the University of Utah surveyed hundreds of men and women on whether they thought the members of their "pool" of potential mates were in general trustworthy, honest and capable of commitment. She also asked them what kinds of tactics they used to attract mates. Cashdan found that the less committed people thought their potential mates would be, the more they themselves pursued short-term mating tactics. For example, if women considered their world to be full of "cads," they tended to dress more provocatively and to be more promiscuous; if they thought that the world was populated by potential "dads"—that is, committed and nurturing men—they tended to emphasize their chastity and fidelity. Similarly, "cads" tended to emphasize their sexuality and "dads" said they relied more on advertising their resources and desire for long-term commitment.

BEAUTY QUEST

The most attractive men and women are in fact those whose faces are most average, a signal that they are near the genetic average of the population and are perhaps more resistant to disease.

These perceptions of what to expect from the opposite sex may be influenced by the kind of home life an individual knew as a child. Social scientists have long known that children from homes where the father is chronically absent or abusive tend to mature faster physically and to have sexual relations earlier in life. Psychologist Jay Belsky of Pennsylvania State University argues that this behavior is an evolved psychological mechanism, triggered by early childhood experiences, that enables a child to come of age earlier and leave the distressing situation. This psychological mechanism may also lead to a mating strategy that focuses on short-term affairs.

The green monster. Whether in modern or ancient times, infidelities can breed anger and hurt, and new research suggests subtle differences in male and female jealousy with roots in the ancient past. In one study, for example, Buss asked males and females to imagine that their mates were having sex with someone else or that their mates were engaged in a deep emotional commitment with another person. Monitoring his subjects' heart rates, frowning and stress responses, he found that the stereotypical double standard cuts both ways. Men reacted far more strongly than

EVOLVED FANTASIES

Eroticism and gender

For insights into the subtle differences between men's and women's mating psychologies, one need look no further than the local bookstore. On one rack may be magazines featuring scantily clad women in poses of sexual invitation—a testimony to the ancient legacy of a male psychology that is acutely attuned to visual stimulus and easily aroused by the prospect of anonymous sex. Around the corner is likely to be a staple of women's erotic fantasy: romance novels.

Harlequin Enterprises Ltd., the leading publisher in the field, sells more than 200 million books annually and produces about 70 titles a month. Dedicated romance fans may read several books a week. "Our books give women everything," says Harlequin's Kathleen Abels, "a loving relationship, commitment and having sex with someone they care about." Some romance novels contain scenes steamy enough to make a sailor blush, and studies show that women who read romances typically have more sexual fantasies and engage in sexual intercourse more frequently than nonreaders do.

Sexual caricature. Since sexual fantasy frees people of the complications of love and mating in the real world, argue psychologists Bruce Ellis and Don Symons, it is perhaps not surprising that in erotic materials for both men and women, sexual partners are typically caricatures of the consumer's own evolved mating psychology. In male-oriented erotica, for instance, women are depicted as being lust driven, ever willing and unencumbered by the need for emotional attachment. In romance novels, the male lead in the book is typically tender, emotional and consumed by passion for the heroine, thus ensuring his lifelong fidelity and dependence. In other words, say Ellis and Symons, the romance novel is "an erotic, utopian, female counterfantasy" to male erotica.

Of course, most men also enjoy stories of passion and romance, and women can be as easily aroused as men by sexually explicit films. Indeed, several new entertainment ventures, including the magazine *Future Sex* and a video company, Femme Productions, are creating erotic materials using realistic models in more sensual settings in an attempt to appeal to both sexes. Still, the new research into evolutionary psychology suggests that men and women derive subtly different pleasures from sexual fantasy—something that even writing under a ghost name can't hide. According to Abels, a Harlequin romance is occasionally penned by a man using a female pseudonym, but "our avid readers can always tell."

---

women to the idea that their mates were having sex with other men. But women reacted far more strongly to the thought that their mates were developing strong emotional attachments to someone else.

As with our evolved mating preferences, these triggers for jealousy ultimately stem from men's and women's biology, says Buss. A woman, of course, has no doubt that she is the mother of her children. For a man, however, paternity is never more than conjecture, and so men have evolved psychologies with a heightened concern about a mate's sexual infidelity. Since women make the greater biological investment in offspring, their psychologies are more concerned about a mate's reneging on his commitment, and, therefore, they are more attentive to signs that their mates might be attaching themselves emotionally to other women.

Sexual monopoly. The male preoccupation with monopolizing a woman's sexual reproduction has led to the oppression and abuse of women worldwide, including, at its extremes, confinement, domestic violence and ritual mutilation such as clitoridectomy. Yet the new research into the mating game also reveals that throughout human evolution, women have not passively acquiesced to men's sexual wishes. Rather, they have long employed a host of behavioral and biological tactics to follow their own sexual agenda—behaviors that have a huge impact on men's behavior as well. As Buss points out, if all women suddenly began preferring to have sex with men who walked on their hands, in a very short time half the human race would be upside down.

With its emphasis on how both men and women are active players in the mating game, evolutionary psychology holds out the promise of helping negotiate a truce of sorts in the battle of the sexes—not by declaring a winner but by pointing out that the essence of the mating game is compromise, not victory. The exhortations of radical feminists, dyed-in-the-wool chauvinists and everyone in between are all spices for a sexual stew that has been on a slow boil for millions of years. It is no accident that consistently, the top two mating preferences in Buss's survey—expressed equally by males and females worldwide—were not great looks, fame, youth, wealth or status, but *kindness* and *intelligence*. In the rough-and-tumble of the human mating game, they are love's greatest allies.

WILLIAM F. ALLMAN

DUELING SPERM

If a couple has been apart for some time, the man's sperm count goes up during sex at their reunion—an ancient, evolved strategy against a female's possible infidelities while away.

The Indispensables: 10 Key Reasons Why Love Endures

Why do some relationships self-destruct, while others stay solid—and sexy—for decades? Get ready for some surprising scientific findings . . .

Catherine Houck

Love tops everyone's wish list. We all want someone to hug a lot, somebody to go to the movies with, a person who *cares* that we just located a Pontiac Grand Am with only three thousand miles. Still, nearly half of all marriages go *poof,* while unmarried liaisons have an even higher mortality rate.

Until recently, we could only speculate why some relationships cool and collapse while others remain redhot *indefinitely.* Now, however, researchers looking into love are beginning to log in some basic truths about this elusive, chaotic emotion. Here, the latest *scientific* findings on what keeps love alive in the long run.

Although people often believe that important differences will go away with time, this is a myth. Marriage does not automatically bring lovers closer.

1. MAGNETS WE'RE NOT

"The belief that opposites attract explains magnets but misunderstands the nature of lasting love," says Atlanta psychiatrist Frank Pittman, author of *Private Lies: Infidelity and the Betrayal of Intimacy.* Instead, "mutuality"—similar values and attitudes, ethnic backgrounds, interests, IQs, religions, customs, life-styles—may be the single most important ingredient in successful relationships, Dr. Pittman and other researchers concluded.

In fact, a high level of mutuality is so vital for a couple's future happiness that, according to David H. Olson, professor of family social sciences at the University of Minnesota, Saint Paul, it's possible to predict as early as the day a couple becomes engaged whether that marriage will last. Questioning a cross section of 164 courting couples on their values, Olson identified more than 100 as seriously mismatched. Three years later, he found that 90 percent of these couples had not been able to produce successful marriages. Fifty-two never *got* married, while thirty-one of those who did had already separated. Another twenty-two described their union as unhappy.

On the other hand, the remaining lovebirds, who started off by sharing key characteristics, *did* settle down harmoniously. "Clearly, love seldom conquers all," says Olson. "Though people often believe that important differences will go away with time, we can now say with some certainty that this is a myth. Marriage does not automatically bring lovers closer."

2. HOW DO I LIKE THEE?

Though rock stars revel in finding new ways to croon "I love you," "I like you" seems to have more to do with lasting

From *Cosmopolitan,* May 1992, pp. 84, 86, 88, 94.

passion. Robert and Jeannette Lauer, authors of *Til Death Do Us Part,* found over 70 percent of the happily married couples they surveyed "strongly agreed" with the statement "I like my mate as a person, "while only 13.2 percent of the miserable twosome could say the same.

"A lover who is also a friend provides us with shored-up self-esteem, shared attitudes and interests, keeps us from feeling lonely, reduces our anxiety, and helps us get the things we want," observes psychologist Elaine Walster, a pioneer researcher on the dynamics of liking and loving. "I love my husband," said one wife of twenty-two years in the Lauers' study, "but it was the *liking* that helped us get through the times I wanted to wring his neck."

Many people think that "love" is simply a stronger form of "like" and that loving would be impossible without liking someone first. Not so, says Pittman. All too often, men and women choose partners who confer the most status, elicit the most envy, or horrify the most relatives. Others can be passionately, desperately in love yet consumed with distrust and rage at their mate.

The best indication of whether a man or women is capable of genuine friendship with a mate, claim social psychologists, is whether he or she has close, nonsexual friends of the opposite sex. Also important, says Pittman, is whether that person is friends with his parents, because a lover who is still at war with his parents is probably not ready for peace and friendship with a romantic partner.

3. INTIMACY: THE ESSENCE OF LOVE

"The need to feel close to another person is probably the most basic of all psychological needs," says psychologist Dan P. McAdams, whose national study of 1,208 men and women is the most intensive look at intimacy to date.

McAdams has found that emotional intimacy is of nearly equal importance for the happiness of both sexes, but its rewards tend to be different for men and women. For a women, feeling close to a man makes her feel happier; for a man, achieving intimacy not only bestows happiness, it seems to provide a springboard to confidence and resilience that encourages worldly achievements. "In relationships lacking intimacy, neither the man nor the women has a secure emotional base," says McAdams, who, along with other psychotherapists, reports seeing more couples than ever before who feel this essential relationship ingredient eludes them.

Perhaps that's because intimacy, once described by the late psychologist Abraham Maslow as "gentle, delicate, unintruding, undemanding, able to fit itself passively to the nature of things as water gently soaks into crevices," is not easily obtained through conscious effort. Instead, say researchers, the surest road to this meeting of two minds *and* hearts is good communication.

Couples who feel free to discuss whatever is deeply important to them—including their relationship—are both happier and more likely to bask in lasting love than less-chatty lovers. Honestly (accompanied by *plenty* of concern about the other person's feelings) is a necessity. "Even the smallest lie can be hopelessly disorienting," says Dr. Pittman. "Lovers usually know when they're being lied to. . . . They just don't know what the truth is. Intimacy seeps away, and the relationship soon follows."

In a study reported in the journal *Social Work,* couples married twenty-four years were asked to describe first their own interests, personality traits, characteristic feelings, and social needs, then those of their spouse. The happiest couples were uncannily able to portray their mates exactly as the mates portrayed themselves. "They were people who knew each other well," writes study author Nina S. Fields. "That sort of familiarity grows out of spending time together, and not only talking but *listening.*"

"Listening well requires a good deal of energy," say the Lauers. A mate "mustn't allow her mind to wander and must be prepared for some unpleasant feelings—she may not want to know about the frustrations or grievances of her lover, or it may be painful to acknowledge that the relationship is anything less than deeply satisfying." But accepting the risks and costs of both self-disclosure and listening are vital for intimacy—and happiness. Otherwise, issues are ignored and fester.

By listening requires more than just sitting quietly. When a mate confides his troubles, many lovers respond by freely sharing their thoughts on the matter. "They correct, judge, and give advice," says the Family Relations Institute's Lori Gordon. "This causes resentment, because it implies you think he isn't intelligent enough to solve his problems himself. Eventually, he may decide not to talk about problems—and good-bye, intimacy." According to Gordon, when your lover opens up, you must be sure to ask "Do you want my opinion, or should I just listen?"

In the movies the leading man and lady may hurl verbal missiles, then fall into each other's arms. But in real life, yelling or sobbing seldom helps solve problems.

Still another way happy couples encourage intimacy is through praise and mutual reinforcement. "Letting a partner know when he's done something that pleases, whether it's leaving a thoughtful phone message or successfully unclogging the pepper mill, helps make him feel loved and confident enough to share further expressions of love," says Robert J. Sternberg, IBM professor of psychology and education at Yale University.

4. BETTER ENEMIES

The difference between a relationship that gets better over time and one in which the lovers grow apart can often be traced to

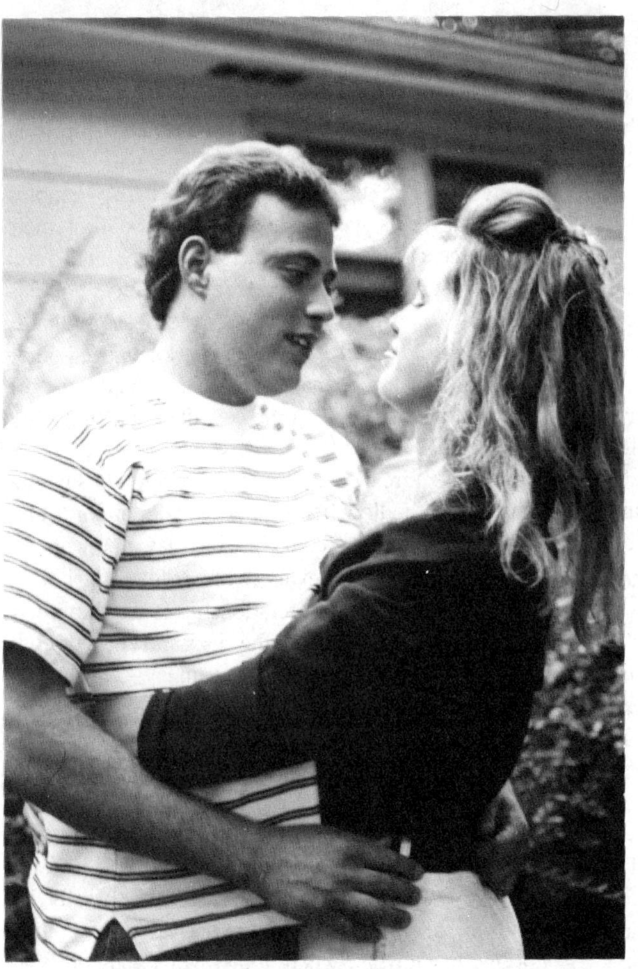
Photo by Marcuss Oslander

For a relationship to grow and develop each partner must trust that the other is dedicated to the union. Without trust, no firmly based relationship can evolve and stand the test of time.

how conflicts are resolved, according to a study by John Gottman, a professor of psychology at the University of Washington, and Lowell Krokoff, a former assistant professor of psychology at the University of Wisconsin at Madison. When Gottman and Krokoff analyzed the actual emotional maneuvers of battling couples, then checked their status again three years later, they discovered that there are three particularly destructive ways certain couples deal with conflicts. In some cases, one or both partners simply refuse to listen to complaints by withdrawing ("I'm not going to argue with you about this"). Another devastating ploy is inaccurate "mind reading," in which the adversary claims to know what the other partner *really* thinks or feels ("You don't need anybody but your mother"). Still a third counterproductive pattern is making contemptuous or insulting remarks rather than asking for a specific behavior change "You know, you're really an exploitive person" instead of "I think you should take me out to dinner more, since I cook for us at home." Or "You're a slob" rather than "It bothers me that you leave your dirty underwear lying around the bathroom").

In a fruitful argument, each partner feels free to explain why he or she is mad while the other one listens—with respect. A particularly effective way some couples demonstrate that the explanation is getting through, the researchers have found, is by one partner's repeating, in his or her own words, the point that the other has just made.

Long-term happy couples also tend to argue calmly and in a normal voice. While in movies the leading man and lady may hurl verbal missiles and then fall into each other's arms, in real life, loss of control—yelling, quaking with fear, sobbing piteously—seldom helps a couple solve problems. "Couples whose relationship has improved over time usually have learned to keep the lid on arguments," says Gottman. "Rather than being swept away by anger, they know how to de-escalate by suggesting a compromise or solution."

5. THE LABOR OF LOVE

"To love somebody is not just a strong feeling—a feeling may come and it may go," wrote the late Erich Fromm in *The Art of Loving,* published several decades ago. "Rather, love is a decision, a judgment, a promise." Today we call this aspect of *l'amour* "commitment," and virtually all researchers report that it's the Elmer's glue of happy relationships. "To know your mate is committed to you—and you to him—is to have a sense of security in a turbulent world," say the Lauers.

"Successful couples view commitment as a task," says Yale's Robert Sternberg. "They don't take each other for granted but work constantly at rejuvenating their good feelings for each other. The most satisfied couples put the kind of thought and energy into their relationship that they put into their children or career."

This sort of commitment is being increasingly viewed as crucial for getting through marriage's most dangerous years: number four. Analyzing divorce data from fifty-eight different countries since 1947, anthropologist Helen Fisher found evidence in *all* societies of a "four-year itch" that made couples dramatically prone to divorce at that point. "Four years happens to be how long it took our ancestors to wean their young," Fisher explains. "It seems nature has a strong interest in keeping humans pair-bonded for four years but provides no similar incentive to keep couples bonded for life. That's why, after an initial period of grace, marriages must be worked on."

Today, more and more stable, loving couples credit professional help of some sort for keeping their marriage out of trouble—and divorce court. Some simply find a good family counselor, while others take courses, such as the sixteen-week program developed by Lori Gordon, director of the Family Relations Institute, in Falls Church, Virginia, which provides "skill training for relationships." There, couples attend seminars on how to share feelings, respond to a mate's criticisms, express affection, offer comfort, and work on problems with sensuality and sex. For still others, skill training has meant working with a therapist to understand the origins of destructive emotional patterns—and how to change them effectively.

6. A PINCH OF TOLERANCE . . .

"At the beginning of a romance, the other person's habits usually don't seem important and may even be endearing, but over the long term, his nightly snoring or her thing about never raising the window shades can begin to grate," says Sternberg. Yet the most successful couples, he finds, have developed a high tolerance for each other's imperfections. They've simply acknowledged that many problems are unsolvable—and learned to work around them.

After interviewing eighty-seven married couples for her book *Married People: Staying Together in the Age of Divorce,* Francine Klagsbrun found "an ability to forgo perfection" to be vital for relationship satisfaction. "Every relationship has sore spots," says Klagsbrun. "Successful lovers are usually able to accept these limitations and get on with life instead of wasting energy." One simple but effective ploy used by many devoted pairs, she found, is determinedly focusing on the relationship's strengths rather than its weaknesses. "With that outlook, they're able to enhance what's good so that it becomes the core of their relationship, while negatives become peripheral."

7. PASSION: LOVE'S SWEET POETRY

Virtually all serious researchers agree that sexual attraction normally peaks within the first year or two of a relationship. But they've also found that the happiest lovebirds still have plenty of sexy feelings left. Says psychologist Paul Pearsall, author of *Super Marital Sex,* "Staying at a peak isn't necessary for a happy union. An enduring attraction *is.* An ongoing sexual relationship with one person is the most intense, fulfilling experience any human can have."

Sternberg agrees but adds that an important component of continued ardor is the woman's appearance. "Men care about a woman's physical attractiveness. The more attractive a man feels his wife is, the more successful their relationship will be over time."

Among the thousands of couples he studied for his book, Pearsall found that those reporting the happiest marriages and sex lives put their relationship first. "Attending to each other came before the lawn, the kids, job, car, or leaky sink." Steven Carter and Julia Sokol, who interviewed 250 men and women for their book *What Really Happens in Bed,* reached much the same conclusion. "In happy marriages, both participants are deeply committed to making it work—and this includes working out a satisfactory sexual relationship," they say.

But research also demonstrates that even the most deliciously blissful couples seldom agree on how often to make love. One partner may feel amorous four times a week, the other once—and they compromise on twice. as long as both partners enjoy the experience, couples who make love infrequently—even once a month—tend to be as happy as those who are more active.

One surprise: Though sex therapists have long lauded spontaneous sex, the most contented couples in all current surveys maintain that spontaneity gets less desirable the longer the relationship. "Women specifically mentioned that they prefer having time to mentally prepare themselves for sex as opposed to just being grabbed without warning," says Sokol. Many also report that making love on a familiar schedule provides something to look forward to.

8. LOVE RESPECTS EQUALITY

Q. Who's better off—the lover who loves more or the one who loves less? **A.** *Neither*. The lovers with the best chance for happiness are those who contribute more or less equally to a relationship, according to psychologist Elaine Walster, who, with colleague Jane Traupmann, interviewed more than six hundred people to find out what happens when one partner gives more than the other. "Lovers who knew they were getting far more than they really deserved felt uneasy and guilty, while those who felt they were getting less were angry and resentful," says Walster. "On the other hand, equitable relationships seem to be unusually solid."

Connell Cowan, coauthor of *Women Men Love, Women Men Leave,* also feels strongly that for a love relationship to flourish, the needs and desires of each partner must be *equally* important. "Healthy love has built-in constraints; it's conditional," he says. "Paradoxically, the happiest lovers are those willing to give up love if their sensitivities aren't respected.

"Women (or men) who give too freely inadvertently press all the wrong buttons in their partners," says Cowen. "Wishing only to please, they push their lovers away, making them determined to give less and less as the partner gives more and more. All chance for a mutually satisfying closeness vanishes, with lasting love soon to follow."

9. OLD-FASHIONED TRUST

"Feelings of love may wax and wane during a relationship, but trust is a constant," says Klagsbrun. Infidelity, of course, is the most devastating betrayal of that trust a couple can experience at *any* time in their relationship. In a survey of twelve thousand couples nationwide for their book *American Couples,* sociologists Philip Blumstein and Pepper Schwartz found that of all couples—whether married or living together, heterosexual or gay—those in which either partner had sex outside the relationship were more likely to break up than others. "Even a little bit of infidelity can set forces in motion that eventually wreck a marriage," says Schwartz.

Dr. Frank Pittman agrees. "It's commonplace for guilt-ridden people, after an infidelity, to distance their unsuspecting mate, whose love makes them feel even guiltier. At the same time, they seek out the only person who can assure them no wrong was done—the accomplice. Guilt therefore undermines the marriage and fuels the affair."

In addition, someone who is having an extramarital affair is clearly not trying to increase the degree of intimacy and mutual understanding in his or her marriage, which bodes badly for lasting love. Says Cowan, "Only when we trust our lover to be faithful and know that he or she can trust us do we feel comfortable and at peace with our own conduct and our relationship."

10. THE PATTER OF FOUR-LEGGED FEET

A recent Indiana University study has shown that adding dogs or cats to your household can make love more likely to endure. Researchers found that pets actually help ease marital conflicts. And their unconditional love for their owners also sets a good example. "Dogs relax people and reduce stress and anger," says Alan Beck, director of the University of Pennsylvania School of Veterinary Medicine's Center for the Interaction of Animals and Society. "A pet in the room makes people like each other better. When we get home and see the dog or cat curled up and content, we, too, relax our guard."

CHOOSING A CONTRACEPTIVE

What's Best for You?

Joseph Anthony

Joseph Anthony is a Contributing Editor at AMERICAN HEALTH.

If you've been frustrated by a lack of contraceptive choices, there's good news: In the last couple of years, several new forms of contraception specifically, the long-lasting, hormone-based products Depo-Provera and Norplant and the female condom have been approved for use in the U.S., which means that we're finally catching up with the rest of the world. Depo-Provera and Norplant have been in use in other countries for years. But much ballyhooed new methods, such as contraceptive "vaccines" and a male birth control pill, are still probably a decade or more away.

Why? Manufacturers worry about boycotts and other protests from the religious right and antiabortion activists. And, says Dr. Michael Policar, vice president for medical affairs at the Planned Parenthood Federation of America, "the threat of litigation has had an incredibly chilling effect on contraceptive development in the last 10 years."

What are in the pipeline are mostly variations on existing themes—a two-capsule Norplant (instead of today's six); redesigned, baggier male condoms that promise greater comfort; intrauterine devices (IUD's) that release hormones; barrier methods that release spermicides, creams or gels with anti-HIV as well as antisperm properties; and perhaps some new injectables. There has also been some movement toward making the Pill available over the counter (without a prescription), although the Food and Drug Administration (FDA) is not currently considering any formal proposals to do so.

Here's a rundown on newly available methods of birth control, followed by more-established and better-known alternatives.

THE FEMALE CONDOM: This device looks like a large, floppy tube closed at one end. Marketed by Wisconsin Pharmacal under the name Reality, the polyurethane barrier (thinner, stronger and a better conductor of heat than latex) was approved by the FDA last May. Like other barrier methods this one can take some time and patience to use correctly. The device has two rings, one around the outer rim and one inside. The inner ring is designed to fit over the cervix, anchored in place behind the pubic bone, like a diaphragm. The outer ring covers the labia and the base of the penis during intercourse. Some women have complained that the condom can rise into the vagina if not sufficiently lubricated; it can also twist around if not inserted properly.

The one-year failure rate with "typical use" is high, estimated at 21% to 26%, which means that about one in four women using it may become pregnant over the course of a year. (The pregnancy rate for "perfect use" would be much lower—about 5%.)

DEPO-PROVERA: This injectable prescription contraceptive, first available in New Zealand in 1969 and subsequently used by 30 million women in 90 countries, was finally approved in the U.S. in late 1992. One injection of this synthetic version of the female hormone progesterone every three months blocks ovulation.

The drug, which provides no protection against sexually transmitted diseases (STD's), may cause irregular periods, and women may not regain fertility until six to 12 months after they stop taking it.

Side effects of Depo-Provera are similar to those of other hormonal contraceptives and may include weight gain, headaches and fatigue. Women usually experience some irregular bleeding or spotting during the first months of use. On the plus side, studies by the World Health Organization have found a link between Depo-Provera use and a reduced risk of cancer of the endometrium (the lining of the uterus).

NORPLANT: This implant of six thin capsules, placed under the skin of a woman's arm, releases the hormone levonorgestrel, which keeps the body from producing the hormones necessary for ovulation. Norplant is effective for up to five years.

The implant was approved after two decades of testing on more than 50,000 women. More than 900,000 American women have received Norplant since it was introduced in February of 1991 by U.S. distributor Wyeth-Ayerst Laboratories. It's not appropriate for women who have liver disease,

From *American Health*, April 1994, pp. 68-71. © 1994 by Joseph Anthony. Reprinted by permission.

blood clots, inflammation of the veins or a history of breast cancer, or for those who are breast-feeding in the first six weeks after delivery. Fertility returns soon after the implant is removed.

The most common side effect of Norplant is irregular menstrual bleeding during the first six months after implantation. Norplant provides no STD protection.

Wyeth-Ayerst Laboratories has been charging $365 for Norplant in the U.S. (With doctor's fees, Norplant generally costs between $500 and $800.) After congressional hearings last year revealed that the drug sells for as little as $23 in other countries, the company announced that the price to public clinics would be lowered in 1995. But company officials won't comment on what the new price will be.

STERILIZATION: Every year more than 600,000 women in the U.S. have their fallopian tubes surgically blocked or severed, thus preventing eggs from reaching the uterus. About 25% of all women at risk of pregnancy (sexually active, heterosexual and fertile) aged 15 to 50 have had this procedure, called a tubal ligation; among such women 35 to 44 the number soars to more than 60%, according to the Alan Guttmacher Institute, a nonprofit group studying contraceptive issues. In addition, each year about half a million American men have vasectomies, in which the tube that carries sperm from the testes is cut and sealed. Vasectomy, which is performed under local anesthesia, carries less surgical risk than tubal ligation, which requires general anesthesia.

Both forms of sterilization are more than 99% effective and virtually permanent. (Though surgical sterilizations can sometimes be reversed—the success rate for such procedures is better for vasectomies than for tubal ligations—but anyone contemplating surgical sterilization is generally advised to consider the operation irreversible.)

ORAL CONTRACEPTIVES: Commonly known as the Pill, oral contraceptives, which suppress ovulation, are the most popular form of birth control for women in the U.S. About 28% of American women at risk of pregnancy between 15 and 44 use oral contraceptives. Fewer than 1% of women using oral contraceptives properly will become pregnant in the course of a year.

Literally hundreds of studies over the past four decades have attempted to analyze the effect of the Pill on women's health. No solid connections between taking the Pill and getting breast cancer have been made. The Pill does appear to increase the risk of blood clots, heart attack and stroke for women over 35 who smoke. The authors of *Contraceptive Technology,* a leading reference manual in the field, characterize the risk for nonsmokers and smokers under 35 as relatively minor.

While the Pill has been linked to circulatory problems in women who have high cholesterol, hypertension or any heart or vascular disease, as well as those who have a family history of heart disease, oral contraceptives also have been associated with several health *benefits.* Some studies indicate that birth control pills can actually reduce a woman's chances of developing ovarian or endometrial cancer, as well as lower her risk of pelvic inflammatory disease. Women taking the Pill also have fewer ovarian cysts and benign breast tumors than other women.

There are more than a dozen side effects attributed to the Pill, including breast tenderness, fluid retention, weight gain and headaches.

BARRIER METHODS: Condoms, diaphragms, cervical caps, sponges and spermicides all operate on the same basic principle: preventing sperm from reaching an egg. Latex condoms have the added benefit of providing the most protection against STD's, although all barrier methods, even spermicides, are thought to provide some protection when used properly.

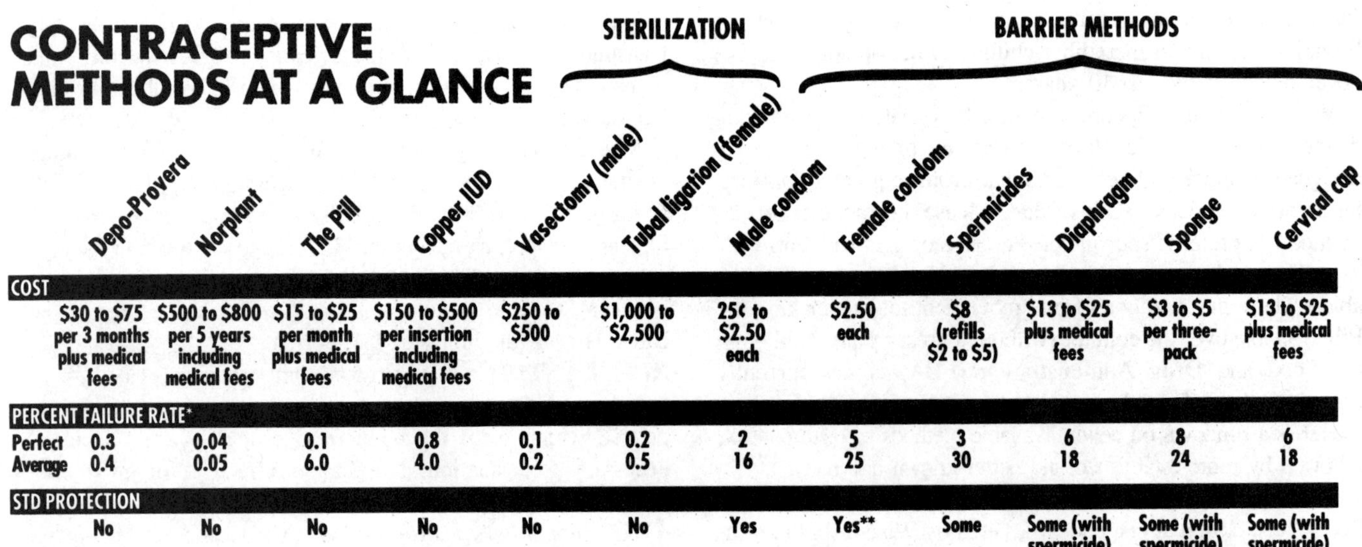

CONTRACEPTIVE METHODS AT A GLANCE

	Depo-Provera	Norplant	The Pill	Copper IUD	Vasectomy (male)	Tubal ligation (female)	Male condom	Female condom	Spermicides	Diaphragm	Sponge	Cervical cap
					STERILIZATION		BARRIER METHODS					
COST	$30 to $75 per 3 months plus medical fees	$500 to $800 per 5 years including medical fees	$15 to $25 per month plus medical fees	$150 to $500 per insertion including medical fees	$250 to $500	$1,000 to $2,500	25¢ to $2.50 each	$2.50 each	$8 (refills $2 to $5)	$13 to $25 plus medical fees	$3 to $5 per three-pack	$13 to $25 plus medical fees
PERCENT FAILURE RATE*												
Perfect	0.3	0.04	0.1	0.8	0.1	0.2	2	5	3	6	8	6
Average	0.4	0.05	6.0	4.0	0.2	0.5	16	25	30	18	24	18
STD PROTECTION	No	No	No	No	No	No	Yes	Yes**	Some	Some (with spermicide)	Some (with spermicide)	Some (with spermicide)

*Estimated percentage of women who get pregnant unintentionally in the first year of use. "Perfect use" is calculated from pregnancies occurring among couples who use the method correctly each time they have intercourse; "average use" combines perfect use figures with pregnancies occurring among couples who use the method sporadically or incorrectly.

**Although the female condom does provide protection against sexually transmitted diseases (STD's), its manufacturer is required by the Food and Drug Administration to note that for "highly effective protection" against STD's, including AIDS, it is important to use latex condoms for men.

FAILURE RATE DATA: ALAN GUTTMACHER INSTITUTE. FEMALE CONDOM FAILURE RATES: WISCONSIN PHARMACAL

RU-486 and MORNING-AFTER TREATMENTS

Women who fear they may have become pregnant because they experienced condom rupture or otherwise engaged in unprotected intercourse have a little-publicized "morning-after," or postcoital, contraceptive option. Take what Dr. Felicia Stewart, director of research for the Sutter Medical Foundation in Sacramento, Calif., calls emergency contraceptive pills as soon as possible after the unprotected intercourse but no later than 72 hours afterward.

The "emergency pills" are regular birth control pills, but taken in two larger-than-usual doses (the second 12 hours after the first). The number of pills per dose depends on the brand: two Ovral, or four Lo/Ovral, Nordette, Levlen or yellow-colored Triphasil or Tri-Levlen (the yellow versions of both are the strongest formulas). By taking a larger-than-normal dose of birth control pills, you'll disrupt your body's natural hormone patterns, thereby reducing your chances of becoming pregnant by about 75%.

Obviously, the morning-after option shouldn't be looked at as a regular birth control method—it's a one-time emergency measure. And the procedure may not be suitable for women suffering from severe liver disease, blood clots or other circulation problems. Up to half of all women using this approach report short-term nausea or vomiting.

The drug RU-486, which prevents a fertilized egg from implanting itself in the uterine wall, might also find a secondary use as a morning-after contraceptive if it's approved for sale in the U.S. A University of Edinburgh study published in *The New England Journal of Medicine* found that if taken within 72 hours of unprotected sexual intercourse, RU-486 also prevents pregnancy. The women surveyed in the study reported much milder side effects than those taking birth control pills as morning-after measures.

Last year RU-486 manufacturer Roussel-Uclaf announced it would grant U.S. rights to the drug to the nonprofit research organization the Population Council, which would market and test the drug. As of the beginning of this year, however, the final details of the agreement had not been ironed out.

The main side effects of barrier methods are allergies or sensitivity to latex or spermicides. (The sponge is off-limits to women who have had toxic shock syndrome.)

INTRAUTERINE DEVICES (IUD's): IUD's are placed in a woman's uterus, where they prevent pregnancy by interfering with sperm transport and egg fertilization. The Dalkon Shield gave IUD's a terrible name in this country during the 1980s. After more than 10,000 lawsuits over pelvic inflammatory disease linked to the shield, IUD's have fallen out of favor. Fewer than 2% of women in the U.S. currently use them, a fact some experts regard as unfortunate.

"Compare that to around 30% of the women in Finland who choose an IUD," says Dr. Daniel Mishell, chairman of obstetrics and gynecology at the University of Southern California School of Medicine. "The IUD is effective and is one of the least expensive forms of long-term contraception, but it is also one of the least used in the U.S. because of the perception that it is dangerous." Recent studies have shown modern copper IUD's present little, if any risk of pelvic inflammatory disease.

The only IUD's currently sold in the U.S. are the Copper T-380A, which can be used for up to eight years, and the Progestasert, which releases progesterone and can be used for up to one year.

What form of contraception is right for you? People who have new or multiple partners have to be concerned about STD's as well as pregnancy. That means they should use condoms for maximum STD protection. A survey of 678 women receiving Norplant in Texas indicated that about half who had previously used condoms intended to keep doing so at least some of the time. "Until the last few years, nobody even *asked* questions about whether women using a hormonal contraceptive like Norplant would also continue to use barrier methods like condoms," says Margaret Frank, a contraceptive researcher at the University of New Haven in Connecticut and coauthor of the Texas study. People in monogamous, long-term relationships shouldn't have to worry about diseases and may focus instead on effective contraception.

But there's no way of saying that any one choice is "best." "Some women are going to get along really well with a particular method, and that's great," says *Contraceptive Technology* coauthor Dr. Felicia Stewart, director of research for the Sutter Medical Foundation, a managed-care organization in Sacramento, Calif. "If you have a method that is a comfortable fit with your hormonal makeup or your anatomy and your habits, then that method is fine for you. Trying, to say there's one best method is just ridiculous."

NEW, IMPROVED AND READY FOR BATTLE

THE ABORTION PILL is finally coming to the U.S., and a breakthrough that eliminates the follow-up shots will make it simpler to use

Jill Smolowe

Abortion is never easy. There is the anguish of the decision, the invasive nature of the procedure, and sometimes an ugly confrontation with right-to-life forces lying in wait outside the clinic door. But imagine if abortion could be a truly private matter. Say, something as easy as visiting a doctor, getting a few pills, returning home to swallow them, then checking back a few days later to make sure that all went as planned.

Science and politics are now conspiring to make that scenario—scary to some, a godsend to others—a reality, one that could allow abortion to be a truly private decision, albeit still not an easy one. Doctors have reported on a pivotal breakthrough in the use of the controversial French abortion drug known as RU 486: a woman who takes the drug will no longer have to go to a clinic for a follow-up injection to induce contractions. Instead, the entire procedure will involve simply taking two sets of pills. Concurrently, President Clinton has firmly signaled a willingness to reconsider the policies of the Reagan and Bush Administrations, which barred RU 486 from the U.S.

> "This new regimen is simpler and potentially allows greater privacy than any other abortion method."
>
> —Dr. Etienne-Emile Baulieu, Inventor of RU 486

The resulting social upheaval could transform one of the nation's most divisive political debates by making abortion far more difficult to regulate. And eventually it could mean abortions will become simpler, safer and more accessible not only throughout the U.S. but also around the world.

Dr. Etienne-Emile Baulieu, the inventor of RU 486, and his French colleagues describe the successful tests of the no-injection method in the *New England Journal of Medicine.* "This new regimen," they conclude, "is simpler and potentially allows greater privacy than any other abortion method." In a tough accompanying editorial, the *Journal* brands efforts to block use of the drug in the U.S. a "disgrace."

Those political barriers, however, are quickly crumbling. Two days after his Inauguration, President Clinton ordered his Administration to "promote the testing, licensing and manufacturing" of RU 486. Until then, the French manufacturer of the drug, Roussel Uclaf, and its German parent company, Hoechst AG, had steadfastly shied away from becoming involved in the American market for fear of infuriating antiabortion activists. But in April, at the instigation of the U.S. Food and Drug Administration, Roussel announced a compromise: it agreed to license RU 486 to the U.S. Population Council, a nonprofit organization based in New York City, which in turn would run clinical tests.

As a result, the abortion pill could become available through a testing program later this year. The Oregon and New Hampshire legislatures have already volunteered their states as test sites, and the FDA is enthusiastic. Says commissioner David Kessler: "If there is a safe and effective medical alternative to a surgical procedure, then we believe it should be available in this country." Although testing a new drug generally takes seven to 10 years, RU 486 has been so widely used in France that U.S. approval could come in as little as two to three years. In the meantime, the testing will enable at least 2,000 women to use the pill.

These developments could change the nature of abortion and even of birth control by eventually permitting the widespread distribution of pills. Though the Supreme Court's *Roe v. Wade* decision of 1973 made abortion legal in the U.S., the ruling was rendered moot in some places by the dearth of doctors willing to perform the procedure and by the fervor of demonstrators who frightened women away from clinics. Now the battleground may shift to the FDA, drug manufacturers and state legislatures.

> "When they invent new ways to kill children, we will invent new ways to save them."
>
> —The Rev. Keith Tucci, Operation Rescue National

"We will not allow anti-choice zealots to deny RU 486 to American women," vows Pamela Maraldo, president of the Planned Parenthood Federation of America. The pro-life forces are no less determined. "When they invent new ways to kill children, we will invent new ways to save them," warns the Rev. Keith Tucci of Operation Rescue National. A coalition of antiabortion forces has scheduled a demonstration in front of the French embassy in Washington on June 18, just three days before Roussel Uclaf holds its annual meeting in Paris.

THE ABORTION DRUG HAS BEEN A source of controversy ever since its invention was announced in 1982 by Baulieu, a French physician who worked as a researcher at Roussel Uclaf. The concept was rather simple: RU 486, an antiprogestin, could break a fertilized egg's bond to the uterine wall and thus induce a miscarriage. An injection two days later of prostaglandin, a hormone-like substance, would force uterine contractions and speed the ejection of the embryo. It took six more years and tests on more than 17,000 women before the French government announced that RU 486 would be made available for public use.

The news spawned furious reaction in the press, an outpouring of outraged letters from Roman Catholic doctors, and a church-sponsored protest through the streets of Paris. A month later, a shaken Roussel Uclaf yanked the drug from the market, saying the company did not want to engage in a "moral debate."

Doctors around the world certainly did. Thousands of physicians had convened that month at a medical congress in Rio de Janeiro, and most of them signed a petition demanding that the French government reverse Roussel's decision. Within 48 hours, Health Minister Claude Evin declared that once government approval had been granted, "RU 486 became the moral property of women," and he ordered Roussel to resume distribution. In 1989 RU 486 was made available to all licensed abortion clinics and hospitals in France. The results proved encouraging, save for a freak incident in 1991 when a woman who was an avid smoker suffered a heart attack while trying to use RU 486 to abort her 13th pregnancy. After that mishap, the government banned use of the pill by heavy smokers and women age 35 and older, who have a greater than usual risk of complications.

Using RU 486 was less painful, carried less risk of infection and gave women greater control over the process than a surgical procedure. Over the next 3½ years, 100,000 Frenchwomen used it successfully. Of those who made the decision early enough, about 85% chose RU 486 over surgery. (The pill is currently used in France only within seven weeks of the first day of a woman's last menstrual period; there is now talk of extending usage to a 10-week interval.) Almost all judged the method satisfactory.

Such promising results persuaded both Sweden and Britain to license RU 486; India is testing the drug. China is manufacturing clones that as yet are not widely available. Other countries, most notably Canada, are waiting for the U.S. to take the lead. "The U.S. is the leader in advanced research, the main source of development funds and the heart of worldwide networks that can allow RU 486 to help women everywhere," explains Baulieu.

HOW RU 486 WORKS

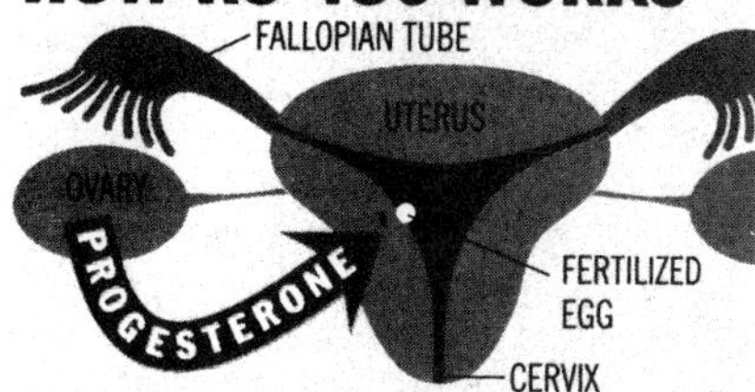

Progesterone, a hormone produced by the ovaries, is necessary for the implantation and development of a fertilized egg.

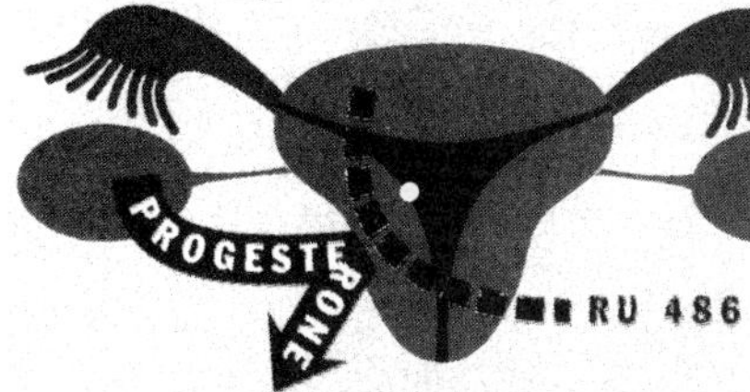

Taken early in pregnancy RU 486 blocks the action of progesterone and makes the body react as if it isn't pregnant.

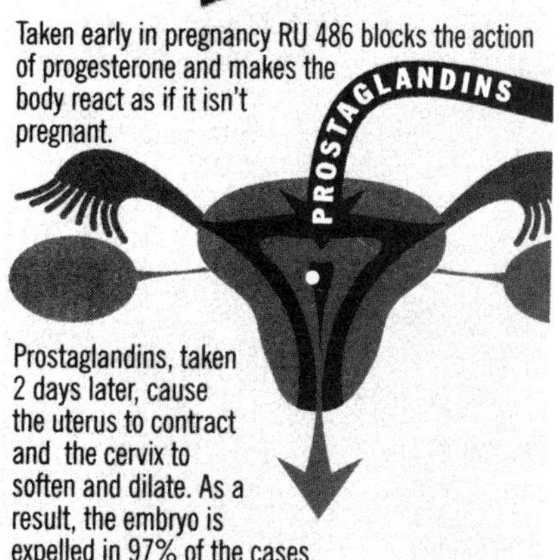

Prostaglandins, taken 2 days later, cause the uterus to contract and the cervix to soften and dilate. As a result, the embryo is expelled in 97% of the cases.

In 1991 the French began testing the new method of using RU 486 that does not require going to a clinic for a follow-up shot. An oral prostaglandin, commercially marketed as Cytotec by the American manufacturer G.D. Searle, enabled women to abort simply by swallowing a combination of pills. The efficiency rate rose from 95.5% to 96.9%, and the speed of the procedure improved. In 61% of the cases, the uterine contents were expelled within four hours after taking Cytotec, in contrast to 47% in the case of prostaglandin injections. Although there were instances of nausea and diarrhea, which are also common side effects with injections, those who took the pills reported considerably less pain. "Women tolerate it much better," says Dr. Elisabeth Aubeny of the Broussais Hospital in Paris, a testing ground for RU 486 in 1984. For French taxpayers, who foot 80% of the bill for each abortion through their national health-care system, there is also an advantage: a dose of Cytotec costs only 72¢, vs. $22 for the prostaglandin shot.

Once again, controversy erupted. When Baulieu first began experimenting with RU 486 in combination with an oral prostaglandin, Roussel balked. As a result, Baulieu had to persuade French public health officials to defray insurance costs. After preliminary trials, the government compelled Roussel to participate, arguing that the proposed testing of an oral prostaglandin was important for women. Although Searle raised no objections, its executives remain uncomfortable about being linked to the abortion business. "Searle has never willingly made [Cytotec] available for use in abortion," a company official wrote in a letter to the *Wall Street Journal* in February. "It is not Searle's intention or desire to become embroiled in the abortion issue." Searle's reservations echo that of Hoechst president Wolfgang Hilger, who has been open about his ethical objections to RU 486.

The uses of RU 486 could extend well beyond dealing with some of the 37 million abortions carried out around the globe each year. European studies have shown that it is an effective morning-after pill, inducing less nausea or vomiting than other drugs used for the same purpose. There are also indications that RU 486 can combat endometriosis, a leading cause of female infertility, and fibroid tumors, a condition that often necessitates hysterectomy. Thus the same drug that can help some women end unwanted pregnancies may enable others to bear children. Assorted studies have found that RU 486 may also combat breast cancer and Cushing's syndrome, a life-threatening metabolic disorder.

Despite the many potential uses for RU 486 and its effectiveness as an abortion method, efforts to legalize it in the U.S. have met with repeated failure. Last year a pro-choice group called Abortion Rights Mobilization decided to force a court challenge of the import ban imposed on RU 486 by the Bush Administration in 1989. The organization helped Leona Benten, a pregnant 29-year-old California social worker, fly to England, obtain a dose of RU 486, then try to bring it into the U.S. through New York City's Kennedy Airport. Customs officials seized the pills. The ensuing legal battle went up to the Supreme Court, which refused to order the government to return the pills. Benten subsequently had a surgical abortion.

The Clinton Administration has not yet revoked the ban, but its significance is minor. Because distribution of the pills is tightly controlled in Europe and they cannot easily be purchased and imported, the real issue is how quickly the Administration will encourage the manufacture and marketing of the drug in the U.S.

When the pill does become available in America, abortion will not be as easy as going to the doctor and taking some of the tablets home—at least not right away. In

France, for instance, a woman is required to pay four visits over a three-week period to one of the country's 800 licensed clinics or hospitals. The first step is a gynecological exam. Doctors make sure the pregnancy is in its early stages, and a social worker or psychologist discusses with her the decision to abort. Then the woman is sent home for a weeklong "reflection" period.

When she returns, she is required to sign a government form requesting the abortion. She must also sign a Roussel form that confirms her understanding that a malformed fetus might result if she does not see the abortion through to completion. (As yet no defects have been found in the small number of babies born to women known to have taken RU 486.) At that point, the woman is given three aspirin-like RU 486 tablets, each containing 200 mg of the drug. After swallowing the pills, she again goes home.

Except in the rare instance where the RU 486 is enough to induce a quick abortion, the woman must take two 200-mg Cytotec pills within the next 48 hours. Because the timing is critical and doctors want to monitor the effects of this contraction-inducing drug, women are required to return to the clinic. They are encouraged to remain for four hours, even if the expulsion happens earlier. Eight to 10 days later, they must pay a final visit for an exam to make sure no part of the egg remains.

Even with all these steps, the procedure seems blessedly simple to most women. "Taking a pill seems far less murderous and violent to the child than using a vacuum cleaner," says a 31-year-old woman who has had both types of abortion. "You feel so helpless when they put you to sleep and you know they're going to be using their tubes and knives on you." Some women, however, become traumatized by the thought of performing an abortion with their own hand. After her experience with RU 486, Joelle Mevel, 34, vows that if there is a next time, she will choose surgery. "I spent the whole time worrying that I would see the child in the basin, that I would be able to discern something human in the blood," she says. "I would rather have gone to sleep and awakened later knowing it was all over."

American abortion-rights advocates talk of boiling France's time-consuming RU 486 procedure down to just two visits to the doctor. It would be possible, though controversial, for the government to let RU 486 be administered in any doctor's office or possibly even by trained nurse practitioners. If that happened, many women could avoid running a gauntlet of protesters outside an abortion clinic. Still, it won't take all the anguish out of the procedure. "It's insulting to women to say that abortion now will be as easy as taking aspirins," says Baulieu. "It is always difficult, psychologically and physically, sometimes tragic."

—Reported by
J. Madeleine Nash/Chicago, Frederick Painton/Paris, Janice C. Simpson/New York and Tala Skari/Paris

IT'S NOT JUST AIDS

UNINFORMED AND MISINFORMED, TEENS FACE AN EPIDEMIC OF SEXUALLY TRANSMITTED DISEASES.

William L. Bergman, M.D.

William L. Bergman, M.D., is the medical director of Hahnemann Health Associates in New York and president of the World Medical Health Foundation.

While the sexually transmitted disease (STD) epidemic is a terrifying reality, in many ways it is a silent epidemic. In the privacy of their offices, doctors are seeing large numbers of STD patients. This new epidemic is a result of the increase in promiscuity that began with the sexual revolution of the 1960s.

One in five Americans between the ages of fifteen and fifty-five is infected with a sexually transmitted disease; 63 percent of the newly infected are under twenty-five.

As pointed out by Dr. Joe McIlhaney, Jr., president for Sexual Health, teenagers tend to think that STDs have always been around in the same numbers they are today. Looking at their parents' generation, who they know from accounts of the sixties have had multiple sexual partners, they may think that these older folk do not look like they were hurt by having sex as single people.

What the younger generation does not realize is that the older generation was not as likely to be infected with STDs as people are today. Centers for Disease Control (CDC) statistics reveal that one in five Americans between the ages of fifteen and fifty-five are infected with an STD, with 63 percent of the newly infected people under twenty-five years of age. The enormous increase in STD infection and of serious STDs makes it dangerous for anyone, especially young people, to have sex outside of marriage.

TRACKING THE INCREASE

Before 1960, syphilis and gonorrhea were the only important STDs, and the existing strains were easily treated. Today, however, Americans face over twenty significant STDs—some fatal, a few relatively harmless, but all contributing to the problem. It is estimated that twelve million people in the United States become infected each year.

The spread of STDs is alarming. In 1976, chlamydia was first reported; now it is the most common STD in the United States. In 1981, HIV was identified; today, between 1 and 1.5 million Americans are estimated to be infected and, in 1992, there were 140,000 deaths. Infection in the teenage population is increasing dramatically. In 1984, herpes became common, and today over thirty million Americans are infected with that virus. In 1985, we began to see an increasing incidence of human papilloma virus (HPV), which causes genital warts and cancers in both sexes.

In 1990, there was a 400 percent increase in the rate of tubal ectopic pregnancy. Not all tubal pregnancies are caused by STDs, but the huge increase is importantly the result of the rising rate of pelvic inflammatory disease (PID), which comes from chlamydia and gonorrhea. Scarred fallopian tubes caused by PID block the passage of fertilized eggs to the uterus; the growing embryo causes the tube to rupture. The April 1989 *Female Patient* reported that teens have the highest death rate from tubal ectopic pregnancy, which also can increase the incidence of infertility and subsequent tubal pregnancies. PID is painful and is the most common cause of hospitalization for women between the ages of fifteen and fifty-five, next to pregnancy.

This article appeared in *The World & I*, October 1993, pp. 151-161. Reprinted with permission from *The World & I*, a publication of The Washington Times Corporation. © 1993.

YOUNG AT GREATER RISK

One reason teens are vulnerable is that people are likely to have more sexual partners the earlier they start having sex, according to a January 1991 study by the CDC.

OB/GYN reported in August 1990 that the lining of the cervix of a teenage girl produces extra mucus that nourishes STDs. As women reach their twenties or have babies, that lining is replaced by a tougher one. Also, during the first two years of menstrual periods, 50 percent occur without ovulation, making the cervical mucus more liquid and a better medium for disease-producing microorganisms.

A recent survey of high school students reveals that knowledge about AIDS or HIV infection and its prevention is not associated with any change in risk behavior.

Contraception (vol. 41, 1990) reports that women are more likely to have chlamydia or gonorrhea-induced PID if they begin having sex early. *Texas Medicine* (1987) reports that teens with PID are more difficult to treat than older patients. Teens have a 14 percent chance of not responding well to antibiotics and requiring major surgery involving the removal of the uterus, tubes, and ovaries. While most women survive tubal ectopic pregnancy, 70 percent who have never had a baby before their ectopic pregnancy will be infertile.

Medical Aspects of Human Sexuality (July 1990) states that "adolescent females appear to be at higher risk for HPV infection than most adult populations. Rates of HPV infection among teenage girls have been reported as high as 40 percent compared with 2 percent to 15 percent among adult women." *Pediatrics* reported in 1988 that teenagers are more likely to have precancerous and cancerous growths resulting from HPV than are adults with the same infection.

To what extent are STDs treatable? Chlamydia and gonorrhea can be cured by antibiotics, but after the microorganisms are killed, scars remain that can cause infertility, ectopic pregnancy, and pelvic pain. In 1990, penicillin-resistant strains of gonorrhea were identified in all fifty states; they can be cured, but only by fairly expensive drugs. Often, patients' inability to comply in taking prescribed medicine results in failure to successfully treat those disease for which there is a cure.

In 1990, syphilis, which is easy to diagnose and 100 percent sensitive to penicillin, reached a forty-year high. Babies are once again being born with syphilis. HIV, which causes AIDS, is, unlike syphilis, a very complex virus that mutates rapidly. The spread of syphilis indicates that any HIV cure may be only temporary if people continue their present sexual behavior.

SEXUAL 'LIBERATION'

What predisposing causes underlie our present patterns of sexual activity?

In the sixties, through an increase in social rebellion, alcohol, drugs, and free sex were increasingly condoned. "Sexual liberation" was justified as a kind of new morality: the idea that people were no longer bound or restricted by the traditional ethical standards of the past. Among the fast-breaking technological advances were new contraceptives that severed the link between sexual intercourse and procreation. In this environment, the sexual revolution was born. The idea that teenage sexual activity was inevitable was increasingly accepted. The popular culture, especially the entertainment industry, encouraged it.

The outcome was a kind of self-fulfilling prophecy in which the results reflected the expectations. With the widespread acceptance of the inevitability of premarital sexual activity, contraceptive-based sex education was embraced by many as a necessity.

A Harris poll found that after comprehensive sex ed emphasizing condoms, teens were 53 percent more likely to have intercourse than those whose sex ed did not discuss contraceptives.

As a result, in the early 1970s federal dollars began flowing into contraceptive approaches. Clinics were opened under Title X to provide birth control to teenagers as well as others. The problem was defined as teen pregnancy and STD, rather than as adolescent premarital sexual activity itself.

CONDOM EDUCATION FAILS

America now has a track record of approximately twenty years of contraceptive-based sex education, where the emphasis has been on knowledge about sexuality, contraceptive methods, and STDs (including HIV). However, during the period in which this knowledge has been disseminated, sexual activity has increased dramatically, and, with it, pregnancy rates and STDs.

A 1989 health risk survey of secondary school students states, "Responses show that nearly all students knew the two main modes of HIV transmission—intravenous drug use and sexual intercourse." *Pediatrics* (May 1992) states, "Knowledge about AIDS or HIV infection and its prevention was not associated with any change in risk behavior, nor were the number of sources of information about the epidemic, acquaintance with those who were infected, estimates of personal risk, or exposure to HIV test counseling."

A 1986 Harris poll reported that only 14 percent of sexually active teens not using contraceptives said they were not using protection due to a lack of knowledge or access. Clearly, knowledge alone has not been very useful in terms of actually making a difference in teenage sexual behavior. Similarly, a study of fourteen nationwide contraceptive-based sex education programs found that none had any impact in decreasing teen sexual involvement, as reported in *Sexuality Education and Evaluation of Programs and Their Effects* (Network Publications, Santa Cruz).

In Virginia, school districts that taught "comprehensive contraceptive-based sex education" experienced a 17.3 average percent increase in teen pregnancies, whereas school districts not offering such programs had a 15.8 average percent decrease, according to 1988 Virginia Department of Health statistics.

The April 1988 *American Journal of Public Health* reported that a study of condom education and distribution in San Francisco schools showed that a yearlong effort resulted in only 8 percent of males and 2 percent of females using condoms every time they had sex.

The overall pregnancy rate at a Dallas high school dispensing condoms was 1.47 times greater than the pregnancy rate at a similar school that did not (11.2 percent versus 7.6 percent), as reported in *Family Planning Perspectives* of January–February 1991.

In Adams High School in Commerce City, Colorado, which has had a condom distribution program since 1989, the pregnancy rate has risen 66 percent, to become 31 percent above the national average.

A Harris poll commissioned by Planned Parenthood in 1986 found that, after exposure to comprehensive sex education emphasizing condoms, teenagers were 53 percent more likely to have initiated intercourse than those whose sex education did not discuss contraceptives.

In spite of these appalling statistics, some still claim that we need to push the condom message even more and start introducing the message at earlier and earlier ages. This is advocated even though we have spent already about $2 billion on this type of education, which seems to have contributed to an increase in teen pregnancies and STDs.

PUSHING PLEASURE

Underlying assumptions of contraceptive-based sex education are that human nature is primarily sexual, that it is unnatural to sacrifice sexual desire, and that teens have a right to choose to be sexually active as long as they do it "properly."

In addition to advocating condoms, a goal of so-called protected sex education is to teach "outercourse," those sexual practices that are considered at low risk for HIV. Deborah Hafner, executive director of the Sex Information and Education Council of the United States (SIECUS), says, "We should teach teens about oral sex and mutual masturbation in order to help them delay the onset of sexual intercourse and its resulting consequences." But HIV can be transmitted during oral sex if infected semen, vaginal secretions, or blood enters the bloodstream of the partner through cuts or sores in the mouth. In a society in which public acceptance of unmarried teenagers having intercourse and confidence in condoms is high, it should be pointed out that "outercourse" also may stimulate the desire for intercourse rather than delay it.

Peggy Brick of Planned Parenthood emphasizes the importance of helping adolescents understand "pleasure, sexual satisfaction and gratification and orgasm," whether carried out in the context of marriage or not.

Based on this mind-set, the Pennsylvania Department of Education includes in its publication "I Deserve Love," from the *Pennsylvania Health Curriculum Guide*, the following passage:

> "My lovers now approve of each other. My mother and father approve of my sex life. My minister approves of my sex life. God approves of my sex life. Christ intended for me to have abundance. I have the right to have multiple sex partners. I do not need to hold back and save my orgasms for someone special. I want to experience them now. . . . Oral stimulation can be very effective and I am delighted about it. I have no resistance to trying oral and anal sex. I have the right to enjoy my own genitals."

The New York City Department of Health has a Teenagers' Bill of Rights, funded by the CDC and the City of New York, which states, "I have the right to think for myself, I have the right to decide whether to have sex and who to have it with."

When parents express reservations about this kind of so-called safer sex education, they are accused of wanting to censor information, possibly due to their own sexual repression.

CONDOM FAILURE RATES

Latex condoms can help prevent the transmission of HIV. However, a significant problem with the contraceptive model of sex education is that while condoms are promoted as protecting against HIV, other STDs, and pregnancy, the facts concerning the high rate of condom failure due to product defects and difficulty of use are often never mentioned. This is justified on the assumption that young people are inevitably going to be sexually active and that some protection is better than none.

This point of view is widely held within the public health community. The April 1993 *American Journal of Public Health* states,

> We should be able to agree that premature initiation of sexual activity carries health risks. Therefore, we must exercise leadership in encouraging young people to postpone sexual activity. Adolescents are bombarded with

> messages encouraging them to "do it." We need to strive for a climate supportive of young people who are not having sex and so help to create a new health-oriented social norm for adolescents and teenagers against sexuality. As we proceed toward this objective, we must be mindful that many will continue to engage in sexual activity. It is essential that these youngsters receive the message that they must practice safer sex and use condoms. The message that those who initiate or continue sexual activity must reduce their risk through correct and consistent condom use needs to be delivered as strongly and persuasively as the message "don't do it."

This approach is complicated by the fact that the risks in so-called protected sex are greater than is often admitted. Apart from moral considerations, why should teenagers be taught to abstain from sex until marriage? Because, quite simply, no other approach will sufficiently protect them. We need to look at the medical facts regarding condoms, since they are currently the centerpiece of educational policy with regard to HIV and other STDs.

Unless the sexually transmitted disease is localized directly beneath the condom, there is nothing separating the healthy teenager from the disease.

According to Dr. William R. Archer III, a former deputy assistant secretary for population affairs at the Department of Health and Human Services (HHS), "One out of three sexually active teenagers will acquire an STD before graduating from high school, and in most cases a condom would have done little to stop it. Condoms have an 18 percent failure rate for pregnancy for teenagers. Low-income adolescents, for reasons not fully understood, have a [much higher rate]. Studies suggest that condoms offer even less protection against STDs. A study which looked at a group of monogamous couples in which one partner was HIV positive found a 17 percent transmission rate of the virus at eighteen months, despite consistent use of a condom. Furthermore, many STDs can be passed by direct contact, even though the couple is using a condom. Unless the disease is localized directly beneath the condom, there is still nothing coming between the healthy teenager and direct contact with disease." Many STD sores are in areas of the genitals not covered by a condom.

A study at Rutgers University found that the rate of chlamydia transmission was exactly the same for couples using condoms as for those not using them.

Because of the mortal consequences of condom failure when one partner is HIV positive, it is crucial to understand how well condoms protect against the HIV virus. Consider that in pregnancy only the woman can become pregnant, but with HIV either partner can become infected. A woman is fertile approximately sixty days per year; HIV can be transmitted every day of the year.

Family Planning Perspectives (January–February 1992) expresses serious concerns regarding condoms. It reports "a sobering level of exposure to the risk of pregnancy and infection with HIV and other sexually transmitted diseases, even for those who most consistently use condoms."

A recent policy statement from the CDC entitled *Prevention of Heterosexual HIV Transmission: The Condom Strategy Reaffirmed* states that the partners of HIV-infected persons may consider the risk of transmission during sexual intercourse unacceptably high even if a condom *is* used:

> On the individual level, it means that the likelihood of acquiring HIV infection because of condom failure is largely dependent on the likelihood that the individual sexual partner is HIV-infected. Therefore, in the special circumstance in which one partner is known to be infected and the other is not, even the estimated 1 percent to 2 percent risk of condom failure [resulting from manufacture or product defect] may be unacceptably high. For this reason, persons in this category may be best advised to consider other expressions of intimacy and other methods of sexual gratification in lieu of intercourse even with condoms.

The April 1988 *Journal of the American Medical Association* reported, "Encouraging the use of condoms may in some circumstances even be harmful if it gives a false sense of security in a high-risk situation. . . . Instead of encouraging such couples where one partner is zero-positive to use condoms, the best advice may be that they should stop having vaginal intercourse."

In other words, authorities are saying that the level of risk is unacceptable if you know your partner is HIV-infected, yet somehow acceptable if you do not. If doctors will not recommend that an infected person or a person with an infected partner use a condom, how can this possibly be the basis of sound medical policy for America's youth?

MANY TEEN VIRGINS

According to studies done by the CDC and HHS, nearly half of all teens are virgins, and many others return to sexual inactivity. It is especially the sexually inactive teens who need to be supported in having made the optimum health choice.

If the schools teach so-called protected sex and the parents do not object, teenagers think they must be able to have sex safely because the adults in their lives are explaining how to do it or expecting them to do it. On the other hand, those students who, for whatever reason, are not sexually active may begin to feel abnormal if it appears that everyone expects them to be sexually active.

If contraceptive-based sex education is not effective, and even highly risky in an age of AIDS, what do we then do? What can be the basis for an effective approach?

A historical perspective may provide some clues. Over the period from 1970 to 1990, the rate of premarital sexual activity increased, except for a brief time in the early 1980s. What changes occurred then?

During that period, federal money going into contraceptive-based programs decreased, and federal funding for programs designed to teach adolescents to abstain from premarital sexual activity, the so-called Title XX funding, was instituted. During the mid and late 1980s, however, these policies were weakened or reversed. Why?

AIDS and the HIV crisis of the mid-1980s caused an increase in efforts to teach "safe" and then "safer" sex. Condoms were advocated as the solution, and, once again, funding for contraceptive sex education increased.

What, then, is the answer? An approach to sex education based on promoting abstinence from premarital sexual activity (that is, from the behavior that causes teen pregnancy and spreads HIV and other STDs) must be instituted. This approach can encourage attitudes that lead to marriage and the formation of stable families. We can teach single people that sex is a wonderful thing but that, like fire, it has a capacity for both constructive and destructive results. Almost all risk of STDs, including HIV, and all risk of out-of-wedlock pregnancy can be avoided by saving intercourse for marriage.

Abstinence education has achieved promising results. Americans need to acknowledge which approach has failed: contraceptive education or abstinence education.

But, some would argue, is teaching premarital abstinence realistic? Isn't it naive to propose delaying intercourse until one is older? About 50 percent of unmarried girls and 40 percent of unmarried boys aged fifteen through nineteen have not yet had intercourse. These people are practicing abstinence. Also, 83 percent of Japanese teenage girls are virgins, and 73 percent of America's highest achieving high school students never have had sexual intercourse. Saving sex for marriage was normal for most people until about thirty years ago and can become normal again.

Teens who have been sexually active can choose to stop. Secondary abstinence is based on the idea that people can start over. Teenagers can protect their health. It is never too late to start saying no to premarital sex.

ABSTINENCE POSSIBLE

What, then, of the track record of premarital abstinence programs? After the San Marcos, Texas, unified school district used the Teen AID abstinence program, reported pregnancies dropped from 147 to 20, an 88 percent reduction. Similar programs—Sex Respect, Best Friends, Free Teens—have shown very promising results.

Students who receive the Sex Respect curriculum show significant changes in attitude over the course of their participation. There are consistent increases in the extent to which students (grades seven through nine) feel that sex among unmarried teens is wrong and that teens who have had sex outside of marriage would benefit by deciding to stop and wait for marriage.

Americans need to look at which approach has failed. Federal funding for contraceptive education per year is approximately $150 million, as opposed to about $2 million for abstinence education, a seventy-five to one ratio. It is time for a new approach.

Even if a perfect mechanical technique were invented that would eliminate the risk of pregnancy, HIV, and other STDs, research indicates still more reasons to support teen abstinence. Having sex as a teenager is linked to the use of drugs, alcohol, and tobacco. The February 1991 issue of *Pediatrics* states: "It is essential for health providers to explore the issue of sexual activity and the other risk factors that are strongly linked to it in adolescence. Engaging in one activity significantly increases the risk for the others, which carry additional biological and psychosocial risk."

Should a teenager's decision to be sexually active be affirmed and supported by the meaningful adults in that young person's life because "it's their decision"? Would we affirm teenagers' decisions to use drugs or drop out of school simply because they decided?

Teaching abstinence fits with what we have learned about drug, alcohol, and tobacco education. When we showed teens drug paraphernalia and let them smell marijuana, student drug use went up. When we started teaching that they should not use drugs, alcohol, and tobacco, use of those substances went down. We gave the teenagers the benefit of adult knowledge, and they listened. The same approach will work for sex education.

Consumer Health

For many people the term "consumer health" conjures up images of selecting health care services and paying medical bills. While these two aspects of health care are consumer health issues, the term consumer health encompasses all consumer products and services that influence the health and welfare of people. The implications stemming from a definition this broad suggest that almost everything we see or do may be construed to be a consumer health issue. Such is the case with media coverage of medical investigations. Over the last three years, millions of Americans have added food products that contain oat bran to their diets. Many of these same individuals have eliminated or are considering the elimination of oat bran products from their diets. Why? The answer is simple. They read reports claiming that oat bran could reduce blood cholesterol levels, and so they went out and bought products containing oat bran. When reports began to surface questioning the value of oat bran as a cholesterol reducer, many of these people stopped using it. The scenario that I have just described is typical of the way American consumers respond to media reports on issues of health. Interestingly enough, reports have once again begun to surface that reaffirm the value of oat bran as a cholesterol lowering agent, and consumers are once again purchasing oat bran products. Clearly, media reports such as this add to the confusion and fuel controversy, but they also sell newspapers, and that is, after all, a newspaper's bottom line. Anthony Schmitz explains why consumers should not believe everything they read in "Food News Blues." This essay provides the reader with some useful tips on how to spot front-page fallacies.

There are a number of government agencies in the United States that serve to protect Americans from consumer health fraud. The agencies and organizations involved in this aspect of consumer protection include the Food and Drug Administration (FDA), the Federal Trade Commission, the U.S. Postal Service, the Office of Consumer Education, the Office of Consumer Affairs, the Public Health Service, the National Institutes of Health, the Health Services Administration, and the Consumer Protection Agency. While these agencies play an active role in protecting the health of consumers, they are not able to keep pace with the number of products and services being marketed and sold. Remember, if the advertised claim sounds too good to be true, it probably is.

Of all the consumer health issues, the one that is the greatest source of confusion and controversy is nutrition. Over the past few years, numerous reports have been issued linking the typical American diet to both cancer and cardiovascular disease. On the basis of these reports, consumers have been encouraged to eat more fiber and reduce their intake of dietary fats, particularly saturated fats and cholesterol. The response of the food industry to these reports and recommendations has been a mixed bag. On the positive side, they have introduced new products and modified their packaging so as to demonstrate their awareness of current dietary recommendations. On the negative side, many of the new products are only marginally better than their predecessors even though the labeling suggests otherwise. Some food manufacturers have even resorted to changing the suggested serving size as listed on the label so that their products appear more nutritionally sound. " 'Nutrition Facts': To Help Consumers Eat Smart" by Paula Kurtzweil discusses how the new labeling regulations will change the labeling format that appears on packaged goods. She also explains how this new format will serve as an educational tool that will help consumers evaluate food products in terms of their own diets.

On November 6, 1991 the Food and Drug Administration, in conjunction with the U.S. Department of Agriculture (USDA), announced proposed changes to existing food labeling laws that for 20 years have confused and deceived the American public. This announcement was unique in that the USDA, which regulates labeling on products such as raw and processed meats and poultry, hot dogs, luncheon meats, and convenience foods that contain meat, for the first time is adhering to the labeling guidelines set forth by the FDA. The new guidelines, which took effect in May 1993, include the following categories: (1) *Health Claims*—are limited to only four areas and these include messages about calcium and osteoporosis, fat and cardiovascular disease, fat and cancer, and salt and hypertension; (2) *Descriptors*—phrases used to describe a product's nutritional level are limited to a list of 22 words selected and clearly defined by the FDA. Under the new guidelines words such as "lite" or "light," regardless of spelling, can only mean reduced calorie and not refer to color, flavor, or texture. Any descriptive term not defined when the regulation went into effect is deemed illegal; (3) *Serving Size*—the serving size is standardized for 131 foods and includes measurements in metric units; (4) *Nutrients*—all product labels must disclose the total calories, calories from fat, protein, and carbohydrate, as well as the information regarding the total amount of fat, saturated fat, cholesterol, dietary fiber, sodium, calcium, vitamins A and C. The labels must also indicate how a particular product meets the "Daily Values" (Daily Values replaced the old RDAs). It should be noted that these rules will apply to all processed foods, but

Unit 9

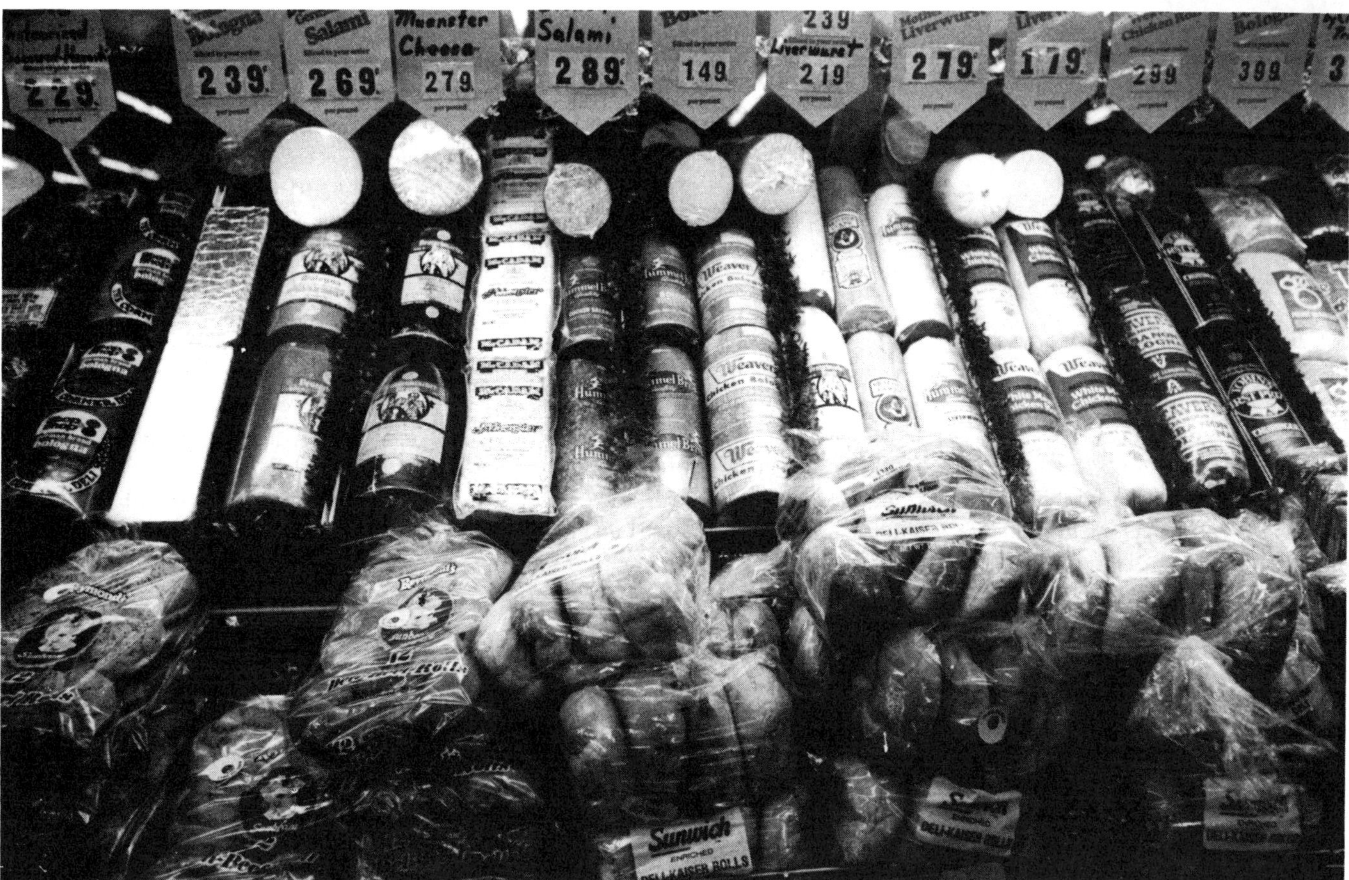

the labeling of fresh meat and poultry will be voluntary.

Despite all the new regulations governing the labeling of processed foods, few regulations exist governing the seafood industry. This lack of regulations has resulted in questionable food handling practices and poor quality control standards. It is ironic that the food industry that has the least amount of regulations governing it, and a high potential for contamination, should be the one we are encouraged to turn to for a supply of fresh fish. In "Something Fishy," Mark Roman examines the seafood industry and discusses why this industry needs tighter controls. He also provides several suggestions for selecting, storing, and cooking fish and shellfish that will preserve their freshness and reduce spoilage.

Other consumer health issues covered by this unit include buying, storing, and using condoms to prevent the spread of AIDS; helpful tips and information about selecting sunscreens and sunglasses; and tips on how individuals can feel in control of their disease rather than allowing the disease to control them. This unit is by no means exhaustive of all the possible topics that could be classified as consumer health issues, but it does demonstrate the diversity of topics that are truly consumer health issues.

Looking Ahead: Challenge Questions

Why should one question the validity of health-related information reported by the media?

What steps could be taken to eliminate deceptive advertising among food manufacturers? What should be done to those found guilty of deceptive advertising?

Is the government doing enough to protect the consumer? If not, what recommendations would you make for changes?

What steps can you take to ensure that the seafood you buy is safe and fresh?

What factors should be considered when purchasing sunscreens and sunglasses?

'Nutrition Facts'

To Help Consumers Eat Smart

Paula Kurtzweil

Paula Kurtzweil is a member of FDA's public affairs staff.

Susan Thom, of Parma, Ohio, knows how important it is for people to know the number of calories from fat they eat each day.

As a registered dietitian, she counsels patients on the need to limit fat consumption to 30 percent or less of total daily calories. As a person with diabetes, and thus at increased risk for heart disease, she strives to do the same for herself.

But, in the past, obtaining that information from the food label has required some mathematical skill—namely, multiplying the total grams (g) of fat in a serving by 9, since 1 g of fat contains 9 calories.

"It does take time," Thom said. "But if you want to feed yourself well, you have to look at the label."

Help is on the way. For Thom and millions of other Americans who seek to restrict their fat intake to recommended levels, a new dietary component is being added to the food label—"calories from fat."

It's just one of many new items of diet-related information manufacturers are required to offer on their food products by 1994. There also will be information on saturated fat, cholesterol, dietary fiber, and other nutrients that relate to today's health concerns, such as heart disease, cancer, and other diseases linked, at least in part, to diet.

There will be more complete nutrient content information because almost all the required nutrients will have to be listed as a percent of the Daily Value. There will be more uniform serving sizes, too, which will make nutritional comparisons between foods easier. And, because nutrition labeling is now mandatory for almost all processed foods, there will be a lot more products with this important information.

"The new information is going to be very helpful for consumers," said Virginia Wilkening, a registered dietitian in FDA's Office of Food Labeling.

"Some of the nutrients—saturated fat and cholesterol—have been allowed on the label before but on a voluntary basis," she said. "Dietary fiber and sugars were not allowed in the nutrition label. With the new label, consumers will soon have information about these and other nutrients, which can help them choose their foods more wisely."

The new requirements for nutrition labeling are spelled out in regulations issued in January 1993 by FDA and the U.S. Department of Agriculture's Food Safety and Inspection Service (FSIS). FDA's regulations meet the provisions of the Nutrition Labeling and Education Act of 1990 (NLEA), which, among other things, requires FDA to make nutrition labeling mandatory for almost all processed foods. FSIS' regulations, which cover meat and poultry products, largely parallel FDA's. (Meat and poultry products were not covered by NLEA.)

FDA has set May 8, 1994, as the date by which food manufacturers must comply with the new nutrition labeling regulations. FSIS requires meat and poultry processors to relabel their products by July 6, 1994. However, some newly labeled products may begin appearing in grocery stores much sooner than the deadlines.

Dietary Components

What can consumers expect? First, they will see a new name for the nutrition panel. It used to go by "Nutrition Information Per Serving." Now, it will be called "Nutrition Facts." That title will

Old Label

NUTRITION INFORMATION	PER SERVING	PERCENTAGE OF U.S. RECOMMENDED DAILY ALLOWANCES (U.S. RDA)	
SERVING SIZE	5 OZ.	PROTEIN	10
SERVINGS PER CONTAINER	4	VITAMIN A	*
CALORIES	250	VITAMIN C	*
PROTEIN	9g	THIAMINE	8
CARBOHYDRATE	19g	RIBOFLAVIN	15
FAT	11g	NIACIN	2
SODIUM	530mg	CALCIUM	20
		IRON	4

*CONTAINS LESS THAN 2% OF THE U.S. RDA OF THIS NUTRIENT

Starting this year, the 'old' nutrition label format above will be replaced by the one on the right. Both labels are for a frozen macaroni and cheese product.

From *FDA Consumer,* May 1993, pp. 22-27. Reprinted by permission of *FDA Consumer,* the magazine of the U.S. Food and Drug Administration.

Key Aspects of the New Nutrition Label

A number of consumer studies conducted by FDA, as well as outside groups, enabled FDA and the Food Safety and Inspection Service of the U.S. Department of Agriculture to agree on a new nutrition label. The new label is seen as offering the best opportunity to help consumers make informed food choices and to understand how a particular food fits into the total daily diet.

New heading signals a new label. →

More consistent serving sizes, in both household and metric measures, replace those that used to be set by manufacturers. →

Nutrients required on nutrition panel are those most important to the health of today's consumers, most of whom need to worry about getting too much of certain items (fat, for example), rather than too few vitamins or minerals, as in the past. →

Conversion guide helps consumers learn caloric value of the energy-producing nutrients. →

Nutrition Facts

Serving Size 1 cup (228g)
Servings Per Container 2

Amount Per Serving

Calories 260 Calories from Fat 120

	% Daily Value*
Total Fat 13g	**20%**
Saturated Fat 5g	**25%**
Cholesterol 30mg	**10%**
Sodium 660mg	**28%**
Total Carbohydrate 31g	**10%**
Dietary Fiber 0g	**0%**
Sugars 5g	
Protein 5g	

Vitamin A 4% • Vitamin C 2%
Calcium 15% • Iron 4%

* Percent Daily Values are based on a 2,000 calorie diet. Your daily values may be higher or lower depending on your calorie needs:

	Calories:	2,000	2,500
Total Fat	Less than	65g	80g
Sat Fat	Less than	20g	25g
Cholesterol	Less than	300mg	300mg
Sodium	Less than	2,400mg	2,400mg
Total Carbohydrate		300g	375g
Dietary Fiber		25g	30g

Calories per gram:
Fat 9 • Carbohydrate 4 • Protein 4

← **New mandatory component helps consumers meet dietary guidelines recommending no more than 30 percent of calories from fat.**

← **%Daily Value shows how a food fits into the overall daily diet.**

← **Reference values help consumers learn good diet basics. They can be adjusted, depending on a person's calorie needs.**

Types of Labels

A tabular format label (top) is allowed on packages, such as this can of tuna, that have less than 40 square inches for nutrition labeling. A simplified nutrition label (bottom), in which information about some nutrients otherwise required in nutrition labeling is omitted, will appear on labels of foods, such as this can of cola, that do not contain significant amounts of certain nutrients.

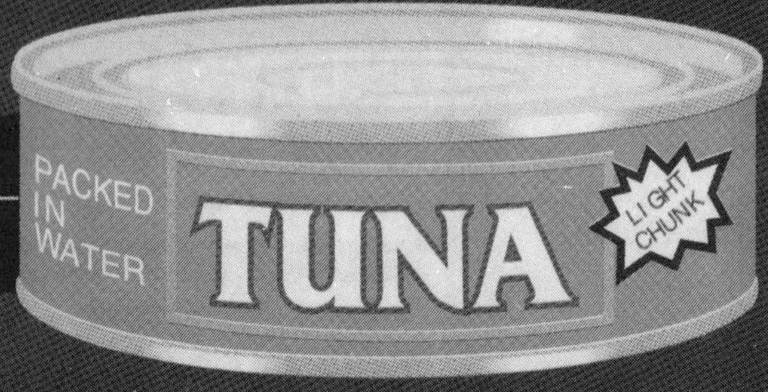

Nutrition Facts	Amount/serving	% DV*	Amount/serving	% DV*
Serv. Size 1/3 cup (56g)	**Total Fat** 1g	**2**%	**Total Carb.** 0g	**0**%
Servings about 3	Sat.Fat 0g	**0**%	Fiber 0g	**0**%
Calories 80	**Cholest.** 10mg	**3**%	Sugars 0g	
Fat Cal. 10	**Sodium** 200mg	**8**%	**Protein** 17g	
*Percent Daily Values (DV) are based on a 2,000 calorie diet.	Vitamin A 0% • Vitamin C 0% • Calcium 0% • Iron 6%			

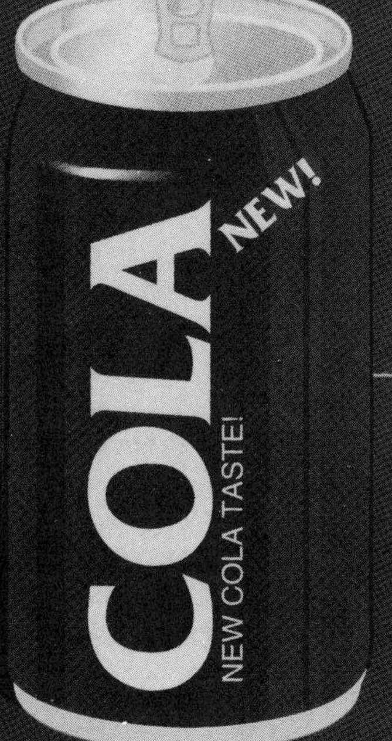

Nutrition Facts	
Serving Size 1 can (360 mL)	
Amount Per Serving	
Calories 140	
	% Daily Value*
Total Fat 0g	**0**%
Sodium 20mg	**1**%
Total Carbohydrate 36g	**12**%
Sugars 36 g	
Protein 0g	**0**%
* Percent Daily Values are based on a 2,000 calorie diet.	

signal to consumers that the product is newly labeled according to FDA and FSIS' new regulations.

The new panel will be built around a new set of dietary components. (See graphic, page 219.) The mandatory (underlined) and voluntary dietary components and order in which they must appear are:

- total calories
- calories from fat
- calories from saturated fat
- total fat
- saturated fat
- stearic acid (on meat and poultry products only)
- polyunsaturated fat
- monounsaturated fat
- cholesterol
- sodium
- potassium
- total carbohydrate
- dietary fiber
- soluble fiber
- insoluble fiber
- sugars
- sugar alcohol (for example, the sugar substitutes xylitol, mannitol and sorbitol)
- other carbohydrate (the difference between total carbohydrate and the sum of dietary fiber, sugars, and sugar alcohol, if declared)
- protein
- vitamin A
- percent of vitamin A present as beta-carotene
- vitamin C
- calcium
- iron
- other essential vitamins and minerals.

If a food is fortified or enriched with any of the optional components, or if a claim is made about any of them, the pertinent nutrition information then becomes mandatory.

These mandatory and voluntary components are the only ones allowed on the nutrition panel. The listing of single amino acids, maltodextrin, calories from polyunsaturated fat, and calories from carbohydrate, for example, may not appear on the label.

The reason, according to Wilkening, is to help consumers focus on nutrients of public health significance. "Too much additional information could clutter the label or mislead or confuse the consumer," she said.

Nutrients required on the label, she pointed out, reflect current public health concerns and coincide with current public health recommendations. She noted that the order in which the food components and nutrients are required to appear reflects their public health significance and the order in which they were specified in NLEA.

On the new food label, the listing of thiamin, riboflavin and niacin will not be mandatory. Under the old nutrition labeling program, these vitamins were required to be listed. But because deficiencies of these are no longer a public health problem in this country, listing them is now optional.

New Format

Consumers also will see a new format, one that calls for many of the macronutrients (such as fat, cholesterol, sodium, carbohydrate, and protein) to be declared as a percent of the Daily Value—a new label reference value. The amount, in grams or milligrams per serving, of these nutrients still must be listed to their immediate right. But, for the first time, a column headed "%Daily Value" will appear.

According to Wilkening, the percent declaration of the Daily Value offers an advantage over amount declaration: The percent Daily Values put the nutrients on an equal footing in the context of a total daily diet.

For example, she said, a food is low in sodium if it has less than 140 mg of sodium. "But people look at that number, 140, and think it's a tremendous amount, when it actually is less than 6 percent of the Daily Value."

On the other hand, she said, a food with 5 g of saturated fat could be construed as being low in that nutrient just because 5 is a small number. Actually, that food would provide one-fourth the total Daily Value of 20 g of saturated fat for a 2,000-calorie diet.

"People are affected by the size of numbers," she said. "That's why percentages are helpful. They put all of the nutrients on a level playing field."

The percent Daily Value listing will carry a footnote stating that the percentages are based on a 2,000-calorie diet and that a person's individual dietary goal is based on his or her calorie needs. Some nutrition labels—at least those on larger packages—will list daily values for selected nutrients for a 2,000- and a 2,500-calorie diet and the number of calories per gram of fat, carbohydrate and protein. The calorie conversion information is required as a general guide about the caloric contributions of fat, carbohydrate and protein.

The content of micronutrients—that is, vitamins and minerals—will continue to be expressed as a percent, although the term "Daily Value" will replace "U.S. Recommended Daily Allowance."

Modifications

Some foods will carry a variation of this format. For example, the label of foods for children under 2 (except infant formula, which is exempt from nutrition labeling under NLEA) will not carry information about calories from fat, calories from saturated fat, saturated fat, polyunsaturated fat, monounsaturated fat, and cholesterol.

The reason, according to Wilkening, is to prevent parents from inadvertently assuming that infants and toddlers should restrict their fat intake, when in fact, they should not. Fat is important during this life stage, she said, to ensure adequate growth and development.

The labels of food for children under 4 cannot include percentages of Daily Values for macronutrients, except protein, nor any footnote information, including the lists of Daily Values for selected nutrients. The reason: Other than protein, FDA has not established Daily Values for macronutrients for this age group. The percent Daily Values for vitamins and minerals is allowed, however. The content of the other nutrients must be expressed as an amount by weight in a separate column to the right of the macronutrients.

Other foods may qualify for a simplified label format. (See bottom label, page 220.) This format is allowed when the food contains insignificant amounts of seven or more of the mandatory dietary components, including total calories. "Insignificant" means that a declaration of "zero" could be made in nutrition labeling or, for total carbohydrate, dietary fiber, and protein, a declaration of "less than 1 g."

For foods for children under 2, the simplified format may be used if the product contains insignificant amounts of six or more of the following: calories, total fat, sodium, total carbohydrate, dietary fiber, sugars, protein, vitamins A and C, calcium, and iron.

When the simplified format is used, information on total calories, total fat, total carbohydrate, protein, and sodium—even if they are present in insignificant amounts—must be listed. Calories from fat and other nutrients must be listed if they are present in more than insignificant amounts. Nutrients added to the food must be listed, too.

Serving Sizes

Whatever the format, the serving size remains the basis for reporting each nutrient's amount. However, unlike in the past, serving sizes now will be more uniform and closer to the amounts that many people actually eat. They also must be expressed in both common household and metric measures. (See accompanying table.)

Before, the serving size was up to the discretion of the food manufacturer. As a result, said Youngmee Park, Ph.D., a nutritionist in FDA's Office of Special Nutritionals, serving sizes often varied widely, making it difficult for consumers to compare nutritional qualities of similar products or to determine the nutrient content of the amount of food they normally ate.

The uniformity also is important, she said, for giving consistency to health claims and words describing nutrient content, such as "high fiber" and "reduced fat."

FDA and FSIS define serving size as the amount of food customarily eaten at one time. It is based on FDA- and USDA-established lists of "Reference Amounts Customarily Consumed Per Eating Occasion."

These reference amounts, which are part of the new regulations, are broken down into 139 FDA-regulated food product categories, including 11 groups of foods for children under 4, and 23 USDA meat and poultry product categories. They list the amounts of food customarily consumed per eating occasion for each food category, based primarily on national food consumption surveys. FDA's list also gives the suggested label statement for serving size declaration.

For example, the category "breads (excluding sweet quick type), rolls" has a reference amount of 50 g, and the appropriate label statement for sliced bread is "__ piece(s) __ (g)" or, for unsliced bread, "2 oz (56 g/__ inch slice)."

The serving size of products that come in discrete units, such as cookies, candy bars, and sliced products, is the number of whole units that most closely approximates the reference amount. For example, cookies have a reference amount of 30 g. The household measure closest to that amount is the number of cookies that comes closest to weighing 30 g. Thus, the serving size on the label of a cookie package in which each cookie weighs 13 g would read "2 cookies (26 g)."

Metric Conversion Chart

Units as they will appear for serving sizes on label

Household Measure	Metric Measure
1 tsp	5 mL
1 tbsp	15 mL
1 cup	240 mL
1 fl oz	30 mL
1 oz	28 g

tsp = teaspoon
tbsp = tablespoon
fl oz = fluid ounce
oz = ounce
mL = milliliter
g = gram

If one unit weighs more than 50 percent but less than 200 percent of the reference amount, the serving size is one unit. For example, the reference amount for bread is 50 g; therefore, the label of a loaf of bread in which each slice weighs more than 25 g would state that a serving size is one slice.

For food products packaged and sold individually, if an individual package is less than 200 percent of the applicable reference amount, the item qualifies as one serving. Thus, a 360-milliliter (mL) (12 fluid-ounce) can of soda is one serving because the reference amount for carbonated beverages is 240 mL (8 fluid ounces).

However, if the product has a reference amount of 100 g or 100 mL or more and the package contains more than 150 percent but less than 200 percent of the reference amount, manufacturers have the option of deciding whether the product is one or two servings.

For example, the serving size reference amount for soup is 245 g. So a 15-ounce (420 g) can can be listed as either one or two servings.

Presentation

There also are rules governing how the nutrition information is displayed. Under existing FDA regulations, nutrition information must appear on the information panel to the immediate right of the principal panel. Thus, on boxed foods, for example, in which the principal panel is on the front of the box, the nutrition information appears on the right side of the box. Packages whose area to the immediate right is too small or not suited for such labeling may provide information on the next panel to the right.

FSIS allows nutrition information to be listed on the principal or information panels.

The new food labeling rules call for one additional variation: For packages that are 40 square inches or less, the nutrition information may be placed on any label panel.

The rules also address size and prominence of the typeface. For example, the heading "Nutrition Facts" must be set in the largest type on the nutrition panel and be highlighted in some manner, such as boldface, all capital letters, or another graphic to distinguish it from the other information. Such highlighting also is required for headings such as "Amount per serving" and "%Daily Value" and for the names of dietary components that are not subcomponents—that is, calories, total fat, cholesterol, sodium, total carbohydrate, and protein.

Exceptions and Exemptions

In some instances, special provisions

exist for providing nutrition information. For example:

• Nutrition information about game meat, such as deer, bison, rabbit, quail, wild turkey, and ostrich, may be provided on counter cards, signs, or other point-of-purchase materials. Because little nutrient data exists for these foods, FDA believes that allowing this option will enable game meat producers to give first priority to collecting appropriate data and make it easier for them to update the information as it becomes available.
• FDA-regulated food packages with less than 12 square inches available for nutrition labeling do not have to carry nutrition information. However, they must provide an address or telephone number for consumers to obtain the required nutrition information.
• Packages with less than 40 square inches for nutrition labeling may present nutrition information in a tabular format (see top label, page 220), abbreviate the names of dietary components, and omit the footnotes with the list of daily values and caloric conversion information but include a footnote stating that the percent Daily Values are based on a 2,000-calorie diet or place nutrition information on other panels.

Some foods are exempt from nutrition labeling. These include:
• food produced by small businesses. (As mandated by NLEA, FDA defines a small business as one with food sales of less than \$50,000 a year or total sales of less than \$500,000. FSIS defines a small business as one employing 500 or fewer employees and producing no more than a certain amount of product per year.)
• food served for immediate consumption, such as that served in restaurants and hospital cafeterias, on airplanes, and by food service vendors (such as mall cookie counters, sidewalk vendors, and vending machines)
• ready-to-eat foods that are not for immediate consumption, as long as the food is primarily prepared on site—for example, many bakery, deli, and candy store items
• food shipped in bulk, as long as it is not for sale in that form to consumers
• medical foods
• plain coffee and tea, flavor extracts, food colors, some spices, and other foods that contain no significant amounts of any nutrients
• donated foods
• products intended for export
• individually wrapped FSIS-regulated products weighing less than half an ounce and making no nutrient content claims.

Although these foods are exempt, they are free to carry nutrition information, when appropriate—as long as it complies with the new regulations.

But, there will be plenty of other foods carrying the new nutrition information. Dietitian Susan Thom sees that as a plus.

"We'll all know exactly what we're putting in our mouths," she said. "So there'll be little room for excuses."

Taking Control of Your Disease

When people learn that they have an illness, they often adopt what anthropologists call "the sick role." In this role, patients are expected to want to recover and to do what they can to get better, but they generally surrender most of their responsibilities to others until they are back in good health. Family and friends usually assume the patients' duties at home and work, while physicians diagnose the condition and prescribe appropriate treatments.

The "sick role" may be a useful adaptation when a disease runs its course quickly, such as in the case of pneumonia, but may not be very helpful and might even be harmful when the ailment is a chronic disease, such as high blood pressure (hypertension), diabetes, angina, and congestive heart failure. Today such chronic conditions are among the greatest challenges for doctors and patients. These chronic conditions are likely to persist for the patient's lifetime; they may be effectively treated but are rarely cured. To live with these conditions and achieve the best possible level of health and function, patients should take an active role with their physician in monitoring the disease and evaluating the benefits of treatments.

Increasingly, many health experts encourage patients to develop a new kind of relationship with their physician — a partnership in which both doctor and patient collect information and discuss choices. This approach, which asks patients to assume substantial responsibility for monitoring their condition, may not be right for every person or every medical disorder. However, by collecting day-to-day or week-to-week information on their condition, patients can help control their disease instead of letting the disease control them.

Tip of the iceberg

For example, consider the typical patient with hypertension. Such a patient rarely experiences any symptoms. In general, people with hypertension feel pretty much the same regardless of their blood-pressure level. They may recognize how well their pressure is controlled only when they visit their doctor — which may be just two or three times a year.

For both the doctor and patient, these rare blood-pressure measurements are just the tip of the iceberg. Blood pressure fluctuates in everyone from minute to minute and day to day. A few drinks the night before might raise a person's blood pressure by 10 points, while exercise could cause an equivalent decline. Also, blood pressure often rises just from the stress of visiting the doctor — a phenomenon called "white-coat hypertension" (see January 1992 *Harvard Heart Letter.*)

If blood pressure is measured only rarely, neither patients nor their doctors can distinguish a normal fluctuation from a real trend. Is a 10-point increase between one reading in January and a second measurement in April significant? Or did the doctor just happen to catch the patient on a stressful day? Sometimes medications are prescribed or increased because of a random "blip" in blood pressure that does not represent a true worsening of hypertension.

Similarly, glucose levels measured during visits to the doctor provide only a little insight into how well a person's diabetes is controlled. On the other hand, a series of glucose measurements obtained via a home glucometer can show whether someone needs more or less medication, or perhaps needs to take it at different times during the day or evening, or needs to adjust his or her diet.

Graphs and charts

Although many patients have monitored their own blood pressures or blood-sugar levels for years, the recent momentum behind teaching patients to chart their medical information has been inspired by the increased emphasis on patients' rights and responsibilities. Consumers in every sphere of society have sought the right to know what service they are purchasing and what effect it will have on their lives. Physicians also increasingly realize that patients are more likely to use a prescribed treatment if they understand the reasons they are being asked to follow a certain regimen.

So it is understandable that in one of the most personal of relationships — that of patient and doctor — both parties should share the responsibility of collecting and analyzing data on the disease. Patients can assist the doctor by charting changes in their condition and by monitoring the effects of therapy. Patients can keep a record of key symptoms or measurements and even log this information onto a graph or chart.

Patients who have erratic blood-pressure levels can monitor themselves with the help of a home blood-pressure unit (see April 1993 *Harvard Heart Letter*). For example, a man with newly diagnosed hypertension might begin by measuring his blood pressure three times a day — upon rising, at lunch while at work, and in the evening (*see illustration*). These readings would show the

Recording Blood Pressure at Home

Sample work sheets on which a hypothetical patient has graphed blood-pressure readings. The notations record unusual circumstances that might be related to the elevated and reduced blood-pressure readings.

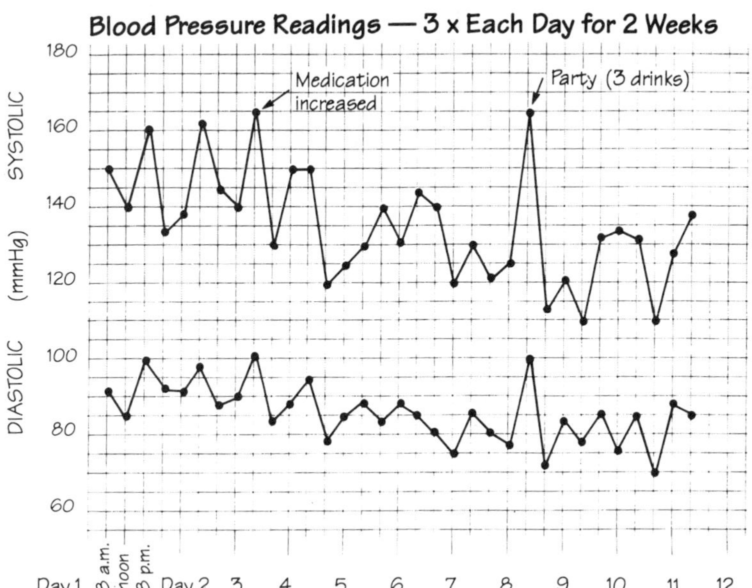

Measurements were taken three times a day for the first two weeks of treatment. The downward trend shows the response of blood pressure to medications and lifestyle changes. The intrinsic random variability of blood-pressure measurements can be distinguished from specific nonrandom events such as exercise, forgetting to take medication, or alcohol consumption.

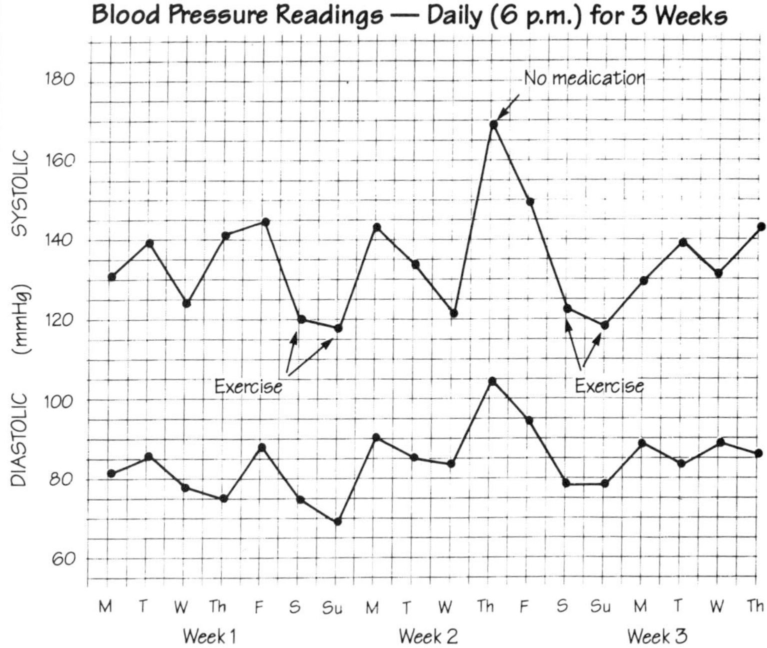

Blood-pressure readings were graphed once daily for three weeks after the blood pressure was stabilized. Lower readings on the weekend show the temporary impact of exercise on blood pressure. A sharp rise occurred when the medications were not taken.

patient how much his blood pressure fluctuates during the day and provide insight into factors affecting the changes. In the hypothetical example shown, the readings suggest that — contrary to the patient's expectations — his blood pressure does not rise with the stress of work, but instead goes up in the evening. The evening increase might result from loss of effect of medications taken in the morning, from stress at home, or from the effects of after-dinner drinks.

Once the patient is on a stable medical regimen, he might shift to daily blood-pressure measurements (*see illustration*). These daily patterns might reveal that his blood pressure was lower on days he went for long walks, but higher when he forgot to take his medication or went to a party.

Eventually, the stable patient would find that the blood-pressure measurements fluctuate within a reasonably predictable range. The patient might also see how a weight-loss program led to a steady decline in blood pressure. But any upward trend that was caused by a worsening of hypertension could be readily identified — well in advance of the next visit to the doctor.

Form and function

Such information is welcomed by most doctors, because it provides them with a more complete view of the patient's blood-pressure condition. This same approach can be extended to other medical conditions. Patients with *angina* (the discomfort that indicates an insufficiency of blood flow to the heart) might record the number of episodes of chest pain per day. Patients with congestive heart failure might monitor their weight daily. Many people with diabetes have been tracking their sugar (glucose) levels for years, and newer insulin regimens make this practice even more important.

The measurements can simply be jotted into a notebook. However, graphs are an effective way of revealing trends, and personal computers can help in what previously may have been an impractical task. The doctor can help to determine the appropriate ranges for systolic and diastolic blood pressure, and the patient can then identify any factors that are associated with major fluctuations or long-term trends.

Not for everyone

This active-participation approach is not right for every patient with cardiovascular problems. Some people do not want to know how they are doing. Others are in danger of becoming overly compulsive about tracking their blood pressure; these people might continue to measure it many times during the day even after such detailed information is no longer necessary. Instead of using this information to gain control of their medical condition, they are at risk of becoming enslaved by the process of monitoring it. There are also many people whose conditions are so stable that the time and effort required to keep a log or make a graph would not be worthwhile. Nevertheless, many patients can gain perspective, increase their knowledge, and improve their care by monitoring their own condition and discussing their findings with the physician.

People who wonder whether this approach might be helpful should discuss the issue with their physician. Some doctors may not be accustomed to having patients play such an active role, but patients should feel free to raise the issue and stimulate an open discussion. If the doctor agrees that more information could help the patient live with and control the disease, then some method for collecting and summarizing the information can be tried. Whether the data are recorded on the back of an envelope or on a chart, the likelihood is that knowledge will be power.

SUNSCREENS: EVERYTHING NEW UNDER THE SUN

After years of impassioned appeals—from public-health officials as well as sunscreen manufacturers—most Americans have resigned themselves to slathering the body with lotion to prevent sunburn, wrinkles, and skin cancer. But last year, in a paper published in the Annals of Epidemiology, California researchers proposed that sunscreen may actually *increase* the risk of cancer.

That heretical notion quickly made headlines. "Does Sunscreen Save Your Skin?" asked Time magazine. Or, as Forbes put it, "Can Sunscreens Kill You?" Mother Jones summed up the depressing situation in two words: "Beach Bummer."

Conflicting reports published since then have added to the dismay and confusion. All that, coupled with the lack of clear Federal guidelines for sunscreens, has left many consumers wondering what to use—and whether to bother.

Let the sun shine?

Two types of ultraviolet light reach the surface of the earth: UVA, the longer wavelengths responsible for tanning, and UVB, the shorter rays that damage the skin. Or at least it used to seem that simple until further research clouded the issue.

Scientists are now finding that the arbitrary classification of UVA and UVB rays into two separate bands of the spectrum may be a distinction without a difference: In particular, studies suggest that UVA rays have many of the same harmful effects as UVB, contributing to sunburn and premature aging of the skin, as well as increasing the risk of skin cancers—perhaps especially the most deadly kind, melanoma.

Sunscreen manufacturers are now scrambling to catch up to the news. Since the 1970's, sunscreens have been formulated specifically to block the burning UVB rays. That's what the familiar SPF, or Sun Protection Factor, rating scale measures. The challenge for manufacturers now is to add effective UVA-blockers to the recipe.

New studies, new sunscreens, and new sun scares have left consumers in the dark.

The controversial paper from the California epidemiologists added urgency to that effort. Citing alarming statistics of increasing skin-cancer rates, the researchers contended that UVB-blocking sunscreens had contributed to that epidemic by disabling the body's natural alarm mechanism: sunburn. By preventing sunburn, they claimed, those sunscreens had actually enabled sunbathers to spend more time exposed to damaging UVA rays.

Other researchers quickly disputed that theory, pointing out, among other things, that the increase in cancer rates predated the widespread use of UVB-blocking sunscreens and was actually the result of unprotected sun exposure from decades earlier. Then, last fall, those critics seemed to get the solid support they had hoped for. A long-awaited Australian study of some 600 people showed that sunscreens can help prevent—and possibly even reverse—precancerous skin lesions, called solar keratoses.

But the rosy glow from that reassuring news quickly faded. By January, the results from another negative study had sun worshipers sweating. Researchers at the University of Texas M.D. Anderson Cancer Center found that, in mice injected with malignant melanoma cells and exposed to artificial ultraviolet light, sunscreen prevented sunburn but not the growth of melanoma tumors. Even sunscreen that blocked UVA rays as well as UVB showed no protective effect.

Once again, various health organizations—including the American Academy of Dermatology and the Skin Cancer Foundation—were compelled to come to the defense of sunscreen, faulting the mouse study for using weak sunscreen and artificial sunlight. Even the Texas researchers themselves, distressed that their study had been interpreted as damning sunscreens, hurriedly released possible explanations for the discouraging findings, noting that the course of cancer in mice differs from humans and that the progression of existing cancer cells does not necessarily reflect the development of new tumors.

Choosing and using sunscreen

Clearly, researchers have a less-than-perfect understanding of the cancer risk from sunlight and the ability of sunscreen to protect against it. But while they may quibble over the specifics, virtually all agree that sunscreens are—despite their limitations—an essential part of "safe sun" practices. There's also general agreement that the majority of sunscreens on the market are not up to the task, since most were formulated to block only UVB rays.

For maximum protection, you should choose a "broad-spectrum" sunscreen that blocks most UVA light as well as UVB. Unfortunately, that's an uncertain business. No rating system yet exists for measuring UVA protection the way the SPF system rates UVB- and sunburn-blocking ability. The U.S. Food and Drug Administration is now in the process of developing guidelines for safe and effective UVA-blocking ingredients—but it's a long process, fraught with intense lobbying from manufacturers and even Congressional supporters. In the meantime, consumers must check the labels for certain ingredients that look promising.

So far, only one of those ingredients has been approved by the FDA specifically for UVA protection: the chemical compound avobenzone (Parsol 1789), now in the broad-spectrum sunscreen *Shade UVAGUARD*. Another chemical that blocks most UVA and UVB light is titanium dioxide, an uncolored relative of zinc oxide, the white stuff you see on a lifeguard's nose. Sunscreens containing titanium dioxide are permitted to claim some UVA protection. Those products include *Clinique Total Cover Sun Block*, *Neutrogena Chemical-Free Sunblocker*, and *TI-Screen Natural*.

Many more products containing certain other ingredients are also allowed to claim UVA protection, but none can say how much. Since each of those chemicals blocks only part of the UVA spectrum, look for a product that contains more than one of them. Check the label for these names:

- dioxybenzone.
- oxybenzone.
- sulisobenzone.
- methyl anthranilate.
- octocrylene.
- octyl methoxycinnamate (sometimes listed as ethylhexyl p-methoxycinnamate).

At least until the Federal regulations for sunscreens are in place sometime during the next few years, most consumers can use any of the UVA-blocking products described above. If you have reason to be especially concerned about ultraviolet radiation—for example, if you have unusually fair skin, a history of skin cancer, or a job that entails long hours in the sun—you might consider paying extra for *Shade UVAGUARD*.

A 4-ounce bottle of *Shade UVAGUARD* costs about $10. Brand-name products containing titanium dioxide can also cost that much or more, but store-brand versions typically cost considerably less. By comparison, for about $6 you can get a 4-ounce bottle of a brand-name sunscreen containing more than one of the other UVA-blocking ingredients—for example, *Coppertone Sunblock* or *Shade Sunblock*. Again, store brands are usually cheaper.

Looking into the sun

Most people know that they must protect their skin from the sun, but few realize how important it is to shield their eyes as well. Prolonged exposure to ultraviolet sunlight—both UVA and UVB rays—can cause cataracts, which cloud the lens of the eye and obscure vision. Sunglasses can neutralize the risk by blocking ultraviolet light.

Any lens—glass or plastic—will block virtually all UVB light. Plastic lenses also block at least 90 percent of UVA rays, enough for most people. But without special coatings, glass lenses won't perform as well. So you'll need to be more careful when choosing glass lenses. Check the label for a pair that filters out at least 90 percent of UVA rays. (If the label doesn't give that information, some eyeglass shops can measure the lenses' UV protection for you.)

In addition, certain people at high risk of eye damage due to UV light should wear sunglasses that provide total protection. That includes people who:

- Spend large amounts of time in the sun.
- Have had cataracts removed without the insertion of an artificial lens.
- Take certain medications that increase sun sensitivity. Such drugs include allopurinol (*Zyloprim*), phenothiazine compounds (*Compazine*, *Thorazine*), psoralen drugs (*Oxsoralen*, *Trisoralen*), tretinoin (*Retin-A*), and the antibiotics doxycycline or tetracycline.

Those high-risk people should look for a label that either indicates 100 percent UV blockage or says "blocks UV up to 400 nm," which means the same thing. Or, if they can't find a labeled pair that suits them, they can ask the salesperson to steer them to an unlabeled pair that provides complete protection—and have it checked.

Even a clear lens can block UV rays, which are invisible; so darkening the lens won't increase protection against cataracts. But darker lenses may help protect against a potential hazard from *visible* light: There's some evidence that lifetime exposure may damage the retina and contribute to blindness. While that threat is not proven, moderately dark glasses may provide an extra margin of safety. (Sunglasses labeled "general purpose," which block 60 to 92 percent of visible light, are best for most people.)

Note that wearing a hat, which protects the skin, also shields the eyes: According to the American Academy of Ophthalmology, a broad-brim hat can cut UV- and visible- light exposure to the eyes by about half.

Despite the current focus on the hazards of UVA light, blocking UVB rays is still as important as ever. In general, choose a sunscreen rated SPF 15, which means it will take 15 times longer for your skin to burn than if you wore no sunscreen. Less protection than that may not last long enough; an SPF greater than 30 is rarely necessary.

Of course, for any sunscreen's UVA- *or* UVB-blocking agents to be fully effective, you have to apply enough of it. Most people use less than half as much as they would need to attain the full SPF rating—which is based on a 1-ounce palmful applied to the entire body. Using that inadequate amount drops an SPF 15 product down below SPF 8.

To give the protective chemicals time to penetrate the skin, apply sunscreen at least 30 minutes before going out in the sun. Reapply if you swim, towel off, or perspire heavily. Note, however, that repeated application ensures only that you get the full SPF protection; it won't extend the amount of time you can spend in the sun without burning.

Beyond sunscreen

If the conflicting research to date proves anything, it's that sunscreens go only so far in protecting against harmful ultraviolet radiation. Limiting your overall sun exposure is just as important. That doesn't mean ducking into a doorway whenever the sun comes out from behind a cloud. (In fact, a little sunshine is good for you, since it helps the body synthesize vitamin D.) But you should take these general precautions against prolonged exposure:

- **Stay out of the noonday sun.** Minimize your exposure during the peak hours of 10 A.M. to 3 P.M., when UVB radiation is generally most intense. Keep in mind, however, that UVA radiation is relatively constant throughout the day.
- **Wear protective clothing.** That includes a wide-brim hat as well as long-sleeved shirts and long pants. (Tight-weave fabrics protect best.)
- **Beware of reflective surfaces.** Sand can reflect most of the sun's rays. So don't rely solely on a beach umbrella. Concrete and white-painted surfaces are also highly reflective.
- **Don't be fooled by clouds.** While thick cloud cover does block most UV light, up to 80 percent of the rays can penetrate high, thin clouds. Starting this summer, the National Weather Service will add a new component to its forecasts—the Ultraviolet Index, which would rate the daily risk from UV radiation on a 15-point scale. In addition to cloudiness, the rating scale would take into account the angle of the sun, the presence of dust or haze in the air, and the depth of the atmosphere's protective ozone layer.
- **Play it safe year-round.** While there may be less of it, winter sunlight can still damage the skin. And skiers take note: Ultraviolet radiation increases with altitude. At 5,000 feet, for example, the sun's UV rays are 20 percent stronger than at sea level. And snow reflects 85 to 100 percent of sunlight.
- **Protect the kids.** Excessive sun exposure during childhood greatly increases the risk of skin cancer. According to one estimate, regular use of an SPF 15 sunscreen before the age of 18 can reduce the lifetime risk by as much as 78 percent. (Don't use sunscreen on infants under six months; just keep them out of the sun.)
- **Examine your skin.** Periodically check for early signs of cancer, such as changes in freckles or moles or new skin discolorations. If you detect anything at all suspicious, see your physician.

A Healthy Tan: Relic from the Dark Ages

For people who want the tan but not the sun, cosmetic manufacturers have created artificial tanning lotions. Most of those products contain dihydroxyacetone, or DHA, a harmless pigmenting agent that produces a reddish-brown color when it binds with amino acids in the outer layers of the skin. The "tan" lasts only a few days until the dead skin cells slough off.

Unlike naturally darker skin, which affords some protection against the hazards of sun exposure, an artificial tan provides no protection at all. That's because the skin pigment melanin works at the cellular level, while tanning agents merely stain the surface of the skin. Spotting an opportunity, some manufacturers now offer products—such as Bain de Soleil's *SPF+Color*—that combine sunscreen and tanning ingredients, so sunbathers can appear to tan while actually blocking sunlight.

Once-popular tanning *pills* are unsafe and illegal—although they still turn up occasionally in health-food stores, tanning salons, and mail-order ads in newspapers and in the back of bodybuilding magazines. The pills contain canthaxanthin, a dye that can build up in the retina and liver, cause skin reactions and itching, and lead to a type of hepatitis.

something fishy

Is Your Seafood Safe Enough to Eat?

Mark Roman

Mark Roman is a health and science writer in New York City.

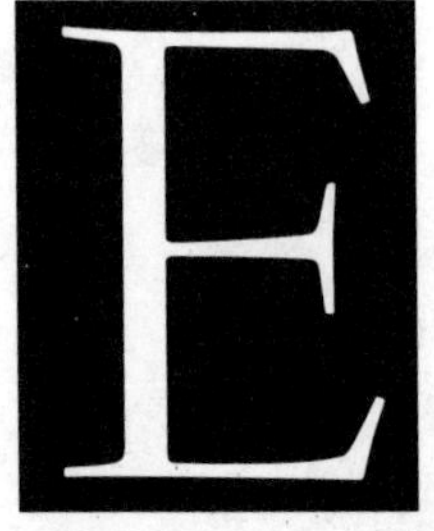

Eric Rosenwald hadn't eaten raw oysters in years. But the Friday night his daughter treated him to dinner at a restaurant near their home in Fort Lauderdale, Fla., he ordered half a dozen.

Monday morning, the 80-year-old man woke up complaining of fatigue and weakness. The flu, he thought. That evening, Rosenwald checked into the hospital with a blistering fever. By 1 a.m., he was dead. "Even the doctors didn't know what was wrong," recalls his daughter, Vicki Peal. "It was an absolute nightmare."

The killer, of course, was Friday night's dinner. Rosenwald had eaten an oyster contaminated with *Vibrio vulnificus,* rare bacteria that sometimes grow in shellfish. In healthy people, V. vulnificus cause little more than stomach cramps. But among cancer patients, diabetics, the elderly and others with weak immune systems, the risk of serious illness is high and the fatality rate is more than 50%.

Again and again in recent years, Americans have heard the mantra, "Eat more fish." And we've heeded the call. During the past decade, annual consumption has risen by almost 25% to more than 15 pounds per person. But at the same time, serious doubts have been raised about not only the safety and quality of the fish we buy, but also the integrity of the seafood marketing industry itself.

Nutritionally speaking, fish is clearly a health food. It's a lean, low-calorie source of high-quality protein. It's rich in minerals and cholesterol-lowering omega-3 fatty acids. But there have been enough reports of seafood-related illness and death in recent years to warrant concern about our fish supply. Three states—California, Florida and Louisiana—now require that notices be posted wherever raw shellfish are sold, warning that they can cause serious illness in people with liver, stomach, blood or immune disorders.

The Food and Drug Administration (FDA) estimates that your overall chance of getting sick anytime you sit down to eat seafood is only one in 250,000. Since thorough cooking destroys most harmful organisms in seafood, avoiding raw fish and shellfish will reduce your chance of illness to one in a million—that's 40 times safer than you are when you eat chicken.

But according to Caroline Smith DeWaal, director of legal affairs at the Public Voice for Food and Health Policy, a Washington advocacy group that seeks tougher regulation of the seafood industry, government estimates are misleading. "Very few seafood-related illnesses are actually reported," she says. "One reason is because the symptoms are often so similar to those of other food-borne illnesses that doctors don't distinguish them."

Seafood takes a desultory path to the consumer, and contamination can creep in at many points. Even in the cleanest waters, fish and shellfish are exposed to naturally occurring marine bacteria along with viruses, pollutants and other potential toxins. Mollusks (oysters, clams and mussels) are particularly susceptible to viral and bacterial contamination because they live close to the shore, where pollution levels are often highest.

 From *American Health,* March 1994, pp. 76-79.

Although V. vulnificus can be deadly for people with weak immune systems, other seafood-borne illnesses occur more frequently. When tainted by human sewage, raw mollusks may carry the hepatitis A virus, which can leave victims with severe liver damage, and the Norwalk virus, which causes acute stomach and intestinal distress.

Although rarely lethal, naturally occurring toxins are responsible for 28% of seafood-borne illnesses. Where the toxins originate is somewhat of a mystery, but they're usually linked to microscopic plant life in the sea. Saxitoxins, sometimes known as red tide, float among ruddy clouds of plankton and contaminate mollusks. The toxins cause paralytic shellfish poisoning, with symptoms that include vomiting, diarrhea, tingling and numbness in the face and extremities, and, if not treated, death. Although the last major outbreak occurred in 1980, several clam beds were closed last year when the toxins turned up along the Georgia coast.

Raw shellfish are the most common source of seafood-borne illness, but finfish also carry contaminants. Ciguatera toxins, organisms found in algae growing along coral reefs in Hawaiian and Southeastern waters, rise through the food chain and accumulate in barracuda, snapper, grouper and other large predators. The toxins, which cause nausea and vomiting within six hours of consumption, are immune to both cooking and freezing.

Scombroid fish poisoning is most commonly associated with bluefish and fresh tuna. Scombroid poisoning occurs when the fish get too warm, a sign of improper handling. In humans who've consumed tainted fish, symptoms range from mild upset stomach to nausea, vomiting and diarrhea.

Pesticides and industrial or household waste products also find their way into the waters where fish swim and can remain active for decades. A 1991 report from the National Academy of Sciences (NAS) revealed chemical residues in lakes, rivers and coastal waters across the country. The following year, *Consumer Reports* magazine uncovered residues of DDT (a pesticide banned in 1972) in catfish and traces of mercury in swordfish from New York and Chicago stores. Lead turned up in clams, and PCB's (pollutants known to cause birth defects) were found in whitefish and salmon. Consumer protection groups worry that even low levels of these contaminants may be dangerous because they accumulate in our bodies over time.

Bacterial contamination of seafood is most directly associated with industry mishandling. Dangerous strains of E. coli from human and animal feces can be transmitted by fish handlers on boats, trucks, piers, loading docks, processing plants and fish markets. Workers who forget to wash after using the bathroom, slide a fish across a contaminated surface or pile bacteria-laden fish on top of uncontaminated fish all contribute to the spread of bacteria-related illnesses.

Guidelines for Seafood Safety

Exercising care in selecting, storing and cooking fish and shellfish will help ensure their freshness and safety.

In the display case at the store:

- Choose whole fish, fillets and steaks that are displayed in a single layer over ice.
- Smell fish before buying. Fresh seafood should remind you of a cool ocean breeze, not dead fish.
- Look for moist steaks and fillets with no drying or browning around the edges. Scales should cling tightly to the skin without feeling slimy.
- Check that a fish's eyes are bright and clear, not cloudy and sunken. Gills should be bright pink or red.
- When choosing mollusks in the shell, pick only those that are still alive. For a quick test, pinch the shells between your thumb and forefinger. If the shells don't budge, it's safe. If the shells move, pick another.

In your refrigerator:

- Store seafood in its original wrapper in the coldest spot—usually the meat drawer or the tray under the freezer. Keep the temperature between 32° and 40° for optimal freshness.
- Keep live mollusks in the refrigerator in a container covered with a moist cloth, not an airtight seal. Don't store in water.

In the kitchen:

- Thaw frozen seafood in the refrigerator on a plate to catch juices.
- Wash plates and cutting boards that have come in contact with raw seafood immediately with soap and hot water to avoid cross-contamination.
- Cook seafood thoroughly. When baking, broiling, poaching, frying or stewing finfish, allow 10 minutes cooking time per one-inch thickness of fish. When properly cooked, fish will flake easily with a fork. For mollusks, boil for three to five minutes, or steam for four to nine minutes. Discard any clam, mussel or oyster whose shell doesn't open during cooking.

At the table:

- Refrain from eating raw shellfish. If you must indulge, the Food and Drug Administration (FDA) recommends that raw shellfish consumption be confined to cold months, when mollusks are less likely to carry toxic organisms. The risk of infection is particularly high for anyone who has liver disease, diabetes or a weakened immune system.
- If you wish to eat sushi or other raw fish dishes, do so only at reputable restaurants. You may want to inquire whether the fish were previously frozen. Freezing reduces the risk of illness by killing the larvae of parasites that may be present in the flesh of raw fish. Even though parasitic infections are the least common of all seafood-related illnesses, the FDA warns consumers not to prepare raw fish dishes at home.
- If you're pregnant or trying to conceive, avoid eating swordfish or any other seafood that is known to accumulate pollutants.

We can't tell when or how often fish is contaminated.

"Bacteria exist everywhere," says Dr. George Hoskin, director of science and applied technology at the FDA Office of Seafood. "So it can come from anywhere." While vacationing in Virginia last summer, he watched fish handlers unknowingly contaminate a load of freshly caught shark. "On the boat, the fish were carefully gutted, headed and covered in ice," he recalls. "But then a dirty hook was used to toss them onto a pier."

That carelessness could lead to several problems, he notes. First, the hook was spreading bacteria like a junkie's needle. Second, piers are laden with bacteria "from dog, cat and seagull droppings and anything else that sticks to the bottom of people's shoes." Finally, the fish were left lying on the pier a long time, allowing bacteria to thrive in the heat of the summer sun. "This is typical of what can happen at so many stages of fish handling," Hoskin says. "And there's no way to know when, where or how often it occurs."

Opportunities for contamination also arise at the retail level. Dirty or poorly cooled display cases in supermarkets and fish stores promote bacterial growth. When merchants display raw fish in piles, the temperatures of the fish on top are often well above the recommended maximum safe storage temperature of 40°, says Hoskin. As their juices trickle down, bacteria spread to the fish at the bottom of the pile.

Bacterial cross-contamination can also occur when raw and cooked seafood are displayed together. Although Styrofoam packaging keeps juices from mixing, it can also insulate fish from the cold, inviting new bacterial growth. Again, Hoskin points out, when packages are stacked, the ones on top may not be cool enough to prevent bacterial growth. In addition, he says, each type of fish has a certain shelf life. Sometimes much of that shelf life has been used up before the fish reaches the market.

Despite all these hazards, the fish industry remains only loosely regulated. The FDA is supposed to have primary responsibility for monitoring fish from sea to supermarket, but limited budgets and small staffs hamper its efforts. No one inspects fishing boats, and retailers are monitored by state and local agencies that also have small staffs. FDA agents inspect only the middlemen—the seafood processors.

Even then, thorough inspections of processing plants may

FREE FACTS ON FISH SAFETY

In response to consumer concern, the FDA has published an informative (and somewhat reassuring) brochure, "Get Hooked on Seafood Safety." To order a free copy, write to the Consumer Information Center, Department 526Z, Pueblo, CO 81009. For recorded messages on seafood purchasing, storage, handling, labeling, nutrition and economic fraud, call the FDA's toll-free seafood hot line, 800-FDA-4010, 24 hours a day. To speak to an operator, call weekdays between noon and 4 p.m. Eastern time.

Buyer Beware

Added to the problem of seafood safety is the opportunity for economic fraud in this loosely regulated industry. Although fraudulent behavior on the part of wholesalers and retailers probably won't hurt your health, it can certainly pinch your wallet.

Unscrupulous fishmongers have ways of adding weight to fish and giving you less for your money. In a technique called overglazing, seafood is sprayed with water before freezing to add weight and increase the price. "We've seen lobster tails on sale that were more than 30% ice," says Mary Snyder, chief of the policy guidance branch of the Food and Drug Administration (FDA) Office of Seafood. She adds that variations on this process, such as "overbreading" ready-to-cook shrimp, are common.

Shellfish such as scallops, shrimp and lobster are sometimes soaked in a phosphate solution to help retain natural moisture. Although this method is FDA-approved, inspectors have uncovered processors who soak shellfish for extended periods of time until they actually gain water weight.

Species substitution, however, is considered the most common type of economic fraud. Because many fish look alike, cheaper or less desirable fish are sometimes passed off as the real thing. Snyder points out that since the differences aren't always obvious, even retailers may unknowingly buy and sell misrepresented products. Consequently, she offers consumers the following tips to help distinguish between some of the more common species:

- **Shark is often substituted for swordfish because the two species look so much alike. Shark has rougher skin, however, and a streak of dark meat in the center.**
- **Red snapper comes only from the Gulf of Mexico and the southern Atlantic Ocean. Ask your retailer where his "snapper" originated.**
- **Skinless cod fillets have a distinct white papery membrane along the belly and a white line of fat along the lateral line of the fillet.**
- **Scrod is not a species of fish. It's a term used to describe a whole cod, haddock or pollock that weighs less than 2½ pounds.**
- **Orange roughy comes only from Australia or New Zealand and arrives in this country frozen. It may be sold thawed and labeled previously frozen but should never be labeled fresh.**

occur only once every two to four years. As a result, Caroline Smith DeWaal says, billions of tons of uninspected seafood reach consumers each year. By comparison, the U.S. Department of Agriculture posts agents in every meat and poultry plant, and each carcass is inspected by sight. "We don't have the manpower or the budget for that," says Hoskin. "And besides, there are over 3,000 seafood processors in this country and only 116 slaughterhouses."

The FDA has proposed use of a program called Hazard Analysis Critical Control Point (HACCP), a quality-control system that would focus on the stages of fish processing where contamination is most likely to happen. HACCP, which is already used by canned food processors, is a self-monitoring system. Under it, storage temperatures, cleaning schedules for equipment, and storage dates would be kept in logs by individual plants. FDA agents would then visit the plants for routine inspections and check the books for errors and inconsistencies.

The FDA claims that with the HACCP system, contamination and fraudulent fish sales would be easier to detect (see "Buyer Beware"). While the seafood industry, the NAS and most consumer groups endorse the HACCP, the program cannot be put into effect immediately. Before the HACCP program is formally adopted, it will be subject to the extensive scrutiny of consumer and industry groups. As a result, Hoskin says, the program may not be approved until 1995, and the industry will probably be given another year to put it into effect.

Scary as it all seems, most experts agree that the nutritional benefits of eating fish still outweigh its risks. While the government and the seafood industry are stepping up their regulatory systems, it's important for consumers to take steps to educate and protect themselves. The FDA estimates that as many as half of all seafood-related illnesses may result from unsafe handling in the home and in restaurants. These dangers can easily be avoided by buying seafood from known, reliable merchants, developing good food safety habits at home and eating only in reputable restaurants.

Clams filter all the dirt, the worst.

Preventing STDs

This article is part of a [continuing FDA Consumer*] series with important health information for teenagers. Unlike previous articles, however, it contains sexually explicit material in an effort to reduce the incidence of STDs among teens. Parents and teachers may want to review the article before giving it to teenagers.*

Judith Levine Willis

Judith Levine Willis is editor of **FDA Consumer.**

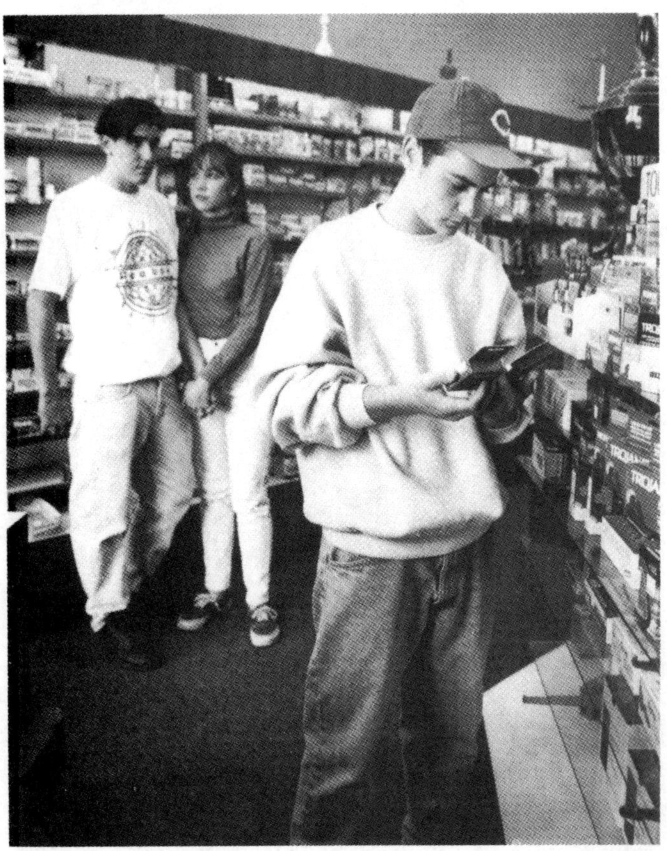

It's important to read the information printed on the package to make sure a condom's made of latex and labeled for disease prevention. The label may also give an expiration date and tell you if there is added spermicide or lubricant.

You don't have to be a genius to figure out that the only sure way to avoid getting sexually transmitted diseases (STDs) is to not have sex.

But in today's age of AIDS, it's smart to also know ways to lower the risk of getting STDs, including HIV, the virus that causes AIDS.

Infection with HIV, which stands for human immunodeficiency virus, is spreading among teenagers. From 1990 to 1992, the number of teens diagnosed with AIDS nearly doubled, according to the national Centers for Disease Control and Prevention. Today, people in their 20s account for 1 out of every 5 AIDS cases in the United States. Because HIV infection can take many years to develop into AIDS, many of these people were infected when they were teenagers.

You may have heard that birth control can also help prevent AIDS and other STDs. This is only partly true. The whole story is that *only one form of birth control—latex condoms* (thin rubber sheaths used to cover the penis)—is highly effective in reducing the transmission (spread) of HIV and many other STDs.

(When this *FDA Consumer* went to press, the Food and Drug Administration was preparing to approve Reality Female Condom, a form of birth control made of polyurethane. It may give limited protection against STDs, but it is not as effective as male latex condoms.)

So people who use other kinds of birth control, such as the pill, sponge, diaphragm, Norplant, Depo-Provera, cervical cap, or IUD, also need to use condoms to help prevent STDs.

Here's why: Latex condoms work against STDs by keeping blood, a man's semen, and a woman's vaginal fluids—all of which can carry bacteria and viruses—from passing from one person to another. For many years, scientists have known that male condoms (also called safes, rubbers, or prophylactics) can help prevent STDs transmitted by bacteria, such as syphilis and gonorrhea, because the bacteria can't get through the condom. More recently, researchers discovered that latex condoms can also reduce

From *FDA Consumer*, June 1993, pp. 33-35. Reprinted by permission of *FDA Consumer*, the magazine of the U.S. Food and Drug Administration.

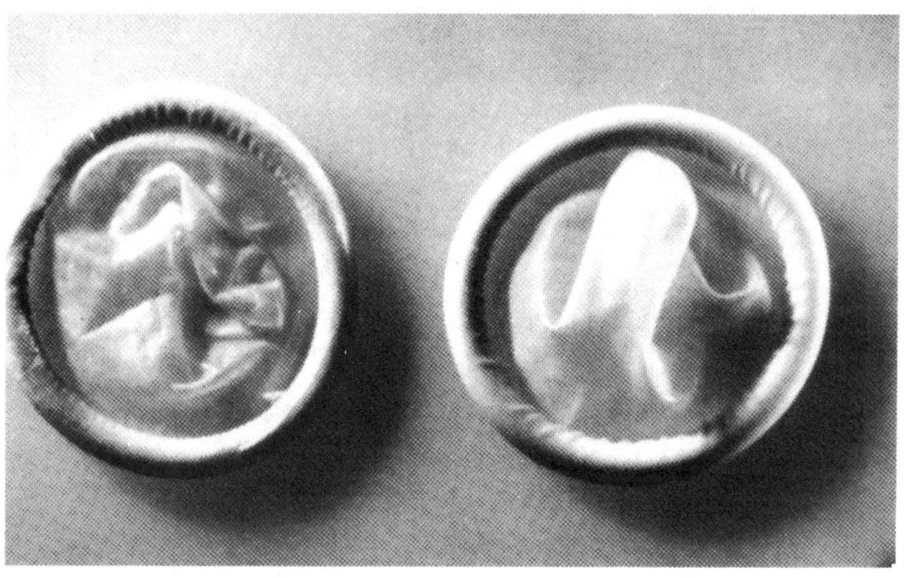

If a condom is sticking to itself, as is the one on the left, it's damaged and should not be used. The one on the right is undamaged and okay to use.

the risk of getting STDs caused by viruses, such as HIV, herpes, and hepatitis B, even though viruses are much smaller than bacteria or sperm.

After this discovery, FDA, which regulates condoms as medical devices, worked with manufacturers to develop labeling for latex condoms. The labeling tells consumers that although latex condoms cannot entirely eliminate the risk of STDs, when used properly and consistently they are highly effective in preventing STDs. FDA also provided a sample set of instructions and requested that all condoms include adequate instructions.

Make Sure It's Latex

Male condoms sold in the United States are made either of latex (rubber) or natural membrane, commonly called "lambskin" (but actually made of sheep intestine). Scientists found that natural skin condoms are not as effective as latex condoms in reducing the risk of STDs because natural skin condoms have naturally occurring tiny holes or pores that viruses may be able to get through. Only latex condoms labeled for protection against STDs should be used for disease protection.

Some condoms have lubricants added and some have spermicide (a chemical that kills sperm) added. The package labeling tells whether either of these has been added to the condom.

Lubricants may help prevent condoms from breaking and may help prevent irritation. But lubricants do not give any added disease protection. If an unlubricated condom is used, a water-based lubricant

New Information on Labels

Information about whether a birth control product also helps protect against sexually transmitted diseases (STDs), including HIV infection, is being given added emphasis on the labeling of these products.

"In spite of educational efforts, many adolescents and young adults, in particular, are continuing to engage in high-risk sexual behavior," said FDA Commissioner David A. Kessler, M.D., in announcing the label strengthening last April. "A product that is highly effective in preventing pregnancy will not necessarily protect against sexually transmitted diseases."

Labels on birth control pills, implants such as Norplant, injectable contraceptives such as Depo Provera, intrauterine devices (IUDs), and natural skin condoms will state that the products are intended to prevent pregnancy and do not protect against STDs, including HIV infection (which leads to AIDS). Labeling of natural skin condoms will also state that consumers should use a latex condom to help reduce risk of many STDs, including HIV infection.

Labeling for latex condoms, the only product currently allowed to make a claim of effectiveness against STDs, will state that if used properly, latex condoms help reduce risk of HIV transmission and many other STDs. This statement, a modification from previous labeling, will now appear on individual condom wrappers, on the box, and in consumer information.

Besides highlighting statements concerning sexually transmitted diseases and AIDS on the consumer packaging, manufacturers will add a similar statement to patient and physician leaflets provided with the products.

Consumers can expect to see the new labels by next fall. Some products already include this information in their labeling voluntarily. FDA may take action against any products that don't carry the new information.

FDA is currently reviewing whether similar action is necessary for the labeling of spermicide, cervical caps, diaphragms, and the Today brand contraceptive sponge.

Looking at a Condom Label

Like other drugs and medical devices, FDA requires condom packages to contain certain labeling information. When buying condoms, look on the package label to make sure the condoms are:

- made of latex
- labeled for disease prevention
- not past their expiration date (EXP followed by the date).

(such as K-Y Jelly), available over-the-counter (without prescription) in drugstores, can be used but is not required for the proper use of the condom. Do *not* use petroleum-based jelly (such as Vaseline), baby oil, lotions, cooking oils, or cold creams because these products can weaken latex and cause the condom to tear easily.

Condoms with added spermicide give added birth control protection. An active chemical in spermicides, nonoxynol-9, kills sperm. Although it has not been scientifically proven, it's possible that spermicides may reduce the transmission of HIV and other STDs. But spermicides alone (as sold in creams and jellies over-the-counter in drugstores) and spermicides used with the diaphragm or cervical cap do not give adequate protection against AIDS and other STDs. For the best disease protection, a latex condom should be used from start to finish every time a person has sex.

FDA requires condoms with spermicide to be labeled with an expiration date. Some condoms have an expiration date even though they don't contain spermicide. Condoms should not be used after the expiration date, usually abbreviated EXP and followed by the date.

Condoms are available in almost all drugstores, many supermarkets, and other stores. They are also available from vending machines. When purchasing condoms from vending machines, as from any source, be sure they are latex, labeled for disease prevention, and are not past their expiration date. Don't buy a condom from a vending machine located where it may be exposed to extreme heat or cold or to direct sunlight.

Condoms should be stored in a cool, dry place out of direct sunlight. Closets and drawers usually make good storage places. Because of possible exposure to extreme heat and cold, glove compartments of cars are *not* a good place to store condoms. For the same reason, condoms shouldn't be kept in a pocket, wallet or purse for more than a few hours at a time.

STD Facts

- Sexually transmitted diseases affect more than 12 million Americans each year, many of whom are teenagers or young adults.
- Using drugs and alcohol increases your chances of getting STDs because these substances can interfere with your judgment and your ability to use a condom properly.
- Intravenous drug use puts a person at higher risk for HIV and hepatitis B because IV drug users usually share needles.
- The more partners you have, the higher your chance of being exposed to HIV or other STDs. This is because it is difficult to know whether a person is infected, or has had sex with people who are more likely to be infected due to intravenous drug use or other risk factors.
- Sometimes, early in infection, there may be no symptoms, or symptoms may be confused with other illnesses.
- You cannot tell by looking at someone whether he or she is infected with HIV or another STD.

STDs can cause:

- pelvic inflammatory disease (PID), which can damage a woman's fallopian tubes and result in pelvic pain and sterility
- tubal pregnancies (where the fetus grows in the fallopian tube instead of the womb), sometimes fatal to the mother and always fatal to the fetus
- cancer of the cervix in women
- sterility—the inability to have children—in both men and women
- damage to major organs, such as the heart, kidney and brain, if STDs go untreated
- death, especially with HIV infection.

See a doctor if you have any of these STD symptoms:

- discharge from vagina, penis or rectum
- pain or burning during urination or intercourse
- pain in the abdomen (women), testicles (men), or buttocks and legs (both)
- blisters, open sores, warts, rash, or swelling in the genital or anal areas or mouth
- persistent flu-like symptoms—including fever, headache, aching muscles, or swollen glands—which may precede STD symptoms.

How to Use a Condom

- Use a new condom for every act of vaginal, anal and oral (penis-mouth contact) sex. Do not unroll the condom before placing it on the penis.
- Put the condom on after the penis is erect and before *any* contact is made between the penis and any part of the partner's body.
- If the condom does not have a reservoir top, pinch the tip enough to leave a half-inch space for semen to collect. Always make sure to eliminate any air in the tip to help keep the condom from breaking.
- Holding the condom rim (and pinching a half inch space if necessary), place the condom on the top of the penis. Then, continuing to hold it by the rim, unroll it all the way to the base of the penis. If you are also using water-based lubricant, you can put more on the outside of the condom.
- If you feel the condom break, stop immediately, withdraw, and put on a new condom.
- After ejaculation and before the penis gets soft, grip the rim of the condom and carefully withdraw.
- To remove the condom, gently pull it off the penis, being careful that semen doesn't spill out.
- Wrap the condom in a tissue and throw it in the trash where others won't handle it. (Don't flush condoms down the toilet because they may cause sewer problems.) Afterwards, wash your hands with soap and water.

Latex condoms are the only form of contraception now available that human studies have shown to be highly effective in protecting against the transmission of HIV and other STDs. They give good disease protection for vaginal sex and should also reduce the risk of disease transmission in oral and anal sex. But latex condoms may not be 100 percent effective, and a lot depends on knowing the right way to buy, store and use them.

FOOD NEWS BLUES

Grapefruit peel lowers cholesterol? Coffee's dangerous again? Here's how to separate the sense from the nonsense in your morning paper.

Anthony Schmitz

Anthony Schmitz is a contributing editor.

Note long ago I set a coffee cup on the table and opened the newspaper to a piece of good news. "New Study Finds Coffee Unlikely to Cause Heart Ills," read the headline. One less thing to worry about, I thought, until I remembered a story from a few weeks before. That morning the headline warned, "Study: Heart Risk Rises on 4, More Cups Coffee Daily." My paper—yours too, most likely—does this all the time. Concerning the latest dietary findings, it flips and flops like a fish thrown to shore.

"Medical research," it declared one Wednesday, "repeatedly has linked the soluble fiber in oats with reductions in serum cholesterol." By Thursday of the next week all that had changed. "Studies Cast Doubt on Benefits From Oat Bran," the headline cried. Once again the paper offered its readers a familiar choice. Which story to believe? This week's, last week's, or none at all?

The paper in question is the *St. Paul Pioneer Press.* It's a respectable provincial daily, not unlike the papers in Houston, Detroit, and dozens of other cities. One day recently the news editor, Mike Peluso, said he'd take a crack at explaining his paper's flip-flops.

Peluso is compact, graying, more grave than jocular. He met me at the newsroom door. "You want a cup of coffee?" he asked, pointing at a vending machine. No, I said, trying to recall whether this week coffee was good or bad. Peluso shrugged and headed for his cluttered cubicle. Beyond its flimsy walls reporters jabbered into phones.

I arranged the coffee and oat bran clippings on a paper-strewn table. Peluso examined them one by one. He grimaced. He sighed. He swallowed black coffee from a paper cup.

"How do you reconcile the conflicting claims?" he asked himself. "One month coffee can't hurt you, the next month quit coffee and your heart will tick forever."

Exactly.

Peluso shook his head. "I don't know. I don't have any answers for that. You've got to talk about the real world here."

For Peluso, the real world looks something like this: News of a hot nutrition study gets beamed into the newsroom from wire services such as Associated Press, the *New York Times,* or the *Baltimore Sun.* Peluso and his staff poke at the story, trying to find flaws that argue against putting it in the paper. By and large it's a hamstrung effort. Never mind that the reporter who wrote the piece is thousands of miles away. She'd defend the story anyway. The paper's own health reporter is scant help; he's been on the beat two months.

Meanwhile, Peluso knows that his competitors—another daily paper, plus radio and television news—won't spend a week analyzing the study. They'll run it today. Which is to say Peluso will, too. But the story the reader sees won't be as detailed as the piece that came over the wire. Compared to the *New York Times* or the *Washington Post,* the *Pioneer Press* is something of a dwarf. Stories get trimmed to fit. Subtleties and equivocations—the messy business of research—don't always make the cut.

"Look," said Peluso, "we're not medical authorities. We're just your normal skeptics. And it's not like we're inventing this research. We're simply reporting on it. We present what's there and let people draw their own conclusions."

"So what should readers make of all the contradictory advice you offer them?"

Peluso sighed again. "I don't know," he said. "You've got to take everything with a grain of salt until the last word comes in. I hate to tell people I don't believe everything I read, but the fact is anybody who believes everything they read is nuts."

RESEARCHERS WHOSE WORK makes news soon learn that the match between science and journalism wasn't made in heaven. Richard Greenberg, a microbiologist who directs the office of scientific and public affairs at the Institute of Food Technologists, has watched what happens when the scientific method collides with journalistic technique.

"The first thing you've got to remember," says Greenberg, "is that science is not fact. It is not truth. It is not holy scripture. It's a compendium of information. You try to put all the research together and come to a consensus. Just because somebody runs a study that comes to a particular conclusion doesn't change everything that's gone before."

Scientists don't generally reach consensus in time for the next deadline. After 30 years of study, coffee's link to heart disease remains an open question. Four-plus cups a day may slightly increase the risk, though some research suggests only decaf is linked to heart problems. Similarly, a decade's worth of oat bran experiments have served only to get a good argument going. Some studies suggest oat bran isn't any better at lowering cholesterol than white bread. If you eat enough of either, the message goes, you won't have room for fatty food. Others say oat bran has innate—though so far inexplicable—cholesterol-lowering properties.

While on their way to answering the big questions about fat or cholesterol or fiber, researchers often pause and dicker merrily about the design flaws in one study or the dicey statistical analysis in another. "Among ourselves," says one epidemiologist, "we're more interested in the detail of how things are done than in saying right now whether oat bran's good for you."

For journalists it's exactly the opposite. The arcana of statistical analysis and research design are boring at best, baffling at worst. The big question is whether oat bran will keep your heart ticking.

"You've got to take everything with a grain of salt until the last word comes in. I hate to tell people I don't believe everything I read, but the fact is anybody who believes everything they read is nuts."

–A NEWSPAPER EDITOR

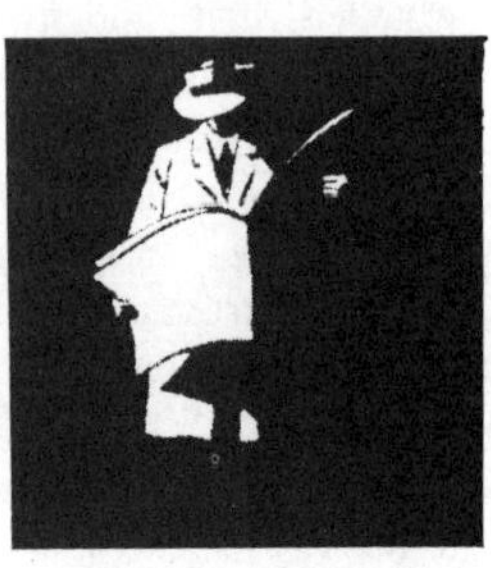

"The reporter and headline writer are trying to distill the meaning of the latest piece of research," says Greenberg. "They're trying to grab the eye of the reader. They're searching for absolutes where there are no absolutes. And this is what happens: One day you read caffeine is bad. Then you read that if you take caffeine out, coffee is okay. Then you hear the solvent that takes out the caffeine is dangerous. Then you find out the caffeine isn't dangerous after all. It so confuses the public they don't know who to believe. And the truth is, there wasn't really any news in any of these studies. Each of them was just another micromillimeter step toward scientific consensus."

For Greenberg, news exists in those rare moments when scientists weigh the evidence and agree to agree—when the American Heart Association, the National Cancer Institute, or the National Academy of Sciences pronounces that you ought to eat less fat, or more vegetables.

But by the terms of journalism, scientific consensus is a dead-letter file. If everybody agrees, there's no conflict. If there's no conflict, there's no news. In comparison, debates such as those about coffee or oat bran are a newsroom gold mine. Contradictions and conflict abound. Better still, almost everyone has oatmeal or coffee in the cupboard.

"You can't convince an editor not to run this stuff," says Howard Lewis, editor of the newsletter *Science Writers.* "My advice is that they do it for the same reason they run the comic strips and the astrology columns. But I feel it's all a hoax. Usually they're not accomplishing anything except sowing panic or crying wolf."

A Purdue communications professor raised a stir a few years back when he suggested that research news might be more harmful than helpful. Writing in the journal *Science, Technology, and Human Values,* Leon Trachtman observed that some 90 percent of the new drugs touted in newspaper reports never reached the market or were driven from it because they were ineffective, too toxic, or both. Readers relying on this information would have made wrong choices nine times out of ten.

So who's served, Trachtman asked, by publicizing these drugs before there's a scientific consensus on them? "When there's no consensus, why broadcast contradictory reports?" Ultimately, he said, readers are paralyzed by the pros and cons. He asked whether the result will be contempt for research, followed by demands to stop wasting money on it.

Not surprisingly, Leon Trachtman got blasted for implying that a scholastic elite ought to be making decisions for us. Among the critics was David Perlman, science editor for the *San Francisco Chronicle,* who writes regularly about health and nutrition. Often, Perlman says, research leads to public debates. Will avoiding fatty foods really lengthen your life? Should government experts try convincing people to change their eating habits? It's debatable. But citizens can hardly take part if they're capable of nothing more than numbly accepting expert advice. "To abdicate an interest in science," says Perlman, citing mathematician Jacob Bronowski, "is to walk with open eyes toward slavery." Perlman trusts people's ability to sort through well-written news.

"It's not just the masses who are confused," says Trachtman. "It's the same for well-trained scientists once they're out of their field. I think people ought to establish a sensible, moderate course of action and then not be deflected from it every morning by what they read in the paper."

"The public doesn't know what to believe anymore. And the truth is, there wasn't really any news on coffee in any of these studies. Each of them was just another micromillimeter step toward scientific consensus.

–A FOOD RESEARCHER

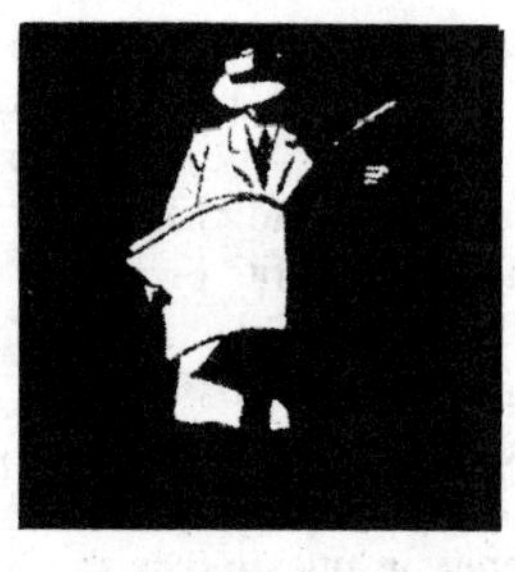

BUT LET'S FACE FACTS: Do you have the resolve to ignore a headline that declares, "Sugar, Alzheimer's Linked"? If you can't help but play the game, you can at least try to defend yourself from nonsense by following these rules:

COUNT THE LEGS. First, ask if the group studied bears any relation to you. Don't let research done only on four-legged subjects worry you. Pregnant rats, for instance, are more likely to bear offspring with missing toes after getting extremely high jolts of caffeine. What's this mean for humans? Probably nothing. There's no evidence that drinking moderate amounts

1. Study: Eating Citrus Can Help Against Cholesterol

Associated Press

MIAMI—Eating citrus can reduce cholesterol plaque in clogged arteries and help reverse atherosclerosis, a leading cause of heart attacks and strokes, researchers said Wednesday.

2. A two-year experiment with pigs found that citrus pectin—the sticky substance that's used to make jelly—reduces the formation of fatty plaque in coronary arteries, said Dr. Sigurd Normann of the University of Florida.

3. "The practical impact of our investigation is that we can tell a patient with severe atherosclerosis all is not lost," said fellow researcher Dr. James Cerda. "Based on this research, I would advise my patients with high cholesterol levels to eat a low-fat diet, get some exercise, and eat at least one grapefruit or several fresh oranges every day."

4. The researchers emphasized that citrus juice doesn't have the same beneficial effects because pectin is found only in the rind and in the pulp.

5. Normann, chief of cardiac pathology at the university's college of medicine, presented the study Thursday to the Federation of American Societies of Experimental Biology in Atlanta.

6. The primary grant for the research came from the Florida Citrus Commission, a state-appointed, industry-funded panel, but the commission played no role in reviewing the results, university officials said.

Normann said the study used pigs because their arteries and susceptibility to atherosclerosis are similar to humans.

7. Dr. Margo Denke, a specialist with the Center for Human Nutrition at the University of Texas's Southwestern Medical Center in Dallas, said she was impressed with the research. The findings fit in with previous studies showing pectin, a type of soluble fiber, can reduce cholesterol levels.

"They saw the change in a very short period of time, which is quite dramatic," she said. "But I think that more research is going to need to be done, and we might not expect such a dramatic effect in humans."

The study indicated as little as one grapefruit a day was enough to show results, but Denke said some other research has suggested that higher amounts might be necessary.

Dr. George Lumb, a scholar in residence at Duke Medical School who has conducted research on heart disease for 30 years, questioned whether people would be willing to eat that much fresh citrus fruit every day. He said his research team is conducting studies on 24 volunteers with high cholesterol levels to test the effects of pectin-enriched fruit punch.

HOW TO SPOT FRONT-PAGE FALLACIES

Your newspaper probably prints some type of food news every day. It may be important, it may be meaningless. Don't count on the paper's editors knowing the difference. You can defend yourself against half-baked findings and wild advice—if you read carefully. Here's how to pick apart a food news piece, one that hit the pages of the *Minneapolis Star Tribune* on April 26, 1991.

1. The bold, beckoning words at a newspaper story's top are usually cranked out by a special headline writer whose familiarlity with the subject can be measured in minutes. If eating citrus can help against cholesterol, your first questions should be: How much citrus? Whom does it help?

2. Now you know they're talking about pigs. Even if you have four legs and a snout, you shouldn't go for the pectin quite yet. The writer left out the study size—seven control pigs, seven pigs on pectin—which is too small to make the results widely applicable *even for pigs.* For humans, the conclusions are shakier still. That's not to say the research is irrelevant. Human arteries harden about the same way pigs' do. But the story doesn't say what else the pigs ate. Pigs are more sensitive to food's cholesterol; we're more sensitive to fat. Animal studies alone can't prove anything about human nutrition and health.

3. Did the pigs eat an amount of pectin that a reasonable pig, or a reasonable person, might eat? The answer (not that it's here) is no. Researchers fed 60-pound Yucatan micropigs half an ounce of pure pectin a day. Changes are you weigh two or three times more than a micropig. To have any hope of a cholesterol drop like that of the pigs you'd have to eat at least *two dozen* grapefruits a day.

4. Great news if you eat grapefruit *rind.* Most people don't.

5. There's a big difference between papers delivered at a conference, such as this one, and papers published in the *Journal of the American Medical Association,* the *New England Journal of Medicine, Science, Nature,* and the like. Journal articles are usually reviewed by experts who help editors toss out the scientific chaff. Presentations at conferences aren't as carefully winnowed and shouldn't be taken as seriously.

6. If the bills are paid by the citrus industry, wouldn't the researchers inevitably find *something* good to say about grapefruits and oranges? Maybe, maybe not. Quaker Oats, for example, recently funded research that showed oat bran has no special cholesterol-lowering effect. But a study of the debate over the drug tolbutamide (a diabetes treatment linked to heart attacks) found that doctors who got drug company funding were four times more likely than were their peers to say that people should keep on using the dangerous drug. You can't jump to conclusions about bias, warns *Washington Post* science writer Victor Cohn. Some crooked researchers *do* get money from corporations, he notes. "But the peddler of a biased point of view is as likely to be an anti-establishment crusader or an academic ladder-climber as a corporate darling." You have to judge each study on its own merits.

7. The last paragraphs are often more helpful than the first. This is usually where outside experts comment, putting the findings in perspective. In this case Margo Denke, a member of the American Heart Association's nutrition committee, makes three good points: This study confirms others showing that soluble fiber lowers cholesterol. Humans, however, aren't the same as pigs. And there ought to be more research done before anyone warms up the citrus bandwagon.

"If you don't like grapefruit," Denke says, "you shouldn't make yourself eat it."

—*A. S.*

of caffeine causes human birth defects.

If research subjects have two legs, read closely to see if they're anything like you. Early research that helped launch the oat bran fad involved only men, most of whom were middle-aged. All had dangerously high blood cholesterol, which reportedly fell after they ate a daily cup-plus of oat bran—enough for a half-dozen muffins. Fine, unless you're female, have low cholesterol already, or can't stand the thought of eating half a dozen bran muffins every day.

CHECK FOR PERSPECTIVE. Even if you're a match for the group being studied, don't assume the results are significant. "Check if the journalist gets the perspective of other people in the field," says Harvard epidemiologist Walter Willett. "People who've watched the overall flow of information are in a good position to say, 'Well, this really nails it down,' or, 'That's interesting, but it needs confirmation.' "

ASK HOW MANY GUINEA PIGS. Quaker Oats research manager Steven Ink, who's written a guide to nutrition studies, says the best research uses at least 50 subjects. By this standard, we should look askance at the recent study showing that eating 17 tiny meals a day lowers cholesterol: Only seven people took part. But rules of thumb don't always work. A small number *can* be meaningful if the effect observed is large and consistent. You don't need to feed 50 people cyanide to figure out that it's going to be bad for everyone.

What's more, Ink advises, subjects shouldn't be fed quantities of food that no one in his right mind would eat. One example is the recent study showing that trans fatty acids such as those in margarine may be bad for your heart. Subjects ate three times more trans fatty acids than the average American.

Finally, any group tested should be compared to a similar group. Early studies that linked coffee to heart disease were skewed because coffee drinkers differed greatly from the control group: The coffee drinkers were more likely to smoke and to eat a high-fat, high-cholesterol diet. Both habits carry bigger heart risks than does drinking coffee.

WAIT FOR CONFIRMATION. "Don't let one study change your life," says Jane Brody, the *New York Times* health writer. She waits for three types of food research to agree before changing her eating habits:

First, she looks for studies of large groups that show a link between a food and good or bad health—Italy's big appetite for olive oil and its low rate of heart disease, for instance. Then she watches for lab evidence in test animals that suggests how the food causes its effect in people. Finally, she considers human experiments in which two groups are compared—one eating the food, the other not eating it, with neither group knowing which is which.

Applying this rule to her own meals, Brody skimps on butter and favors olive oil. She eats plenty of fruits and vegetables, lots of potatoes, rice, beans, and pasta, and modest amounts of lean meat. "This plan won't make you sick, has a good chance of keeping you well, and is immune to these fads that are here today and gone tomorrow," Brody says.

HUNT FOR HOLES. No matter how carefully you read, you'll have to rely on the information your newspaper chooses to supply. If the big mattress ad on an inside page gets dropped at the last minute, the editors may suddenly have room for an exhaustive treatment of the latest coffee study. But if a candidate for national office gets caught with his pants down, the space required for a thorough exposé may mean the coffee piece gets gutted.

When editors at the *St. Paul Pioneer Press* got hold of a wire service report debunking oat bran, they found room for the first two-thirds. The third that didn't fit held a stern critique by other experts. They charged that the study contained too few people (20 female dietitians), didn't control the rest of what they ate, and started with subjects who had unusually low cholesterol.

"The reader really has to be skeptical," says Frank Sacks, the Harvard researcher whose oat bran study was under attack. "Take my case, for instance. The reporter really ought to say that this is a new finding, that it needs to be replicated. This is a warning sign that you have to wait a while. Reporters hate that when you say it. They call it waffling. But the truth is your hot new finding might not be confirmed down the line. You hate it when that happens, but it happens time and again.

"The real conservative advice is not to take any of this stuff in the newspaper with a whole lot of credence," says Sacks. "You could just wait for the conservative health organizations like the American Heart Association to make their recommendations and then follow their advice."

"WE DON'T HAVE an opinion," said John Weeks somewhat plaintively. I'd called the American Heart Association to get its line on oat bran and coffee.

"We get calls every day from the media," said Weeks. "They want to know what we think about every new study that comes out. And we don't have an opinion. We don't try to assimilate every new study. Our dietary guidelines would be bouncing all over the place if we did. Once the evidence is there, we move on it. Until then, we don't."

The Heart Association is sticking with the same dietary advice it's dispensed since 1988, when it last revised its model diet. Eat less fat. Eat more grains, vegetables, and fruit. The evidence that oat bran lowers cholesterol is so limited that the association makes no specific recommendation about it. Concerning coffee, the group has nothing to say.

Weeks's advice for whipsawed newspaper readers has a familiar ring. "What people need to keep in mind," he said, "is that one study does not a finding make."

"You mean," I asked, quoting Mike Peluso's newsroom wisdom, "I'm nuts to believe everything I read?"

Said Weeks, "That's exactly correct."

Index

Credits/ Acknowledgments

Cover design by Charles Vitelli

1. America's Health and the Health Care System
Facing overview—Photo by EPA-Documerica.

2. Contemporary Health Hazards
Facing overview—Photo by the American Cancer Society.

3. Stress and Mental Health
Facing overview—Photo courtesy of Louis P. Raucci.

4. Drugs and Health
Facing overview—Photo by the American Cancer Society.

5. Nutritional Health
Facing overview—WHO photo.

6. Exercise and Weight Control
Facing overview—Photo by the New York State Department of Commerce, Albany.

7. Current Killers
Facing overview—Photo by the New York City Department of Health.

8. Human Sexuality
Facing overview—WHO photo.

9. Consumer Health
Facing overview—Dushkin Publishing Group/Brown & Benchmark Publishers photo.

PHOTOCOPY THIS PAGE!!!*

ANNUAL EDITIONS ARTICLE REVIEW FORM

■ NAME: ______________________ DATE: ______________________

■ TITLE AND NUMBER OF ARTICLE: ______________________

■ BRIEFLY STATE THE MAIN IDEA OF THIS ARTICLE: ______________________

■ LIST THREE IMPORTANT FACTS THAT THE AUTHOR USES TO SUPPORT THE MAIN IDEA:

■ WHAT INFORMATION OR IDEAS DISCUSSED IN THIS ARTICLE ARE ALSO DISCUSSED IN YOUR TEXTBOOK OR OTHER READING YOU HAVE DONE? LIST THE TEXTBOOK CHAPTERS AND PAGE NUMBERS:

■ LIST ANY EXAMPLES OF BIAS OR FAULTY REASONING THAT YOU FOUND IN THE ARTICLE:

■ LIST ANY NEW TERMS/CONCEPTS THAT WERE DISCUSSED IN THE ARTICLE AND WRITE A SHORT DEFINITION:

*Your instructor may require you to use this Annual Editions Article Review Form in any number of ways: for articles that are assigned, for extra credit, as a tool to assist in developing assigned papers, or simply for your own reference. Even if it is not required, we encourage you to photocopy and use this page; you'll find that reflecting on the articles will greatly enhance the information from your text.

We Want Your Advice

Annual Editions revisions depend on two major opinion sources: one is our Advisory Board, listed in the front of this volume, which works with us in scanning the thousands of articles published in the public press each year; the other is you—the person actually using the book. Please help us and the users of the next edition by completing the prepaid article rating form on this page and returning it to us. Thank you.

ANNUAL EDITIONS: HEALTH 95/96

Article Rating Form

Here is an opportunity for you to have direct input into the next revision of this volume. We would like you to rate each of the 52 articles listed below, using the following scale:

1. Excellent: should definitely be retained
2. Above average: should probably be retained
3. Below average: should probably be deleted
4. Poor: should definitely be deleted

Your ratings will play a vital part in the next revision. So please mail this prepaid form to us just as soon as you complete it.
Thanks for your help!

Rating	Article	Rating	Article
	1. Wasted Health Care Dollars		27. The New Thinking about Fats
	2. The Future of Medicine: New Anatomy Lesson, Please		28. Taking Vitamins: Can They Prevent Disease?
	3. Heal Thyself		29. The Salt Shake Out
	4. When Doctors Jump the Gun		30. Snack Attack
	5. Timing Is Everything		31. Revive Sore Muscles
	6. Do Health Care Costs Matter?		32. The 10 Most Common Sports Injuries
	7. Beach Bummer		33. Which Exercise Is Best for You?
	8. Uninvited Guests		34. Losing Weight: What Works, What Doesn't
	9. Allergies: Nothing to Sneeze At		35. The Best Shape of Your Life
	10. Return of the Germ		36. Body Mania
	11. Sleeping with the Enemy		37. Trace Your Family Tree
	12. What Every Woman Needs to Know about Personal Safety		38. Cholesterol
	13. Stress		39. Rating Your Risks for Heart Disease
	14. Does Tension Cause Hypertension?		40. Stopping Cancer in Its Tracks
	15. Energy!		41. Confronting the AIDS Pandemic
	16. Out of the Blues		42. The Mating Game
	17. Depression: Way Beyond the Blues		43. The Indispensables: 10 Key Reasons Why Love Endures
	18. One Pill Makes You Larger, and One Pill Makes You Small . . .		44. Choosing a Contraceptive
	19. OTC Drugs: Prescription for Danger?		45. New, Improved and Ready for Battle
	20. Placebo Effect Is Shown to Be Twice as Powerful as Expected		46. It's Not Just AIDS
	21. Kicking Butts		47. 'Nutrition Facts': To Help Consumers Eat Smart
	22. Alcohol and Tobacco: A Deadly Duo		48. Taking Control of Your Disease
	23. Alcohol in Perspective		49. Sunscreens: Everything New under the Sun
	24. Does Moderate Alcohol Consumption Prolong Life?		50. Something Fishy
	25. How's Your Diet?		51. Preventing STDs
	26. The Mediterranean Diet		52. Food News Blues

(Continued on next page)

ABOUT YOU

Name ___ Date ___
Are you a teacher? ☐ Or student? ☐
Your School Name ___
Department ___
Address ___
City ___ State ___ Zip ___
School Telephone # ___

YOUR COMMENTS ARE IMPORTANT TO US!

Please fill in the following information:

For which course did you use this book? ___
Did you use a text with this Annual Edition? ☐ yes ☐ no
The title of the text? ___
What are your general reactions to the Annual Editions concept?

Have you read any particular articles recently that you think should be included in the next edition?

Are there any articles you feel should be replaced in the next edition? Why?

Are there other areas that you feel would utilize an Annual Edition?

May we contact you for editorial input?

May we quote you from above?

No Postage Necessary if Mailed in the United States

ANNUAL EDITIONS: HEALTH 95/96

BUSINESS REPLY MAIL

First Class Permit No. 84 Guilford, CT

Postage will be paid by addressee

DPG

Dushkin Publishing Group/
Brown & Benchmark Publishers
Sluice Dock
Guilford, Connecticut 06437